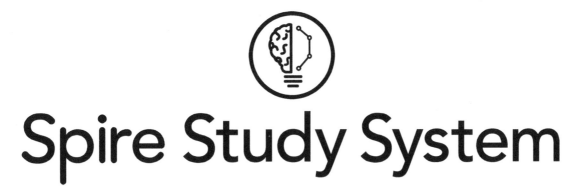

Spire Study System

CAPTURE. CROSS-TRAIN. CONQUER.

HESI A²
2018-2019

STUDY SYSTEM + TEST PREP GUIDE + PRACTICE WORKBOOK

Proudly Printed in the United States of America

ISBN: 978-0-9998764-1-1

HESI® is a registered trademark of Health Education Systems, Inc., which is neither affiliated with nor endorses this book.

Disclaimer: This publication is produced using strict quality control measures to match current HESI A^2 exam guidelines and requirements. As these standards are updated, new editions of this book will reflect those changes. The publisher assumes no liability or responsibility for any damage resulting from any use of the material contained within this book.

ABOUT US

Spire was founded by individuals who wanted to drastically improve the quality of educational materials. Our goal was to create a paradigm shift in the test prep industry, just like modern technology and innovative companies have done for smartphones and computers.

To do that, we assembled a team of seasoned educators, creative professionals, and young entrepreneurs. The end result was a specially formulated study system that outperforms traditional study guides in every way.

See, just about every study guide company supplies you with a daunting volume of information, with no real instructions on how to dig through it. After you purchase their product, you're on your own.

Spire is with you every step of the way. With a 30-day system based on scientific study principles designed to increase retention, you'll know what, when and how to study. This translates into less study time, a better understanding of the material and a more prepared you on test day.

No more cramming. No more wasted studying time. No more guessing at answers and hoping for good luck.

You don't need luck.

You've got **Spire**

CONTENTS

INTRODUCTION

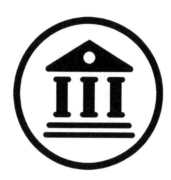

Since there have been schools, there have been tests, and there have been superstitions and myths about the best way to study for them. Maybe you've heard – or currently believe – some of these ancient yarns: "Study somewhere quiet where you won't be easily distracted." "Focus on one subject at a time." "The longer you study, the better your score will be."

These sound like good advice – in fact, they are so ingrained in us that they sound intuitively correct. The problem is that they are dead wrong.

In the last half-century, researchers and psychologists have upended a lot of conventional wisdom about the way humans learn and how we can get the most out of studying. Their discoveries have suggested a number of ways that students can study smarter, not harder.

However, these research findings have been slow to make their way into the school systems, if at all, and they are virtually nowhere to be found in most study guides on the market. That means that there are too many people out there working too hard for too little gain.

It's time to change that – and that's why we invented the Spire Study System. First, we assembled an experienced team of editors, educators, writers, test designers and graphic artists. Then, we built a system around findings from decades of scientific research. Lastly, we refined and designed it for intuitive use and maximum simplicity. The result is what you hold in your hands: Not a study guide, but a study system that makes preparation for any test simpler, easier and more effective.

The Spire Study System operates on the following principles:

1. Study multiple subjects in the same session.

You have to answer questions about multiple topics in the same test session – so why study one subject at a time? By interleaving multiple subjects in the same session, you will strengthen your powers of discrimination – which are crucial to passing a multiple-choice test! That's why this book is organized into a system of study modules, each containing multiple short chapters spanning a variety of subjects.

2. Change your environment often.

The more often you change your studying conditions, the better off you'll be on test day. That means studying in different locations, at different times of day, and even while listening to different kinds of music. The Spire Study System makes this easy, by providing a schedule and framework for changing your environment often enough to achieve maximum gains from your studies.

3. Don't study for too long.

More studying does not necessarily equal a better score. There is a point of diminishing returns that, once crossed, may actually make studying counterproductive. Come the big day of the test, you're going to want to be an expert at retrieving and re-engaging the material that you've memorized. The Spire Study System trains those skills by breaking up study sessions and spacing them out over a longer overall period of time.

4. Give yourself breaks.

Most of us were repeatedly told, all throughout our childhood, to "pay attention" to lectures that were much longer than our attention spans. Well, trying to pay attention is usually as effective as trying to relax or trying to fall asleep. It isn't. That's why the Spire Study System incorporates regular breaks,

timed to the average person's studying speed, to help recharge the innate capacity for focus and jumpstart subconscious synthesis processes.

5. Start studying a month before the test.

In the time-management nightmare known as modern life, how are you supposed to carve out entire nights to devote to studying? The answer: you can't, until it's too late, when that most primal and effective of motivators – fear – sends you into a cramming frenzy the week before the test. The Spire Study System breaks up studying into short, maximally effective sessions. Rather than trying to find hours upon extra hours to study huge reams of material, you revisit small chunks of the subject matter many times, enabling more reinforcement in less overall study time.

6. Self-testing is very strong.

Once you've thoroughly studied the material, self-testing is your strongest tool for reinforcement. That's why this book has three practice tests. Taking the practice tests, making flash cards to test yourself, and getting someone else to quiz you are all stronger methods to build retention than an equal amount of studying.

There's so much more – but we invented the Spire Study System so you wouldn't have to become an expert in advanced learning theories. All you have to do is stick to the following 30-day schedule, and follow the directions in the book. Easy peasy.

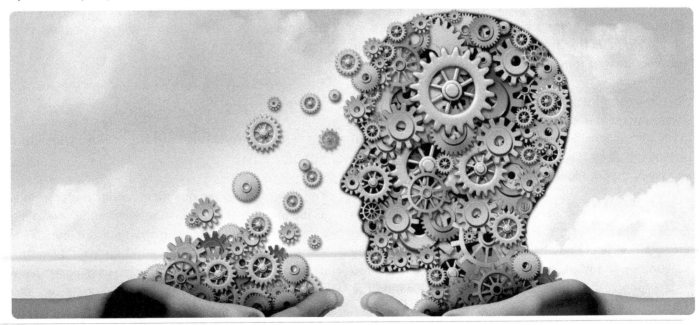

HESI A² - Spire Study System

CALENDAR

Day 1 Pre-Test	**Day 2** Study Module 1	**Day 5** Review Module 1	**Day 6** Study Module 2	**Day 8** Review Module 2
Day 9 Study Module 3	**Day 11** Review Module 3	**Day 12** Study Module 4	**Day 13** Review Module 4	**Day 15** Practice Test 1
Day 16 Targeted Self-Study	**Day 19** Review Module 1 Self-Test	**Day 20** Review Module 2 Self-Test	**Day 22** Review Module 3 Self-Test	**Day 23** Review Module 4 Self-Test
Day 26 Targeted Self-Study	**Day 27** Targeted Self-Study	**Day 28** Review Modules 1-4 Practice Test 2	**Day 29** No Studying Allowed - Celebrate	**Day 30** Take the Test!

TARGETED SELF-STUDY
study your notes
and focus on your
weakest areas

SELF-TEST
flashcards
or a friend

CELEBRATE
reward yourself with a day off,
filled with your favorite activities
and foods!

EDUCATION IS LEARNING WHAT YOU DIDN'T EVEN KNOW YOU DIDN'T KNOW

FAQ

Q: When I try to make plans, life always throws me a curveball. What should I do if I can't stick perfectly to the schedule?

A: Dwight Eisenhower once said, "Plans are useless, but planning is indispensable." If you miss a session or have to cut one short because, you know, life, the first order of business is: Forgive yourself. What you have (or haven't) done is irrelevant. What matters is what you are doing. Get back to your book and stick to the schedule as best as you can.

Q: I fear change, and want to keep my bad habits. Can I still use this book?

A: Of course you can. This book contains all of the information you need to pass your test, regardless of whether you follow the Spire Study System or want to do it on your own.

Q: Should I do anything specific when I take my breaks?

A: Yes: don't study. Don't think about the material. Don't talk about the material. Do some light activity like taking a walk, or dancing in the living room (well, that's what we do – don't judge us.) The least productive activities are those designed to distract, so avoid playing video games or anything involving your smartphone, if possible. However, if answering texts or checking the comments on your latest Instagram post are going to free your attention for more studying, then do what you gotta do.

Q: What are some other bad study habits I can break?

A: We got you. Here's a handy list: Don't rewrite your notes, don't work from any test outline, and don't restudy subject material from the same module twice in one session.

Q: Should I take notes?

A: Yes. Keep them brief and focused on the main points of the subject matter, and be sure to review them during Targeted Self-Study on days 16, 26 and 27.

Q: AAAAAAAGGGGGGHHHHH! I don't have 30 days! I just got this book and the test is tomorrow!

A: Hey. Take a deep breath, Lucky. We hate to break this to you, but you're in for a long, anxious night of that time-tested torture technique: Cramming. The good news is that even if you don't gain the distinct studying advantages of long-term spacing and luxurious breaks, you'll still benefit from the interleaved content and the self-testing included in the practice tests at the back of the book. Now quit reading this FAQ and turn to Practice Test 1, ASAP!

That's it! You've got a command of the basics and you understand how the Spire Study System works: Just follow the calendar and the directions in the book. Now, your first task is to head to the next section, where the Pre-test is.

That's right: Before you read any of the modules, you take the Pre-test. That may sound counterintuitive, but the science is clear: Testing on the material before you start studying yields drastically better results. So don't even peek at the content – just get ready to take the first test.

About the HESI A²

Congratulations! You've decided to enter the world of nursing. You're in for a long journey ahead, but you've chosen an excellent profession. Your study partners at Spire wish you the best of luck in your new career.

The first order of business is to successfully pass the HESI A² exam. The HESI A² is an admissions exam used by many nursing schools to assess potential students and their likely future success. Nursing students who take the HESI A² must be prepared to complete reading, math, science, and English language sections on the exam.

Scoring

If you want to pass the HESI A², you need to know how well you have to perform. Some nursing programs require that you score a certain percentage in each exam category, while others evalutate your overall score and compare it with your qualifications and credentials.

Although different nursing schools will require different minimum scores, here are some general guidelines:

- English Language 80%
- Mathematics: 75%
- Science: 75%
- Personality Profile: used for non-scoring purposes

Minimum scores are dependent on the nursing programs you apply to, so be sure to contact the appropriate admissions offices for specific scoring requirements.

Exam Breakdown

Now that you know the score you need to get, let's talk about the actual HESI A² exam. The HESI A² evaluates your aptitude in the following categories and subtests:

Section	Questions/Time
ENGLISH LANGUAGE	
Reading Comprehension	55/60 minutes
Vocabulary & General Knowledge	55/50 minutes
Grammar	55/50 minutes
MATHEMATICS	
Basic Math Skills	55/50 minutes
SCIENCE	
Biology	30/25 minutes
Chemistry	30/25 minutes
Anatomy & Physiology	30/25 minutes
PERSONALITY PROFILE	
Personality Profile	15/15 minutes
Learning Style	14/15 minutes
Total	**339/5.25 hours**

HESI A^2 - Spire Study System

PRE-TEST

As you read in the FAQ, with the Spire Study System, you take the Pre-test before you look at any other material in this book.

Here's a little secret: the Pre-test is actually Practice Test 1. That's right, it's the same exact test. But there's a reason for that! Because the Spire Study System will allow you to better retain and recall the information in this book, you can compare your Pre-test and Practice Test 1 scores to see how much you've learned since you started.

After you complete the first practice test, you'll want to take a look at the answer key. That way you can establish a baseline for your current knowledge.

Then, after you work through the Spire Study System – according to the 30-day schedule – you'll take Practice Test 1...again.

Later on – according to the 30-day schedule – you'll take Practice Test 2. Because you will have never seen these questions before, the second practice test will be a bit more challenging than the first.

But don't stress out! As long as you followed the Spire Study System, you'll do great. In fact, you'll be surprised at just how well you do.

But let's not get ahead of ourselves. Once you're ready to experience the magic of the Spire Study System, turn to the back of the book to begin the first test.

MODULE 1

DAY, LOCATION, MUSIC

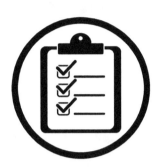

1 MONDAY, OCTOBER 12

COFFEE SHOP ON MAIN STREET

MY FAVORITE BAND

2

3

VOCABULARY

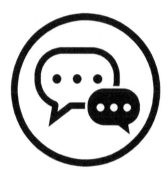

EXPANDING YOUR VOCABULARY

The best, most natural way to expand your vocabulary is to read everything you can get your hands on. That means blogs, articles, social media, physical books, posted signs and even the labels on your shampoo bottle. Start looking for opportunities to read a little bit more every day, from now until the day of the test.

Of course, you do have that test coming up quick, so you don't have much time to go *au naturale.* We got your back. Here is your first and most crucial vocabulary hack: identifying root words.

WHAT IS THE WHAT?

Many words are little stories in and of themselves, which is to say that they have a beginning, middle and end. These parts are, respectively, the prefix, the root word and the suffix.

Not all words have all three parts. Sometimes it's just the prefix and root, sometimes just the root and suffix, and sometimes there are multiple roots. But—and this is important—a word is never just prefixes and suffixes. There is always at least one root word, because that's the main idea of the word. You can't have a complete, grammatically correct sentence without a subject, and you can't have a complete word without a root word.

For example, here's a word that's close to your heart lately: *reviewing.* It means viewing something again. Here are its parts:
Prefix = re
Root = view
Suffix = ing

Re is a prefix that means "again." *View* means "look." *Ing* is a suffix that denotes tense; it tells you the root word is happening in the present. So, if you're reviewing, you're currently viewing something again. The root word, or main idea of the word, is "view.

Let's get concrete: If you went up to one of your friends and just said, "Again," they would give you a funny look and say, "What again?"

It's the same idea if you went up to them and said, "Doing." They would say, "Doing what?"

If you went up to them and just said, "Look," they would get the point and try to see what you're seeing. They may not know what to look for, but they get the gist of what your trying to communicate to them. That gist is the root of the word.

Almost every vocabulary word on the test will be some combination of prefixes, roots and suffixes. If you run into one that you don't know, the first question to ask yourself is, "What is the what?"

Here is another example: *unemployment*
Prefix = un
Root = employ
Suffix = ment

You can't just say "un" or "ment" and expect to be understood, but when you add the main idea, *employ*, the word makes sense. It means the state of not having a job.

Where It Gets Messy

Of course, we speak the English language, which is a marvelous, madcap collage of many other languages, but mostly Latin, German and Greek. That means many root words are not English words. On top of that, there are no hard-and-fast rules for how prefixes and suffixes will change root words, so each root may look a little different depending on which prefixes and suffixes are used.

However, you can usually get the gist by breaking off the parts that you know are prefixes and suffixes and asking yourself what the remaining part reminds you of.

In order to break things down, you need to have a grasp of the most common prefixes, suffixes and root words you'll encounter on the test (these are outlined below).

Common Root Words
If you can't identify a word because it seems like it's in another language, that's most likely because it is. This isn't always true, but a good general rule is that our longer, more academic words tend to have their roots in Latin and Greek, while our shorter words tend to have their roots in German. For example, *amorous* and *loving* are synonyms, but one has its roots in the Latin *amor* and the other in the German *lieb*.

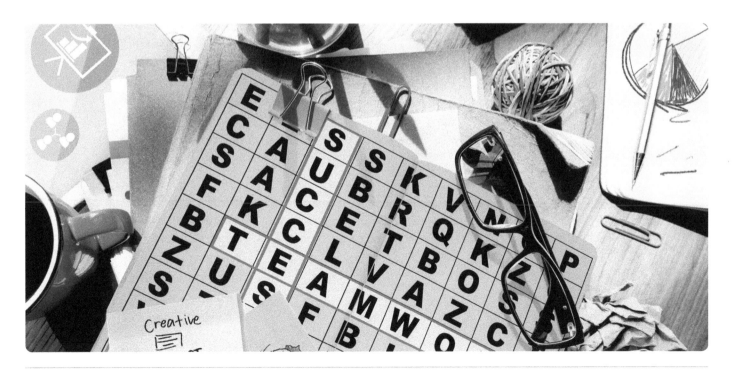

LATIN/GREEK - Because vocabulary words on the test tend toward the longer, more academic variety, you'll get the most out of studying some common Latin and Greek roots:

Root	Variations	What it Means	Examples
Aster	Astro	Star	Astronomy, disaster
Aqua		Water	Aquatic, aquarium
Aud		Hear	Auditorium, audience
Bene		Good	Benevolent, benign
Bio		Life	Biology, autobiography
Cent		Hundred	Century, cent (money)
Chrono		Time	Chronological, synchronize
Circum	Circa	Around	Circumspect, circumnavigate
Contra	Counter	Against or conflict	Contraband, encounter
Dict		Speak or say	Dictate, dictation
Duc	Duct, duce	Lead or leader	Produce, conduct
Fac		Make or do	Manufacture, facsimile (fax)
Fract	Frag	Break	Fraction, defragment
Gen		Birth or create	Genetics, generate
Graph		Write	Telegraph, calligraphy
Ject		Throw	Inject, projection
Jur	Jus	Law	Juror, justice
Log	Logue	Concept or thought	Logo, dialogue
Mal		Bad	Maladaptive, malevolent
Man		Hand	Manuscript, manual
Mater		Mother	Maternal, material
Mis	Mit	Send	Mission, submit
Pater	Pat	Father	Paternal, patriot
Path		Feel	Sympathy, empathetic
Phile	Philo	Love	Philosophy, anglophile
Phon		Sound	Telephone, phonetic
Photo		Light	Photograph, photosynthesis
Port		Carry	Transport, portable
Psych	Psycho	Soul or spirit	Psychiatrist, psyche
Qui	Quit	Quiet or rest	Acquittal, tranquility
Rupt		Break	Rupture, interrupt
Scope		See, inspect	Telescope, microscopic
Scrib	Script	Write	Describe, transcription
Sens	Sent	Feel	Sensory, consent
Spect		Look	Spectate, circumspect
Struct		Build	Construct, obstruction
Techno	Tech	Art or science	Technical, technology
Tele		Far	Teleport, television
Therm		Heat	Thermometer, thermal
Vac		Empty	Vacation, evacuate
Vis	Vid	See	Visual, video
Voc		Speak or call	Vocal, vocation

HESI A² - Spire Study System

PREFIXES - Here are your opposite prefixes, which you'll encounter a lot on the test:

Prefix	Variations	What it Means	Examples
Anti-	Ant-	Against or opposite	Anti-inflammatory, antagonist
De-		Opposite	Decontaminate, deconstruct
Dis-		Not or opposite	Disagree, dis (slang for insult)
In-	Im-, Il-, Ir-	Not	Incapable, impossible, illegitimate, irreplaceable
Non-		Not	Noncompliant, nonsense
Un-		Not	Unfair, unjust

Here is a quick list of some other common prefixes:

Prefix	Variations	What it Means	Examples
En-	Em-	Cause	Enlighten, empower
Fore-		Before	Foresee, foretell
In-		Inside of	Inland, income
Inter-		Between	Interrupt, interaction
Mid-		In the middle of	Midair, midlife
Mis-		Wrong	Mistake, misdiagnose
Pre-		Before	Pregame, prefix
Re-		Again	Review, recompress
Semi-		Half or partial	Semitruck, semiannual
Sub-		Under	Subconcious, subpar
Super-		Above	Superimpose, superstar
Trans-		Across	Translate, transform

SUFFIXES - Here are some common suffixes you'll encounter on the test:

Suffix	Variations	What it Means	Examples
-Able	-Ible	Can be accomplished	Capable, possible
-Al	-Ial	Has traits of	Additional, beneficial
-En		Made of	Molten, wooden
-Er		More than	Luckier, richer
-Er	-Or	Agent that does	Mover, actor
-Est		Most	Largest, happiest
-Ic		Has traits of	Acidic, dynamic
-Ing		Continues to do	Reviewing, happening
-Ion	-Tion, -Ation, -Ition	Process of	Occasion, motion, rotation, condition
-Ity		The state of	Ability, simplicity
-Ly		Has traits of	Friendly, kindly
-Ment		Process/state of	Enlightenment, establishment
-Ness		State of	Happiness, easiness
-Ous	-Eous, -Ious	Has traits of	Porous, gaseous, conscious
-Y		Has traits of	Artsy, fartsy

VOCABULARY PRACTICE TEST

For items 1-5, try to identify the root and write an English translation or synonym for it. We did the first one for you as an example.

#	Word	Root	Translation/Synonym
Ex	Description	Script	Something written
1	Irresponsible		
2	Entombment		
3	Professorial		
4	Unconscionable		
5	Gainfully		

For items 6-10, identify the prefix and write an English translation or synonym for it.

#	Word	Prefix	Translation/Synonym
Ex	Prepare	Pre	Before
6	Proceed		
7	Misapprehend		
8	Antibiotic		
9	Hyperactive		
10	Cacophony		

For items 11-15, identify the suffix and write an English translation or synonym for it.

#	Word	Suffix	Translation/Synonym
Ex	Lovable	Able	Can be accomplished
11	Tedious		
12	Absolution		
13	Cathartic		
14	Merriment		
15	Inspector		

Now, it's time to test your current vocabulary:

16. Achromatic most nearly means:
a. full of color
b. fragrant
c. without color
d. vivid

17. Cursory most nearly means:
a. meticulous; careful
b. undetailed; rapid
c. thorough
d. expletive

18. Hearsay most nearly means:
a. blasphemy
b. secondhand information that can't be proven
c. evidence that can be confirmed
d. testimony

19. Magnanimous most nearly means:
a. suspicious
b. uncontested
c. forgiving; not petty
d. stingy; cheap

20. Terrestrial most nearly means:
a. of the earth
b. cosmic
c. otherworldly/unearthly
d. supernatural

ANSWER KEY

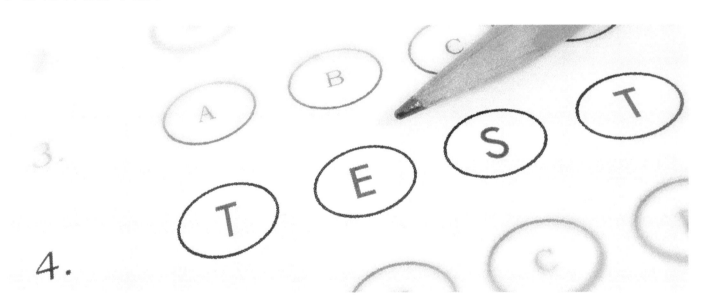

1. response	6. pro-	11. -ious	17. (b) undetailed; rapid
2. tomb	7. mis-	12. -tion	18. (b) secondhand information that can't be proven
3. profess	8. anti-	13. -tic	
4. conscience	9. hyper-	14. -ment	19. (c) forgiving; not petty
5. gain	10. caco-	15. -tor	20. (a) of the earth
		16. (c) without color	

CRITICAL READING

FINDING THE MAIN IDEA

Many of the reading comprehension questions you will encounter on the exam are structured around finding the main idea of a paragraph. The last section on root words was all about finding the main idea of a word – notice a theme developing here?

In this section, you will need to find the main idea of a paragraph. Luckily, that's nice and simple once you know what to look for.

First of all, we're going to re-define a few terms you might think you already know, so don't rush through this part:

PARAGRAPH

A paragraph is a tool for organizing information. It's simply a container for sentences in the same way that a sentence is a container for words. Okay, maybe you knew that already, but you'd be surprised how many

professional writers get their minds blown when they realize that almost all books are structured in the same way:

Books are made of...
Chapters, which are made of...
Sections, which are made of...
Paragraphs, which are made of...
Sentences, which are made of...
Words

It's a simple hierarchy, and smack in the center is the humble paragraph. For the purposes of the test, you need to be able to comb through given paragraphs to find two kinds of sentences: topic and detail.

TOPIC SENTENCE

A well-written paragraph, which is to say all of the paragraphs that you'll find on the test, contains just one topic. You'll find this in the topic sentence, which is the backbone of the paragraph. The topic sentence tells you what the paragraph is about. All of the other sentences exist solely to support this topic sentence which, more often than not, is the first or last sentence in the paragraph. However, that's not always the case, so use this foolproof method: Ask yourself, "Who or what is this paragraph about?" Then find the sentence that answers your question.

DETAIL SENTENCE

Detail sentences exist to support the topic sentence. They do so with all kinds of additional information, such as descriptions, arguments and nuances. An author includes detail sentences to explain why they're writing about the topic in the first place. That is, the detail sentences contain the author's point, which you'll need in order to find the main idea. To easily spot the author's point, just ask yourself, "Why is the author writing about this topic?" Then pay close attention to the detail sentences to pry out their motivations.

Got it? Good. Now, let's do some really easy math: The topic + the author's point = the main idea.

Now, let's put that in English:
What + Why = Main Idea

IN THE REAL WORLD

All right, you've got the abstract concepts nailed down. Now, let's get concrete. Imagine a scenario where a friend is explaining the movie *Toy Story* to you. Also, imagine that she has already picked her jaw up off the floor, because seriously, how have you not seen *Toy Story*? You should fix that.

She tells you what the movie is about: There are these toys that get lost, and they have a bunch of adventures trying to get back to their owner. Then she tells you why you should see it: It's cute and funny, and it's a classic.

Two sentences: The topic (what the movie is about) and the author's point (why she's telling you about it.) And now you have the main idea: Your friend thinks you should see the movie Toy Story because it's a cute, funny classic about toys having adventures.

ILLUSTRATING THE MAIN IDEA

Here is a paragraph similar to one you might encounter on the test, followed by the types of questions that you will need to answer:

EXAMPLE 1 – FROM *THE ART OF CONVERSATION* BY CATHERINE BLYTH:

"Silence is meaningful. You may imagine that silence says nothing. In fact, in any spoken communication, it plays a repertoire of roles. Just as, mathematically speaking, Earth should be called Sea, since most of the planet is covered in it, so conversation might be renamed silence, as it comprises 40 to 50 percent of an average utterance, excluding pauses for others to talk and the enveloping silence of those paying attention (or not, as the case may be.)"

This one is relatively easy, but let's break it down:

Who/What is the paragraph about? Silence.

Why is the author writing about this topic? It is often overlooked, but it's an important part of conversation.

What is the main idea? Silence is an important part of conversation. Or, put it another way: "Silence is meaningful" - it's the first sentence!

Okay, you've seen the technique in action, so now it's your turn. Read the following paragraphs and determine the topic sentence, the author's main point, and the main idea.

EXAMPLE 2 – FROM *LOVE, POVERTY AND WAR* BY CHRISTOPHER HITCHENS
"Concerning love, I had best be brief and say that when I read Bertrand Russell on this matter as an adolescent, and understood him to write with perfect gravity that a moment of such emotion was worth the whole of the rest of life, I devoutly hoped that this would be true in my own case. And so it has proved, and so to that extent I can regard the death that I otherwise rather resent as laughable and impotent."

1. The main topic of this paragraph is:
a. gravity

b. adolescence

c. death

d. love

2. The author's main point about this topic is that:

a. it is something to be resented

b. it is something to laugh at

c. it makes life worth living

d. it is brief

3. The final sentence is:

a. the topic sentence

b. the author's main point

c. detail sentence

d. the beginning of a new topic

4. The main idea of the paragraph is that:

a. a moment of love is worth all of life's woes

b. adolescence is something to laugh at

c. Bertrand Russell is very wise

d. death is something to be resented

EXAMPLE 3 – FROM *RIVER OF DOUBT* BY CANDICE MILLARD

"Theodore Roosevelt, one of the most popular presidents in his nation's history, had vowed never to run again after winning his second term in the White House in 1904. But now, just eight years later, he was not only running for a third term, he was, to the horror and outrage of his old Republican backers, running as a third-party candidate against Democrats and Republicans alike."

5. The topic of this paragraph is:

a. Teddy Roosevelt

b. early 20th century politics

c. independent presidential candidates

d. the election of 1912

6. Why does the author mention "old Republican backers?"

a. Roosevelt's backers were all elderly

b. Roosevelt used to be a Republican

c. Roosevelt used to be a Democrat

d. they backed Roosevelt eight years ago

7. Where is the topic sentence?

a. the last sentence

b. the first sentence

c. it is likely stated before the chosen selection

d. it is likely stated after the chosen selection

8. The main idea of the paragraph is:

a. Roosevelt was a popular president

b. Roosevelt ran for a third term as a third-party candidate

c. early 20th century politics had three parties

d. the election of 1912 had three candidates

EXAMPLE 4 – FROM *LOVE IN THE TIME OF CHOLERA* BY GABRIEL GARCÍA MÁRQUEZ

"To him she seemed so beautiful, so seductive, so different from ordinary people, that he could not understand why no one was as disturbed as he by the clicking of her heels on the paving stones, why no one else's heart was wild with the breeze stirred by the sighs of her veils, why everyone did not go mad with the movements of her braid, the flight of her hands, the gold of her laughter. He had not missed a single one of her gestures, not one of the indications of her character, but he did not dare approach her for fear of destroying the spell."

9. The main topic of this paragraph is:

a. a beautiful woman

b. fear

c. love

d. seduction

10. The author uses many details to:

a. show that the man is obsessive

b. show the vividness and intensity of love

c. make people admire his writing ability

d. show that the woman is unique

11. The topic sentence:

a. is the final sentence

b. is the initial sentence

c. also contains many details

d. is not present in this paragraph

12. The main idea of the paragraph is that:
a. the man is afraid of the woman he loves
b. the woman doesn't even know the man is alive
c. love is vivid and intense
d. there is no main idea because this is fiction

EXAMPLE 5 – FROM *ON LOOKING* BY ALEXANDRA HOROWITZ

"Part of human development is learning to notice less than we are able to. The world is awash in details of color, form, and sound – but to function, we have to ignore some of it. The world still holds these details. Children sense the world at a different granularity, attending to parts of the visual world we gloss over; to sounds we have dismissed as irrelevant. What is indiscernible to us is plain to them."

13. The main topic of this paragraph is:
a. what humans notice or don't
b. human development
c. the world's details
d. children

14. The author's main point about the topic is that:
a. children see more details than adults
b. adults see more details than children
c. aging inevitably results in wisdom
d. the world is very complicated

15. The first sentence is:
a. the topic sentence
b. the author's point
c. a detail sentence
d. the beginning of a new topic

16. The main idea of the paragraph is:
a. children and adults live in different worlds
b. as you age, your experience of the world gets richer
c. what is indiscernible to children is plain to adults
d. as you age, you notice less than children do

Answer Key

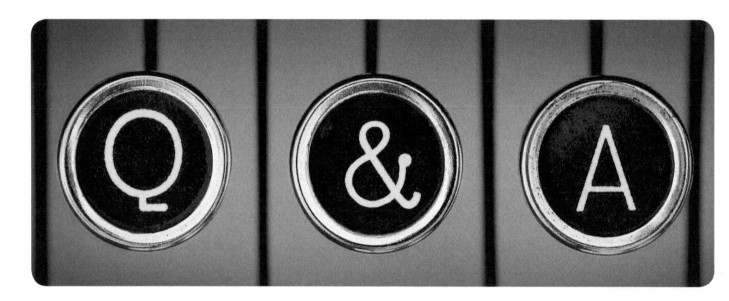

1. d

2. c

3. b

4. a

5. c

6. a

7. d

8. a

9. a

10. c

11. b

12. c

13. a

14. a

15. b

16. a

ARITHMETIC BASICS

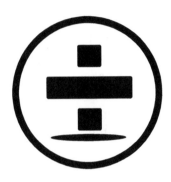

Before you begin studying for the arithmetic section of the exam, let's talk basics. Many math exams will test your memory of basic math definitions, vocabulary, and formulas that have become so distant that the questions on this type of exam may feel unfair. You likely don't refer to quotients and integers in your day-to-day life, so testing your recall of high school math class vocabulary and concepts doesn't exactly feel like a valid way to gauge your mathematical reasoning abilities. Well, as the French say, "C'est la vie!" or "That's life!" Perhaps the most appropriate English expression would be, "You gotta do what you gotta do."

In this section, it's best for you to begin with a refresher list so that you can master basic math terminology quickly.

INTEGER: Any whole number, i.e. any number that doesn't include a non-zero fraction or decimal. Negative whole numbers, positive whole numbers, and 0 are all integers. 3.1415 is not an integer. ½ is not an integer. -47, -12, 0, 15, and 1,415,000 are all integers.

POSITIVE AND NEGATIVE NUMBERS: A positive number is any number greater than zero. A negative number is any number less than zero. Zero is neither positive nor negative. Adding a negative number is the same as subtracting the positive value of that number. Subtracting a negative number is the same as adding a positive number.

EVEN AND ODD NUMBERS: An even number is any number that can be evenly divided by 2, with no remainder left over. -4, 2, 6, 24, and 114 are all even numbers. An odd number has a remainder of 1 when it is divided by 2. -19, 1, 3, 5, 17, and 451 are all odd numbers. Another way to think about even/odd is that even numbers are all integers that are multiples of two, and odd numbers are any integers that are not multiples of two.

FACTORS AND MULTIPLES:
The factors of a number (or a polynomial) are all of the numbers that can be multiplied together to get the first number. For example, the following pairs of numbers can be multiplied to get 16: 1 * 16, 2 * 8 and 4 * 4. Therefore, the factors of 16 are 1, 2, 4, 8, and 16. Note: a polynomial is an expression that can have constants, variables and exponents, and that can be combined using addition, subtraction, multiplication and division.

PRIME NUMBER:
An integer that only has two factors: 1 and itself. There are two things to remember: (1) out of all of the infinite integers in existence, there is only one prime number that is even, and that is the number 2 — that's it, and (2) you can handle almost any prime number question on the test by memorizing all of the primes between 0 and 100. This is not required, but you will save time and mental anguish if you do this. Here they are:

2, 3, 5, 7, 11, 13, 17, 19, 23, 29, 31, 37, 41, 43, 47, 53, 59, 61, 67, 71, 73, 79, 83, 87, 89

PRIME FACTORIZATION:
The prime numbers you have to multiply to get a number. Take the number 24. First, you should find the factors of 24: 1, 2, 3, 4, 6, 8, and 12. Then, you need to pull out all the numbers that are not prime: 1, 4, 6, 8, and 12. What's left? 2 and 3 are the prime factors of 24! Now, that's a simple example, but the concept remains the same, no matter how large the number. When in doubt, start working from the number 2 (the smallest prime), which will be a factor of any number that ends with an even number. Be on the lookout for sneaky questions. For example, if the exam asks you for the prime factors of the number 31, for instance, recall that 31 is a prime number (but 1 is not!) so the only prime factor it can possibly have is itself — 31. The same goes for all prime numbers.

SUM:
Add — the number you get when you add one number to another number.

DIFFERENCE:
Subtract — the number you get when you subtract one number from another number.

PRODUCT:
Multiply — the number you get when you multiply one number by another number.

QUOTIENT:
Divide — the number you get when you divide one number by another number.

EXPRESSIONS

An expression is made up of terms that are numbers, variables, and operators which are added together. If that sounds complicated, expressions are simply made up of the basic symbols used to create everything from first-grade addition problems to formulas and equations used in calculus. The individual terms of the expression are added to each other as individual parts of the expression. Remember that expressions may stand for single numbers, and use basic operators like * and ÷. However, a single expression does not suggest a comparison (or equivalency). But an equation does and can be represented by a simple expression equal to a number. For example, 3 + 2 = 1 + 4 is an equation, because it uses the equal sign. So, think of 3 + 2 and 1 + 4 as building blocks — they are the expressions that, when joined together by an equal sign, make up an equation. Another way to think of an expression is that it is essentially a math metaphor used to represent another number.

ORDER OF OPERATIONS

An operation is what a symbol does. The operation of a + sign, for instance, is to add. That's easy enough, but what happens if you run into a problem like this?

$$44 - (3^2 * 2 + 6) = ?$$

You have to solve this equation by simplifying it, but if you do it in the wrong order, you will get the wrong answer. This is an incredibly important concept. This is where the Order of Operations comes in — here's what you have to remember.

1. Parentheses
2. Exponents

3. Multiplication and division (from left to right)
4. Addition and subtraction (from left to right)

You must do these operations in order, starting with parentheses first and addition/subtraction last, in order to get the correct answer.

$$44 - (3^2 * 2 + 6) = ?$$

Start by focusing on the expression in parentheses first. Inside the parentheses, you will find an exponent, so do that first so that you can do the operation within the parentheses:

$$3^2 = 3 * 3 = 9$$

then the expression becomes $(9 * 2 + 6)$

To complete the operation within the paragraph, you need to remember to do the multiplication operation first:

$$9 * 2 = 18$$

$$(18 + 6) = 24$$

You don't need the parentheses anymore because there are no operations left to complete inside of them. Now the problem looks like this:

$$44 - 24 = ?$$

$$20 = ?$$

You can use the phrase, Please Excuse My Dear Aunt Sally as a useful mnemonic. It has the same first letters as parentheses, exponents, multiplication, division, addition, subtraction.

However, the most common mistake involving the order of operations is the following: doing division after multiplication and subtraction after addition, which results in the wrong answer. You have to do multiplication and division as you encounter it from left to right, and the same goes for addition and subtraction. Remember to do what is inside parentheses first, and that might require you to do exponents, multiplication/division, and addition/subtraction first.

Here's another example of this concept:

$$(4^2 + 5^3 - 120) * 3 = ?$$

$$4^2 = 4 * 4 = 16$$

$$5^3 = 5 * 5 * 5 = 125$$

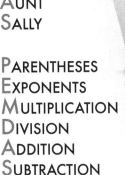

PLEASE
EXCUSE
MY
DEAR
AUNT
SALLY

PARENTHESES
EXPONENTS
MULTIPLICATION
DIVISION
ADDITION
SUBTRACTION

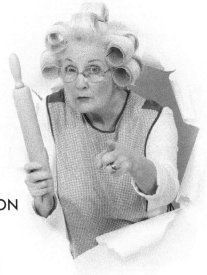

$$(16 + 125 - 120) * 3 = ?$$

$$21 * 3 = ?$$

$$63 = ?$$

If you didn't understand this example, you should go back and review the Order of Operations again.

Occasionally, you may encounter an equation that uses brackets. You should think of brackets as super parentheses, i.e. it's at the top of the list, and so you do that first, before anything else.

EQUATIONS

Equations relate expressions to one another with an equal sign. In algebra, they can get pretty complicated, but in arithmetic, equations often center around finding the equivalent of a single expression. For instance,

$$3 + 2 = 5$$

It may seem pretty simple to say $3 + 2$ expresses 5 because they have a clear and simple relationship — they are equal. Other kinds of equations, i.e.

relationships, include symbols like > (greater than) and < (lesser than), which can join two expressions together. These are often called inequalities since they are not equal. The greater than or less than relation is a sign of inequality.

Remember that equations can be rearranged by doing the same operations to each side of the equivalency. Here's an example of subtracting 6 from both sides of the equation:

$$34 - 23 = 6 + ?$$

$$34 - 23 - 6 = 6 + ? - 6$$

The number 6 subtracted on both sides of the equation cancel each other out. The equality of the relation remains unaffected.

$$11 - 6 = ?$$

$$5 = ?$$

GREATEST COMMON FACTOR
Sometimes the term Greatest Common Factor is called the Greatest Common Divisor, but either way, the concept is the same - it's the largest factor that two (or more) numbers share.

To use this concept, you should first work out all of the factors for each number and then find the largest factor they have in common. For example, find the Greatest Common Factor of 18 and 30:

The factors of 18 are: 1, 2, 3, 6, 9 and 18
The factors of 30 are: 1, 2, 3, 5, 6, 10, 15 and 30

The highest number in both sets, i.e. the highest number that are common to both sets, is 6, so that's your Greatest Common Factor.

LEAST COMMON MULTIPLE

Sometimes the term Least Common Multiple is called the Lowest Common Multiple or the Smallest Common Multiple or the Lowest Common Denominator when used in a fraction, but in any case, the concept is the same - without knowing this term, you can't compare, add, or subtract fractions, and that's important.

The least common multiple is the smallest number that can be divided by two (or more) given numbers. To get this number, first write out the multiples for each number and then find the smallest multiple that they share.

For example, find the Least Common Multiple of 3 and 7:

The multiples of 3 are: 3, 6, 9, 12, 15, 18, 21, 24, 27...
The multiples of 7 are: 7, 14, 21, 28, 35, 42, 49, 56...

The lowest number in both sets is 21, so that's your Least Common Multiple. Notice that there are other multiples, but we are interested in the lowest or least of the common multiples.

EXPONENTS AND ROOTS

EXPONENTS
An exponent is an algebraic operation that tells you to multiply a number by itself.

For example, 4^2 is the same as 4 * 4, and 4^3 is the same as 4 * 4 * 4. The exponent tells you how many times to multiply the number by itself.

Exponents have a few special properties (you can think of them as shortcuts or even helpful tricks if you want):

1. If two numbers with exponents share the same base number, you can multiply them by adding the exponents:

$$2^5 * 2^3 = 2^8$$

2. If two numbers with exponents share the same base number, you can divide them by subtracting the exponents:

$$2^5 \div 2^3 = 2^2$$

3. A number with an exponent raised to a negative power is the same as 1 over or the reciprocal of that number with an exponent raised to the positive power:

HESI A^2 - Spire Study System

$$5^{-2} = 1/5^2$$

$$1/5^2 = 1/25 \text{ or } 1 \div 25 = 0.04$$

4. A number raised to a fraction power is the same as a root, or radical:

$9^{1/2} = 3$ (the square root indicated by the two in one half)   Remember that the root of a number x is another number, which when multiplied by itself a given number of times, equals x. For example the second root of 9 is 3, because $3 * 3 = 9$. The second root is usually called the square root. The third root is usually called the cube root. Because $2 * 2 * 2 = 8$, 2 is the cube root of 8. Two special exponent properties are explained more in the two examples below.

1. 1 raised to any power is 1; for example:

$$1^2 = 1$$
$$1^{-4} = 1$$
$$1^{912} = 1$$

2. Any number raised to the power of 0 equals 1 — sounds crazy, but it's true! Here's an example:

$$253^0 = 1$$

If you can remember these six properties, you'll be able to simplify almost any problem with exponents.

ROOTS AND RADICALS

Roots and radicals are sometimes held up as cliché symbols for difficult math problems, but in the real world, they're easy to understand and use to solve equations.

A radical is an expression that has a square root, cube root, etc; the symbol is a $\sqrt{\ }$. The number under that radical sign is called a radicand.

A square is an expression (not an equation!) in which a number is multiplied by itself. It is often said that the given number is raised to the power of 2. Here's an example: 4^2 is a square. $4 * 4$ is the same square, expressed differently.

The square root of a number is a second number that, when multiplied by itself, will equal the first number. Therefore, it's the same as squaring a number, but in the opposite direction. For example, if you want to find the square root of 25, we have to figure out what number, when squared, equals 25. With enough experience, you will automatically know many of the common square roots. For example, it is commonly known that 5 is the square root of 25. Square and square root are operations that are often used to undo or cancel out each other in problem-solving situations. A mental image, kind of like a numerical mnemonic, that helps some people is to think of the given number and the square root (in the above case, 25 and 5) as the tree and its much smaller roots in the ground.

The previous example uses the number 25, which is an example of a perfect square. Only some numbers are perfect squares – those that are equal to the product of two integers. Here's a table of the first 10 perfect squares.

It is helpful to remember that if you find that the square root of any radicand is a whole number (not a fraction or a decimal), that means the given number is a perfect square.

To deal with radicals that are not perfect, you need to rewrite them as radical factors and simplify until you get one factor that's a perfect square. This process is sometimes called extracting or taking out the square root. This process would be used for the following number:

$$\sqrt{18}$$

First, it's necessary to notice that 18 has within it the perfect square 9.
$$18 = 9 * 2 = 3^2 * 2$$

Therefore, $\sqrt{18}$ is not in its simplest form. Now, you need to extract the square root of 9

$$\sqrt{18} = \sqrt{9} * 2 = 3\sqrt{2}$$

Now the radicand no longer has any perfect square factors.

$\sqrt{2}$ is an irrational number that is equal to approximately

1.414. Therefore, the approximate answer is the following:

$$\sqrt{18} = 3 * 1.414 = \text{approximately } 4.242$$

Note that the answer can only be an approximate one since $\sqrt{2}$ is an irrational number, which is any real number that cannot be expressed as a ratio of integers. Irrational numbers cannot be represented as terminating or repeating decimals.

Factors	Perfect Square
1 x 1	1
2 x 2	4
3 x 3	9
4 x 4	16
5 x 5	25
6 x 6	36
7 x 7	49
8 x 8	64
9 x 9	81
10 x 10	100

FACTORIALS

If you have ever seen a number followed by an exclamation point, it's not yelling at you – it's called a factorial. Simply put, a factorial is the product of a number and all of the positive integers below it, stopping at 1. For example, if you see 5!, its value is determined by doing the following example:

$$5! = 5 * 4 * 3 * 2 * 1 = 120$$

Factorials are typically used in relation to the fundamental principle of counting or for the combinations or permutations of sets.

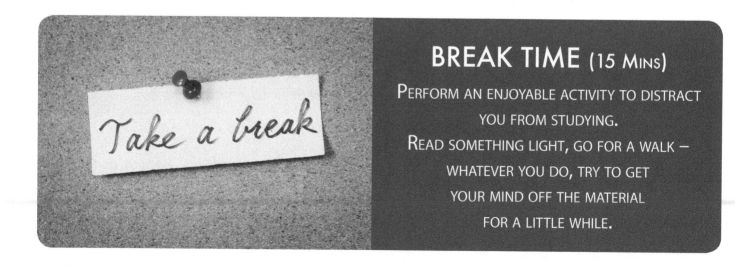

BREAK TIME (15 Mins)

PERFORM AN ENJOYABLE ACTIVITY TO DISTRACT YOU FROM STUDYING.
READ SOMETHING LIGHT, GO FOR A WALK – WHATEVER YOU DO, TRY TO GET YOUR MIND OFF THE MATERIAL FOR A LITTLE WHILE.

ALGEBRA CONCEPTS

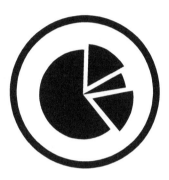

Algebra is a branch of Mathematics with symbols, referred to as variables, and numbers, as well as a system of rules for the manipulation of these. Solving higher-order word problems is a valuable application of the Algebra properties described in this chapter.

EXPRESSIONS

Algebra uses variables, numbers and operations as the basic parts. Variables are typically represented by letters and may have any number of values in a problem. Usually the variable is the unknown quantity in a problem. All letters can and often are used, but x, y, and z are letters that appear most often in algebra textbooks. In a testing situation, letters other than x, y, and z are often used to mislead test takers. Algebraic expressions are variables and numbers with operations such as addition, subtraction, multiplication and division. The following are all examples of algebraic expressions:

x	y	a	(letters)
7u	$\frac{1}{2}$ q (or $q/_2$)	3.9 p	(product of a variable and number)
s + 5	u+v	2.3+r	(sum of a variable and number)
z − 3.5	k-n	t − 1.3	(difference of a variable and number)
m/6	$(z/_2)$	3.9 /p	(quotient of a variable and number)
c^2	$b^{0.5}$	√3	(variable or number with an exponent)

Finally, the sum, difference, product or quotient of these items are also expressions.

Equations

Equations are defined as algebraic expressions that are set equal to a number, variable or another expression. The simplest identifier of an equation is the equal sign (=). When an equation is written to express a condition or represent a situation for problem solving, the solution is normally completed by manipulating the equation correctly so that a variable or unknown quantity is on one side of the equal sign and the numerical answer(s) are on the other side of the equal sign. Let's review some problem-solving methods in the following examples.

If the simple equation is written in word form, the first step must be to write the equation that represents that written question. The simple problem of ages of individuals is a common example:

Example 1: Jane is 8 years older than Nancy. In 5 years, she will be 27 years old. What is Jane's age now?

The variable J will represent Jane's age and the expression J+5 will represent Jane's age in 5 years. In this example, we read that this expression is equal to a number, in this case 27. Our equation becomes:

$$J+5 = 27$$

In the words of the problem, we have the correct expression set equal to a number. Our basic principle is to perform algebraic operations until the "J" is alone on one side of the equation and the numerical answer is on the other side. This type of solution involves the opposite of the addition (+5) so 5 is subtracted from both sides.

$$
\begin{aligned}
J+5 &= 27 \\
-5 &\quad -5 \\
J+0 &= 22
\end{aligned}
$$

Therefore, the answer says that the variable J, Jane's age, is now 22 years.

If the simple equation involved multiplication, the steps would involve an opposite operation that in this case would be division.

$$
\begin{aligned}
7J &= 84 \\
7J\,/7 &= 84/7 \\
J &= 12
\end{aligned}
$$

These examples are typical of "one-step solutions" since a single operation is involved to solve the problem.

Of course, there are multiple step solutions in more involved problems. But the rules are still the same, i.e.

1. Opposite operations are performed to solve
2. The same operations must be performed on both sides of the equation
3. The solution is complete when a variable is on one side and the answers are on the other side

Example 2: Jane is 8 years older than Nancy. In 5 years, she will be twice as old as Nancy. What is Jane's age now?

The first step to solving this type of problem is to identify the variable. In this solution, we will select the variable "J" to represent Jane's age and "N" to represent Nancy's age.

The two equations from the word description, become:

$$J - 8 = N$$

and

$$J + 5 = 2(N+5)$$

Dividing both sides of the second equation by 2 means that it becomes

$$(J+5)/2 = N+5$$

Adding 5 to the original equation we have

$$J - 8 + 5 = N + 5$$

In this method, there are two expressions which contain "J" that are both equal to "N + 5" so therefore, they must be equal to each other. So:

$$J - 3 = (J + 5)/2$$

Multiply both sides by 2 (same operation on both sides) and the equation is:

$$2J - 6 = J + 5$$

Subtract J and add 6 to both sides and the answer becomes:

$$2J - 6 = J + 5$$
$$-J + 6 \quad -J + 6$$
$$J = 11$$

By this solution, the problem is completed and the following statements are clarified:

1. Now, Jane is 11 years old, and Nancy is 3 years old.
2. In 5 years, Jane will be 16 years old, and Nancy will be 8 years old.

We are able to answer the question, "What is Jane's age now?" and all the other ages in the question because of an algebra principle that requires two equations for two unknowns. In the problem, there are two variables (J and N) and two relationships between them (now and 5 years from now). If we are able to formulate two equations with the two unknowns, then algebra principles will allow for the solution of a complex problem.

QUADRATIC EQUATIONS

Quadratic equations are algebraic equations where the largest variable exponent is equal to two. This is often referred to as a "second degree" equation. If there are multiple terms, it can also be referred to as a second degree polynomial, where polynomial indicates that there are multiple terms in the equation. Quadratic equations are valuable in higher-order problem solving situations, with particularly important application in Physics problem solving. Examples are depicted below:

$$7x^2 = 0$$

$$\tfrac{1}{2} (9.8) t^2 = 27$$

$$ax^2 + bx + c = 0 \text{ where a, b and c are real numbers}$$

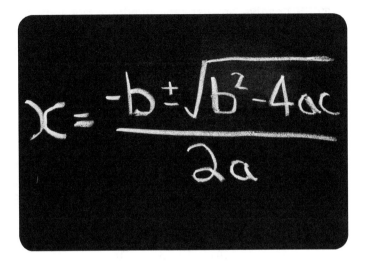

Note that all quadratic equations can be written in the form of the last example because coefficients can be zero and algebra operations can be performed so that the 0 is on the right side of the equation. This last statement is the standard form and is of great importance. Every quadratic equation in this form can be solved with the quadratic formula. It is presented here with a qualifying statement. In a timed testing environment, the use of the following formula is typically used when factoring is not feasible, since it is a time consuming option.

The quadratic formula for equations in the standard form states:

$$x = \frac{-b +/- \sqrt{(b^2 - 4ac)}}{(2a)}$$

Due to the complexity of the quadratic formula, it will normally be used when the term

$$(b^2 - 4ac) / (2a) = 0$$

$$(b^2 - 4ac) / (2a) = \text{a perfect square}$$

Since the use of technology is not allowed, any more intricate application of the quadratic formula will be too time consuming to be useful. Note that the operations before the square root sign are both correct. The plus and minus signs indicate that every quadratic equation has the possibility of two answers. It does not say that both answers will be valid to the multiple-choice word problem that is in quadratic form. This is easily explained with a simple statement. Since two negative numbers and two positive numbers multiplied together give a positive answer, any quadratic equation may have two possible correct answers. When answering questions about quadratic equations in multiple-choice problems, that statement should be considered.

FOIL – POLYNOMIAL MULTIPLICATION

Polynomial multiplication is routinely taught with a method described as FOIL, which stands for First, Outside, Inside and Last. In a binomial multiplication problem, the form will usually look like this, with A, B, C, D whole number coefficients:

$$(Ax + B) * (Cx + D)$$

- The "First" means that Ax and Cx are multiplied together to equal ACx^2
- The "Outside" means that Ax and D are multiplied together to equal ADx
- The "Inside" means that B and Cx are multiplied together to equal BCx
- The "Last" means that B and D are multiplied together to equal BD

  The polynomial answer becomes:
  $ACx^2 + (AD + BC)x + BD$

In testing conditions, this method can be cumbersome, confusing and unreliable because mistakes are too common.

A simplified alternative is called the Box Method, and it is simpler for multiple reasons.

1. There is a box that provides the organization for the multiplication.
2. The box also provides organization for the addition of like terms.
3. This method is expandable for use with longer polynomial multiplication.

To use the Box Method for polynomial multiplication, follow these steps:

1. Create a box that has a row and column for each term in the multiplication problem.
2. Perform the multiplication of each pair of terms.
3. Place the answers in the cells of the box.
4. Add the like terms that are aligned diagonally.
5. Write the polynomial.

The following diagram explains the outcome with the previously noted example:

$$(Ax + B) * (Cx + D) \text{ becomes:}$$

The diagonal boxes in the upper right and lower left are always the "like terms" so there are no questions as to which terms must be added. This is true if you have ordered the binomials correctly with the "x term" of the binomials on the left and on top, respectively.

The final outcome is the same as the FOIL answer previously noted:

$$ACx^2 + (AD + BC)x + BD$$

Notice also that the Box Method has the additional benefit of separating the addition and multiplication operations completely.

In a multiple-choice problem such as this, there is a significant benefit in using the box method as a time saving technique.

Example: $(x + 6) (4x + 8) =$ (choose a correct answer below)

A	$4x^2 + 32x + 48$
B	$4x^2 + 32x + 32$
C	$4x^2 + 32x + 14$
D	$4x^2 + 14x + 48$

The lower right box entry means that the last term in the answer must be $6 * 8$, or 48. So, both answers B and C can be eliminated because the last term is not 48.

The upper right and lower left box entries are added and the middle term must be 24x + 8x = 32x. So, answer D can be eliminated because the middle term is not 14x.

	Ax	B
Cx	ACx^2	BCx
D	ADx	BD

The correct answer must be A, a choice that can be made logically by looking at the box entries. Eliminating choices is expedited with the Box Method because the box entries can be easily compared to coefficients in the answer choices.

SUBSTITUTE VARIABLES

Many mathematics applications involve using equations and then substituting variables. This terminology means that the algebra equation will typically have a single variable with all other parameters defined as whole, decimal or fractional numbers. Then to solve a specific problem, the value of the specific variable will be uniquely defined (in some cases, multiple values may be supplied for comparison) and the variables used to determine a problem solution. For example, let's use the equation that was previously discussed, for a car traveling 70 miles per hour:

Distance traveled equals 70 mph multiplied by time in hours

Without the words, in strictly algebraic terms:

$$D = 70t \text{ (t in hours)}$$

To find the amount of distance traveled, solve the equation by substituting the value of time that is appropriate for the problem. If the problem stated that the time traveled was two and one-half hours, then the equation would be solved with the following:

$$D = 70 * 2.5$$

After multiplying, the answer for the distance traveled is 175 miles.

In some equations, you may be asked to evaluate an equation that involves a second-degree variable. For example, a word description might read as follows:

Distance traveled is equal to one-half 9.8 m/sec^2 multiplied by the time squared

Again, without words, in strictly algebraic terms the equation would be:

$$D = \tfrac{1}{2} * 9.8 * t^2$$

Evaluating this equation for a time of 2 seconds becomes:

$$D = \tfrac{1}{2} * 9.8 * 2^2 = \tfrac{1}{2} * 9.8 * 4 = 2 * 9.8 = 19.6 \text{ meters}$$

The answers have distance units that are determined by the units of measure that are given in the word problem.

Miles per hour multiplied by hours will provide distances in hours. Meters per second per second will provide distances in meters. The units of time and distance within the problem must be consistent. Substituting variables will be simple if the variables are consistent.

INEQUALITIES – GREATER THAN AND LESS THAN

Inequalities are an algebra topic that is often misrepresented and taught in a more difficult manner than necessary. When we find solutions to algebra equations there is a single number (or two numbers in the case of a quadratic equation) that represents the set of all numbers that are equal to the algebraic expression on the other side of the equal sign.

Inequalities represent the set of all numbers that are either greater than or less than that specific solution. If the number 3 represents the solution of an algebra equation, then the following number line diagram may help visualize what the inequalities may look like:

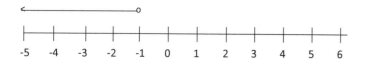

The arrow on the left side of the "o" is the less than inequality, and the arrow on the right side of the "o" is the greater than inequality. Of course, the "o" represents the exact solution of the inequality. This simplicity tells us that the simplest way to solve the inequality is to first solve the equality and then find out which arrow is required. The solution with quadratics will be discussed at the end of this section.

The inequality $7x + 2 > -5$ will be solved by first solving the equality:

$$7x + 2 = -5$$

Following the steps discussed in section 2, the first step is to subtract 2 from both sides and divide both sides by 7. The solution of the equality says:

$$x = -1$$

To see which way the arrow points, we will use the value of $x = 0$ in the inequality to see if it is true. If it is true, then the arrow pointing to the right is correct ($>$), which is what we would expect. If $x = 0$ is not true then the arrow must point the other direction ($<$). The test helps by ensuring that the point at $x = 0$ is or is not in the solution set of the inequality, allowing the correct answer to be chosen.

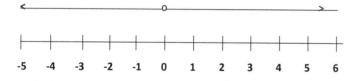

Therefore, substituting $x = 0$ means:

$$7(0) + 2 = 2$$

Since 2 is greater than negative 5, the answer looks like the following diagram:

The arrow does not include the point "0" on the number line because the "Zero Test" tells us that that point does not satisfy the inequality. If the "0" is not included then the arrow must point to the left of the point at -1, which was the answer to the equality. If our test showed that the "0" satisfied the equality, then the arrow would have pointed to the right. For this reason, both "Greater Than" and "Less Than" are addressed in this section. They are determined the same way, specifically:

First, find the solution to the equality.

Second, test to see if $x = 0$ is true for the inequality.

If the test is true, the solution must include the point $x = 0$.

If the test is not true, the inequality goes the opposite direction.

There may be the question as to why the value of $x = 0$ is chosen for the test. Simply, it represents the simplest solution for evaluating algebra equations with variables. Any term which has an "x" (or x^2 or higher order) simply disappears when $x = 0$, leaving only the constant numerical terms.

If there is a need to solve an inequality where the equality solution is $x = 0$, then the inequality test can be performed with $x = 1$. The test is almost as simple as the zero test, and it applies if the equality solution is 0. The same logical decision process used for the zero test also applies here.

HESI A² - Spire Study System

MODULE 2

DAY, LOCATION, MUSIC

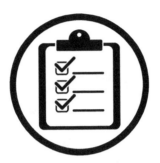

1 MONDAY, OCTOBER 12

COFFEE SHOP ON MAIN STREET

MY FAVORITE BAND

2

3

PHYSICS & GENERAL CHEMISTRY

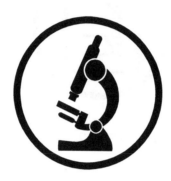

The questions contained in the science sections of the HESI are designed to evaluate one's level of knowledge of the chemical basis of life, cellular biology, human anatomy and human physiology. This includes virtually the entire range of content of a full year of introductory high school level biology and general chemistry. Additionally, the HESI will likely include questions that test for knowledge of topics that are often not well covered by the introductory high school level courses in biology and general chemistry. In particular, these question topics may include material that is usually addressed in higher level courses such as organic chemistry biochemistry, cell physiology, human physiology, human anatomy, human embryology and human genetics.

It is obviously not practical to provide a complete science review within a single manual that includes the entire range of material that is covered in multiple years of science coursework at a high school and/or college level. No study manual can claim that is covers everything in the HESI. The information provided in this manual is - in our opinion - likely to be high-yield. In other words it is material that is very likely to be encountered as topics

of actual HESI science questions. We also present the material as a logical progression of topics - as a storyline that makes sense and is (we hope) reasonably interesting. It is also our judgement that by far most of lower yield science information that is actually encountered on HESI science questions is likely within this section of the manual.

We also - when necessary - may introduce concepts that are unlikely to be directly tested for on the HESI, but which greatly clarify and simplify the explanation of high-yield information. This material will allow one to avoid the need to use rote memorization of a large amount of high yield facts as preparation for the HESI. It will also provide a deeper level of understanding of a large amount of otherwise confusing information and allow us to introduce much of the more advanced science topics in an efficient and more easily grasped manner. Although we cannot guarantee that this manual will prepare you for every possible HESI science question we are confident it will prepare you to succeed at the highest levels of the HESI Science section.

Physics & General Chemistry

A discussion of the physical and life sciences is virtually impossible without providing the basics of physics. Although there are few if any purely physics type questions on the HESI, one is at a huge disadvantage without an understanding of several basic topics in physics. This understanding begins with the fact that the physical universe consists of essentially four things, space, time, matter and energy. These four things have various measurable properties. The properties are measured in standardized units called metric or SI units.

Space

There are three spatial dimensions on our universe and one may define these as length, width and height. The SI unit of measurement for space is the **meter**. The abbreviation for a meter is "m". If we define two points in space we can measure the **linear distance** between the two points. The magnitude of this distance can vary greatly, from the incredibly small to the unimaginably large. At a human level the meter (m) is often used since many of the things we encounter as humans are in the meter scale. The height of an average adult male in the U.S is about 1.7 meters. For larger scales, we often use 1000 meter units called **kilometers** (km).

The circumference of the earth is about 40,000 km. For very large distances we use scientific notation in meters or kilometers. The distance from the earth to the sun is about 1.5×10^8 km. For the largest distance scale, we use the distance that a beam of light would travel (in a vacuum) in one year - a light year. One light year is equal to 9.46×10^{12} km. For small human-scale distance we use **centimeters** (cm) which are 1/100th of a meter and **millimeters** - which are 1/1000th of a meter. At the microscopic scale, we use **micrometers** (μm) which are one millionth of a meter or 1×10^{-6} m. For the atomic scale, we often use **nanometers** (nm) which are 1×10^{-9} m.

Area

A 2-dimensional region in space can be defined as an area or a surface. The simplest of these is a is a flat or planar rectangular surface with a length "L" and a width "W" The resulting area is equal to the product of the length and the width. For instance, a flat rectangular surface with a length of 4 m and a width of 5 m has an area (A) of

$$A = (4 \text{ m})(5 \text{ m}) = 20 \text{ m}^2$$

Notice that the units "m" or meters are multiplied in the equation to give a new metric - meters-squared (m^2) or "**square meters**". Meters-squared" is a distance squared and areas in general have units of distances squared.

In the life sciences, square meters is usually too inconveniently large a scale. More often surface areas are defined as square centimeters. One centimeter is equal to 100 centimeters but 1 square meter is not equal to 100 square centimeters. A square with sides of 1 meter has an area of 1 m^2. This means it has sides that are 100 cm in length, so the area of the square in square centimeters is (100 cm)(100 cm) = 10,000 cm. While 1 meter is equal to 100 centimeters, one square meter is equal to 10,000 square centimeters

Volume

A 3-dimensional region in space can be defined as a volume. The simplest of these volumes is a rectangular volume with a length "L", a width "W" and a height "H". The resulting volume is equal to the product of the length, width and height. For instance, a rectangular volume (V) with a length of 4 m, a width of 5 m and a height of 6 m has an volume of

$$V = (4 \text{ m})(5 \text{ m})(6 \text{ m}) = 120 \text{ m}^3$$

the units "m" or meters are multiplied together three times in the equation to give a new metric - meters-cubed (m³) or "**cubic meters**". Meters-cubed" is a distance cubed and volumes by definition have units of distances cubed. Notice that 1 cubic meter can be the volume of a cube with sides each equal to 1 meter in length, width and height. This means the cube can also be said to have sides equal to 100 centimeters in length, width and height. Therefore the volume of the 1 m³ cube in centimeters is (100 cm)(100 cm)(100 cm) = 1,000,000 cm³. A Volume of 1 m³ is equivalent to a volume of one million or 1×10^6 cm³.

A common non-SI unit of volume particularly in the laboratory is the **liter** (L). The liter is defined as a volume of exactly 1,000 cubic centimeters (cm³). One milliliter (mL) is 1/1000th of a liter or 1×10^{-3} L. The milliliter scale is also a very common volume scale for the life sciences.

Circular Metrics

A linear distance in space often is a displacement distance. Displacement represents the shortest distance between a starting point and ending point location of an object when moves from one location to another object. An object may travel any arbitrary distance in a circle and end up exactly where its motion began. The object will have no overall or net displacement but the object has traveled a distance. This distance - if it is a complete circle - is equal to the diameter of the circle "D) times a constant called pi (π). This is the circumference (C) of the circle.

$$C = \pi D$$

The value of pi is a transcendental number - a number that has no exact value but can be calculated to any arbitrary level of preciseness beyond the decimal point. For our purposes, we will use the value of pi to two places to the right of the decimal point, this value is 3.14.

A **circular area** (A) is calculated by multiplying the

square of the radius (r) of the circle by pi

$$A = \pi r^2$$

A **spherical volume** (v) is given by the formula

$$V = 4/3\, \pi r^3$$

Frequently in the laboratory, volumes are measured in **cylinders**, the formula for the volume (V_c) of a cylinder is height (h) of the cylinder times the cross-sectional area of the cylinder (πr^2)

$$V_c = h(\pi r^2)$$

Constants

Notice that circular surface areas also have units of distance squared. The circular radius is directly proportional to the distance squared. The constant pi converts the proportional value into a precise value. Pi is a purely mathematical constant. Physical properties and processes are often related by physical constants.

Examples of such physical constants include the speed of light in a vacuum "c", the universal gravitational constant "G" , the ideal gas law constant "R" and the chemical reaction equilibrium "Keq" . Universal physical constants are independent of external factors. Most physical processes are dependent on various external factors, so the physical constants associated with these processes are not constant unless they are defined for a precise set of external conditions. These constants are usually required to convert proportional relationships to precise numerical values with the correct units of measurement

Mass

Nearly everything in the universe relevant to the HESI can be defined as matter or as energy. Matter is essentially everything that has mass. Nearly all matter on earth is composed of atoms, and atoms are composed of three basic subatomic particles, the proton, the neutron and the electron. All three of these subatomic particles have a fundamental physical property called mass.

Any physical object on earth should be thought of as being composed entirely of atoms. All physical objects on earth therefore have mass. This mass is the sum of the mass of all of the atoms that comprise the object. The mass of the atoms of the object is the sum of the masses of all of the protons, neutrons and electrons that compose the atoms of the object.

For macroscopic objects such as a rock, a glass of water, or a balloon full of helium gas, The SI units of mass is the **kilogram** (kg). In the laboratory, it is more common to work with smaller units of mass than kilograms. The most common of these mass units are **grams** and **milligrams**. Grams (g) are 1/1000th of a kilogram and milligrams (mg) are 1/1000 that of a gram. It is unusual that the kilogram is the standard SI unit for mass since a kilogram is by definition equal to 1000 grams.

At the atomic scale masses are incredibly small. The mass of a proton is 1.6726×10^{-27} kg, the mass of the neutron is slightly more than the mass of a proton but the mass of the electron is 1827 times lighter than the mass of the proton. For atomic scales, masses are given in **atomic mass units** (AMUs). The AMU unit is vastly smaller than a kilogram unit. The mass of a proton in AMUs is approximately 1.007 AMU. The mass of the electron is so small that it can be approximated as zero for most cases likely to be encountered in the HESI.

Density

In addition to mass, all matter also has a volume. For any given sample of matter, that volume is the volume of space that the sample occupies. The mass of a sample of matter divided by the volume of the sample of matter is the mass per unit volume of the sample (m/V). This property of matter is defined as the density of matter. The scientific symbol for density is the greek letter rho (ρ). There are no commonly used specific SI units of density, density is by definition units of mass divided by units of volume. Density is usually given in units of grams per liter (g/L) or in SI units of kilograms per cubic meter (kg/m^3) or grams per cubic centimeter (g/cm^3). **The density of liquid water at a temperature of 4 C is equal to 1 gram per cubic centimeter (1 g/cm^3)**

Weight

The physical quantities of weight and mass are often misunderstood. Mass is an intrinsic property of matter that is determined by the type and number of atoms that comprise a given sample of matter. **Weight is a force that acts on matter in a gravitational field**. On earth this force is equal to the mass of an object times the acceleration that the object experiences due to the strength of the Earth's gravitational field. This acceleration is 9.8 m/s^2. For instance, the weight of a 20 kg object on the surface of the earth will be

$$(20 \text{ kg})(9.8 \text{ m/s}^2) = 196 \text{ kg-m/s}^2.$$

The units "kg-m/s^2" are defined as the SI units of force - the "newton (N)". One newton equals 1kg-m/s^2, therefore the weight of a 20 kg mass on earth is 196 Newtons (N). When samples of substances are weighed in the laboratory the "weight is usually given in units of mass. Since mass is directly proportional to weight this is an acceptable but technically inaccurate description of the sample weight.

Almost always in experiments, a sample weight is given in mass units, but in reality, what is measured is the weight of the mass due to earth's gravity. And the correct units are not units of mass (i.e kilograms) but units of force (i.e. Newtons). One way to keep this distinction in mind is to consider that in an environment where there is no significant force of gravity, one could not "weigh out" a sample of a substance on a scale. The sample mass would exert no force of the scale and would be literally weightless. Most scientific instruments are calibrated to give the mass of objects even though they are actually measuring the weight of samples.

Of course, this mass measurement will only be accurate in a gravitational field equal to the gravitational force that the earth exerts at the surface of the earth (at sea level). The exception is a scale that balances an unknown mass against a standard mass such as a triple beam balance. These types of balances will be accurate in any gravitational field (but not in environments with no net gravitational field).

Atomic and Molecular Weights

The terms atomic and molecular weights are often used in science and should be considered to be equivalent to the terms atomic mass and molecular mass where the units of mass in grams is substituted for the number of AMU units. If, for example, an atom has an atomic mass of is 10 AMU then the corresponding atomic weight is 10 grams. This is actually equivalent to the number of atoms, that as a sample, would have a mass total mass of 10 grams. We have discussed that a single atom's atomic mass is approximately the sum of the masses of the protons and neutrons contained in the atom's nucleus. The unit of mass at the atomic level is the atomic mass unit (AMU). When the term atomic weight is used it is referring to the average mass of an atom of an element.

Elements

An element is the group of all atoms that have the same number of protons in their nucleus. For instance, the element carbon refers to all atoms that have exactly four protons in their atomic nuclei. Most carbon atoms also have four neutrons in their nuclei so most carbon atoms have an atomic mass of approximately 8 AMU (4 protons + 4 neutrons). Some carbon atoms have more than 4 neutrons in their nuclei so these carbon atoms

have a mass larger than 8 AMU. On average the mass of a carbon atom is somewhat larger than 8 AMU due to the existence of the carbon atoms that have nuclei with more than 4 neutrons. The actual average value depends on the naturally occurring percentages of heavier carbon atoms. This average elemental atom mass is defined as the element's atomic mass - but also is frequently described as the element's atomic weight.

In the laboratory, the term atomic weight is considered to be the equivalent to the element's atomic mass in grams. This is a very important definition to understand because it is used as a scientific basis for designing almost all chemical experiments. The reason for this is because the atomic masses of all of the elements have been determined experimentally. The absolute values of these elemental masses are less important than the fact that we also know what the elemental masses are relative to the other elemental masses. For instance, the atomic mass (average mass) of a carbon atom is approximately 12 AMU (21.01) and the atomic mass of an oxygen atom is approximately 16 AMU.

Molar Mass

We cannot work with individual atoms in the laboratory but since we know what the relative values of the masses of carbon and oxygen atoms are (12-to-16 or 12:16), then we can weigh out 12 grams of carbon and 16 grams of oxygen and since this is the ratio of the masses of carbon and oxygen atoms we know that there are theoretically exactly the same number of carbon atoms in the 12 gram sample of carbon as there are oxygen atoms in the 16 gram sample of oxygen.

This knowledge allows scientists to conduct experiments and make measurements that reveal import and detailed information about chemical reactions. This knowledge of the relative masses or mass ratios of elements is so useful that scientists have adopted a working version definition of an element's atomic mass as being the element's atomic weight in grams.

Molecular weights are defined in the same manner as atomic weights, for instance the mass of one molecule of water (H_2O) is the sum of the atomic masses of two hydrogen atoms and the atomic one oxygen atom. This is (2)(1)+16=18 AMU. The molecular weight of H_2O is the molecular mass of H_2O in grams, so the molecular weight of H_2O is 18 grams. This mass in grams of an atomic or molecular mass is also called the **molar mass** of the atom or molecule.

An example is a single molecule of oxygen which consists of two chemically bonded oxygen atoms. The atomic mass of oxygen is 16 AMU so the atomic weight of oxygen is 16 grams. The molar mass of oxygen atoms is also 16 grams. The oxygen molecule O_2 contains two oxygen atoms so it has a molecular mass of 32 AMU (16+16) and a molecular weight of 32 grams and a molar mass of 32 grams. This can also be stated as "the atomic weight of oxygen is 16 grams per mole (g/M)" or "the weight of one mole of oxygen atoms is 16 grams."

Avogadro's Number

For the molecule of O_2, one can say "the molecular weight of O_2 is 32 grams per mole (g/M)" or "the mass of one mole of O2 is 32 grams". The mole is actually a number without units. It is equivalent to the number 6.022×10^{23}. This number is also called Avogadro's number. This is the number (1 mole) of particles present in any sample of a pure molecular substance where the mass of the sample of the substance is equal to the molecular weight of the substance. It is an awkward concept to express in words but easier to show by example.

Scientific Methods and Reasoning

Suppose that a student is in chemistry lab and is asked to measure out 5 moles of liquid ammonia. First the student must determine what the molecular formula for

ammonia is. It is NH_3 meaning that individual ammonia atoms consist of three hydrogen atoms and one nitrogen atom. Next the student must determine the molecular mass of an ammonia molecule. This can be determined by referring to the periodic table of the elements which generally will list the atomic mass of every element beneath the atomic symbol for the element. For nitrogen (N) this is 14 AMU and for hydrogen this is 1 AMU. The molecular mass of ammonia is therefore 14+(3)(1)=17 AMU. The molecular weight or the molar mass of ammonia is therefore 17 grams.

The student can weigh out a sample of liquid ammonia on laboratory scales such as a triple beam balance scale or on an electronic scale. The scales will give values in grams. It is true that grams is a mass unit not a weight unit, but this is usually not relevant because metric or SI unit scales are calibrated so that the weight the scale indicates for the sample in grams is actually the true mass of the sample in grams. (The true weight of the sample would be $(17g)(9.8 \text{ m/s}^2) = 166.6$ newtons). This 17 gram sample of ammonia is equivalent to one mole of ammonia. The number of ammonia molecules in the sample is 6.022×10^{23} molecules.

Next the student is asked to obtain a 3 mole sample of carbon tetrachloride. The molecular formula for carbon tetrachloride is CCl_4 meaning one molecule of carbon tetrachloride contains one atom of carbon (C) and four atoms of chlorine (Cl). The atomic masses of a carbon atom and a chlorine atom according to the periodic table of the elements is 12 AMU for carbon and 36.45 AMU for chlorine. The molecular mass of CCl_4 is therefore 12+(4)(36.45)=157.8 AMU. This means 1 mole of carbon tetrachloride will "weigh"157.8 grams on a laboratory scale. The molar mass of CCl_4 is 157.8 grams/mole (g/M). Notice that this one molar mass is equal to the mass of 6.022×10^{23} molecules of CCl_4. Since not one, but three moles of CCL_4 are required, the student must weigh out (3 moles)(157.8

grams/mole) = 473.4 grams of CCl_4

The concept of the mole (M) and molar mass is encountered continually in the physical and life sciences. It is more common to think of a chemical reaction as representing the reaction of moles of molecules rather than individual molecules. For instance the chemical equation $2H_2 + O_2 \rightarrow 2H_2O$ can be interpreted as two molecules of hydrogen (each molecule consisting of two atoms of hydrogen) reacting with one molecule of oxygen (the "2" in O_2 indicating the molecule consists of two atoms of oxygen) to produce two molecules of H_2O (the molecular formula "H_2O" indicates that one molecule of H_2O consists of two atoms of hydrogen and one atom of oxygen).

It is often more useful, however, to think of this reaction as being one where two moles of molecular hydrogen (H_2) react with one mole of oxygen molecules (O_2) to produce two moles of H_2O molecules. Molar masses are often inconveniently large for research purposes and it is frequent that experimental procedures use millimolar (mM) units which are equal to 1/1000th of a mole.

Concentrations

Molar masses are almost always the units used to describe concentrations. Nearly all biochemical reaction occurs in liquids. The concentration of chemicals in a liquid is the number of molecules dissolve in the fluid per unit volume of the liquid. The dissolving liquid is called the "**solvent**" and the dissolved molecules are called the **solute** or solute particles. Together, the solvent and dissolved solutes are called a "**solution**". **A one molar solution of a molecular substance contains one mole of the substance dissolved in one liter of solution** (1Mol/L) The term "**molarity**" is closely related - it is the molar concentration of a solution phrased as "the molarity of the solution is". For example, a solution a given molecular substance with a concentration of 0.45 moles/liter (M/L) has a molarity

of 0.45, or equivalently - a molar concentration of 0.45. Millimolar concentration units are also frequently used in the life sciences. A one millimolar solution of a chemical has 1/1000th of a mole of molecules dissolved in one liter of solution.

The Four Fundamental Forces

All matter interacts through space by one or more of the four fundamental forces. These forces are the strong force, the weak force, the electromagnetic force and the gravitational force.

The Strong Force

The strong force is the force that interacts between protons and neutrons in the nucleus of atoms to bind the the individual protons and neutrons tightly together within the nucleus. The strong force is significant for the HESI because it is the force that is acting during the fusion of hydrogen nuclei into helium nuclei at the center of the sun. This fusion reaction produces unimaginable amounts of energy that reaches the earth in the form of photons.

This energy is the energy that is used to power nearly every physical and chemical reaction That occurs on our planet. It is the energy that raises the temperature of the planet to a level that can support the chemical processes of life and it is the energy in the form of photons of visible light that is absorbed by plants to convert carbon dioxide and water into carbohydrates and oxygen. this process - called photosynthesis - is the reaction that allows plants to form the base of the food chain upon which nearly all other forms of life depend and it is the process that continually replenishes the atmospheric oxygen that is essential to all multicellular forms of life including humans.

The Weak Force

The weak force is the force within an atomic nucleus that can induce the radioactive decay (or breakdown) of an atomic nucleus. These radioactive decay products are of two types; alpha particles which are helium nuclei consisting of two protons and two neutrons, and beta particles (previously called beta rays) rays, which are very high energy electrons (or positrons). The weak force is significant for the HESI because it is process that generates many of the harmful types of radiation that humans encounter that can cause damage to human cells. The radiation hazard from radon gas is an example.

The Electromagnetic Force

The electromagnetic force is the force that interacts between charged particles. Charge is a fundamental property of subatomic particles. Electrons have an electric charge of -1, protons have an electric charge of +1 and neutrons have zero charge. Particles with opposite electric charges are attracted to one another by the electromagnetic force and particles with the same electric charge repel each other. It is the electromagnetic force that attracts electrons to an atom's positively charged nucleus.

When an atom contains the same number of electrons and protons, the positive charge due to the protons in the nucleus and the negative charge of the electrons surrounding the nucleus cancel out. As a result, the atom has a net electric charge of zero. When this is the case, the atom is called a neutral atom.

Ions

Atoms can have fewer or more electrons than protons. When the number of electrons exceeds the number of protons, the atom has a net negative charge. When the number of protons exceeds the number of electrons, the atom has a net positive charge. The net charge is equal to the sum of the positive charges due to protons and negative charges due to electrons. For instance, if an atom has eight electrons and six protons, then the net charge of the atom is (-8)+(6)= -2.

Atoms (and molecules) with net charges are called ions.

Negative ions are called anions and positive ions are called cations.

Larger particles such as molecules and even macroscopic objects can have a net charge, but this net charge always is due to an unbalanced number of electrons and protons within the particle or object

We will discuss the electromagnetic force at the atomic and molecular level in greater detail in the chemistry review section, but it is important to note that nearly all of the macroscopic mechanical forces such as mechanical friction, air resistance and the pressures exerted by fluids and gases are actually due to the repulsive electromagnetic force at the atomic level between the electrons of different atoms.

The Electromagnetic Force Equation

The mathematical formula that describes the electromagnetic force between charged objects is as follows:

$$F_e = k_e(q_1q_2)/r^2$$

Where F_e is the magnitude (amount) of the electrical force between two charged objects, q_1 and q_2 are the magnitude of the charge on the two objects and r is the distance between the two charged objects. Is the electric force constant that converts the right side of the equation into the SI units of force - the **Newton** (N).

The Gravitational Force

The gravitational force is a purely attractive force between objects separated in space. The gravitational force between objects depends on the mass of the objects and the distance between the the centers of mass of each of the objects

$$F_g = G(m_1m_2)/r^2$$

Notice that the gravitational force equation is very

similar to the electromagnetic force equation. F_g Is the force of gravity (in Newtons) between two objects with masses m_1 and m_2 respectively, r is the distance between the centers of mass of the twoobjects and G is the universal gravitational constant that converts the right side of the equation into Newtons (the SI unit of force).

General Features of Forces

We have defined the electromagnetic and gravitational forces but we still need to explain what these forces are and how they interact with matter. The nature of a force is best explained using **Newton's second law of motion**. This law describes what a force is in general, rather than describing a particular type of force, such as the electromagnetic force or the gravitational force.

To understand this second law, we must describe three other physical concepts; the concepts of motion, velocity and of acceleration. This is because Newton's second law states that force (F) equals mass (m) times accelerations (a) or F=ma. It is unlikely that you will be asked questions that require calculations as given in the following discussion, but the concepts of a force, of velocity and acceleration are so fundamental it is very difficult to explain human physiology at the level of complexity expected by the HESI without this essential background information

Motion

Physical objects at any instant in time have a precise location in the three spatial dimensions. If an object's spatial location does not change over time, the object is said to be at rest or translationally motionless. If an object continuously changes its spatial location over time it is said to be in translational motion.

When an object moves from one spatial location to another spatial location, this motion is called translational motion. The simplest type of translational motion is motion in a straight line. This is called linear motion.

Objects can have zero or no net translational motion but can have vibrational and/or rotational motion. An example is the particles that comprise a solid substance. Although the individual particles do not change three-dimensional position relative to adjacent particles, they will vibrate or oscillate at their fixed positions. The amount of vibration corresponds to the Temperature of the substance. Many types of molecules in the liquid and gaseous state can have segments that rotate relative to other segments of the molecule.

Velocity

When an object is undergoing linear motion, the linear distance that the object travels during a given period of time is defined as the speed of the object. A car that travels 100 meters in 10 seconds has a speed of 100 meters/ 10 seconds or 10 meters per second (10 m/s).

The velocity of an object includes not only the speed of the object - which is the magnitude (size or amount) of the object's velocity - but also the direction in which the object is traveling. For instance, a car traveling 10 m/s due north has a different velocity than a car traveling 10 m/s due south. For the HESI one usually does not need to consider the direction of an object's motion. And therefore, an object's speed may be considered to be the same as the object's velocity.

The exception to this may be when one is considering velocity in one direction vs. velocity in the opposite direction. For instance, an object that is traveling due north at 10 m/s can be assigned a positive velocity of 10 m/s. In this case, another object that is traveling due south (the opposite direction) at 10 m/s would be assigned a negative value velocity of -10 m/s.

The general equation to determine an object's linear velocity is

$$V = \Delta d/\Delta t$$

V is the object's velocity. The character "Δ" indicates "the change in". Δ d is the linear distance the object has traveled over a certain period of time and Δt is "that certain period of time". This is also called the change in position divided by the change in time.

Acceleration

Acceleration is the change in an object's velocity per unit time. If an object's linear velocity remains constant the object's acceleration is zero. If an object is increasing its velocity at a constant rate it is undergoing a constant acceleration. The general formula for the acceleration of an object is:

$a = \Delta v / \Delta t$

An example is a car that has an initial velocity of 10 m/s. Assume the car begins to accelerate at a constant rate. After 5 seconds the car's new velocity is 60 m/s. The change in the car's velocity, Δv, is (60 m/s) - (10 m/s) = 50m/s. The time span over which this change of velocity occurred - the change in time - or "Δt" - is 5 seconds (5 s). The car's acceleration is therefore:

$a = (50 \text{ m/s}) / (5 \text{ s}) = 10 \text{ m/s}^2$

This "second squared" or s^2 term is commonly called seconds per second - it means that, in the case above, the car is increasing its velocity by 10 m/s for every second that the car is traveling.

One aspect of acceleration to remember for the HESI is that acceleration can be negative. In the example above, if the car had an initial velocity of 60 m/s and slowed down at a constant rate resulting in a final velocity of 10 m/s after a time span of 5 seconds, the car would be accelerating in the opposite direction of its initial velocity. Under these circumstances, the car has a negative acceleration equal to -10 m/s^2.

Forces in Action

At the macroscopic (large scale) level the forces that act on an object resulting in changes in motion of the object are usually mechanical forces or the gravitational force. Mechanical forces at the microscopic level are the result of interactions of matter through the electromagnetic force. Mechanical forces at the macroscopic (large) scale can be generated, for example, by muscle contractions resulting in pushing and pulling mechanical forces that can be applied to an object. Another common means of applying a mechanical force is through chemical reactions such as the combustion of gasoline to exert a mechanical force on the pistons in an internal combustion engine.

Net Force

A force has a magnitude and a direction just as velocity and acceleration have magnitudes and directions. There are usually a number of different forces acting on an object, such as air resistance and surface frictional forces. Depending on their magnitude and direction, all of these forces added together can produce a net force; a single force of a specific magnitude that acts in a specific direction on the object. Often, all of the forces acting on an object cancel each other out and the net force acting on the object is zero.

If a net force is applied to an object the object will begin to accelerate in the direction in which the force is applied. This is given by the general formula

$F = ma$

An example is an object with mass m = 20 kg, that is experiencing an unknown net force. As this net force is exerted upon the object, it experiences an acceleration of 5 m/s^2. We can calculate the force acting on the object by substituting these values into the general force equation

$F = (20 \text{ kg}) (5 \text{ m/s}^2); F = 100 \text{ kg·m/s}^2$

The units kg·m/s^2 are the SI units for force. 1 kg·m/s^2 is equal to 1 Newton (N). Therefore, the object in the example above is experiencing a net force of 100 newtons (100 N)

We can rearrange the general force equation to determine an unknown mass or unknown acceleration of an object. For instance, if a 50 N force is applied to a 25 kg object, we can calculate the object's acceleration by rearranging the force equation to

$a = F/m$
$a = 50 \text{ N} / 25 \text{ kg}$
$a = 2 \text{ m/s}^2$

Notice that by definition, an object at rest has no net force acting upon it. Additionally, and often overlooked, is the fact that an object that has a constant velocity is also experiencing no net force. If a net force was acting on the object, as the equation F=ma shows, the object would be accelerating. An object with a constant velocity is not accelerating.

Pressure - Force Per Unit Area

Pressure is a physical quantity that is defined as the amount of force that is exerted by a substance per surface area (F/A). For example, gases that are confined in a sealed container will exert a pressure against the walls of the container. The individual gas molecules exert a force on the container walls when they collide with the interior surface of the container. The amount of force exerted per unit area by the gas on the container walls depends on how many gas molecules are inside of the container and how much force the average gas molecule exerts on the container wall when it strikes the container walls.

The SI unit of pressure is the **pascal** (Pa). One pascal is defined a **1 newton per square meter** (1N/m or 1 kg-m/s^2). Atmospheric pressure is the pressure that the earth's atmosphere exerts on surfaces exposed to the atmosphere. At sea level this is defined as 1 **atmosphere** (atm) of pressure. One atmosphere of pressure is equal to approximately 1×10^5 pascals (the precise ratio is 1 atm = 101325 Pa). pressure is often measured in a barometer by the displacement height of mercury (Hg) within a U-shaped tube. The pressure unit as measured in this manner is the torr, 1 **torr** of pressure is equal to 1 mm displacement of mercury. One atmosphere will register in a barometer as a displacement height of 760 millimeters of mercury (760 mm Hg), therefore, 1 atm = 760 torr.

In human physiology, pressures effects are important factors in the respiratory system, the circulatory system, the renal or kidney excretory system. There are numerous other instances where pressure or pressure differences are a critical factor in a wide variety of physiological processes. In particular pressure effects are encountered in several physiological processes that involve **diffusion** of substances. **Osmotic pressure** is an important phenomenon that is produced when diffusion is occurring across semipermeable membranes within the body.

Energy

Energy is a fundamental quantity that - along with time and space - defines the physical universe. Energy and matter are intimately related. Matter is a form of condensed energy that has acquired the property of mass. Matter can be created from energy and matter can be converted to energy. This relationship is expressed mathematically by Einstein's famous equation E=mc^2, where E is a quantity of energy, m is a quantity of mass and "c" is the universal constant of the speed of light in a vacuum.

Still we are left with the question "what IS energy?" and that is a very difficult question at the fundamental level but it can be generally understood as a substance that can be absorbed by matter and emitted by matter and can be transferred between material objects. This interaction can change the properties of matter by increasing or decreasing the velocity of matter or by altering the interactions of matter in the form of chemical bonds between atoms and electromagnetic bonds between molecules and other larger particles of matter.

Electromagnetic Energy

Pure energy exists everywhere in the universe in the form of electromagnetic radiation. This energy consists of fundamental subatomic particles called photons. At the atomic level the notion of a particle as a solid object with a definite size and location is no longer valid. Photons can behave as if they are solid particles under certain conditions, but they more often behave as if they are waves of energy. The energy of a photon is related to its wave-like nature. Waves have a wavelength and a frequency. The energy of a photon can be almost zero or almost any higher value. The higher the energy of a photon the shorter the photon's wavelength and the higher the photons frequency. This range of energy wavelengths is referred to as the **electromagnetic energy spectrum.**

Electromagnetic waves are unique compared to other types of waves in that they do not require a medium within which to travel. Sound waves and all other waves must travel through matter in the form of a continuous gas, liquid or a solid medium. Electromagnetic waves can and do travel through the vacuum of empty space.

Beginning at the lowest energies and therefore the longest photon wavelengths (and lowest frequencies) of the electromagnetic spectrum are the radio waves followed with increasingly high energies by microwaves, infrared radiation, wavelengths of the visible light spectrum, ultraviolet wavelengths, x-rays and gamma rays. **Infrared radiation** is also referred to as thermal or heat radiation because it is emitted by all objects in proportion to the temperature of the objects and the absorption of infrared radiation generally results in an increase in the temperature of the substance that absorbs the infrared radiation. This type of transfer of energy in the form of heat is called radiation or radiative heat transfer (the other modes of heat transference are conduction and convection). Excessive heat transference to the body can of course cause thermal injury to cells ranging from mild 1st degree burns to 3rd or 4th degree burns resulting in permanent injury and frequently fatal injury.

The visible light spectrum is significant in that these are the photons that are detected by the human visual system. The light receptors of the eye - the rod and cone cells- actually absorb visible light and convert this energy to electrical signals that are relayed to the brain. Visible light photons are also absorbed by chlorophyll molecules in chloroplast in plant cells and are used as a source of energy for converting carbon dioxide and water into carbohydrates and oxygen.

The ultraviolet spectrum in significant in that photons at ultraviolet energies are emitted by the sun are able to damage DNA in the skin and are a primary cause of skin cancer including the extremely deadly form of skin cancer - malignant melanoma. Prolonged exposure of unprotected skin to sunlight dramatically increases the risk for the development of malignant melanoma. **X-rays and gamma rays** are even more damaging to DNA and even brief exposure can cause severe and widespread cell injury and - at high enough levels - rapid death from radiation poisoning.

In chemical reactions photons are absorbed and emitted by electrons as electrons rearrange themselves within and among the atoms that are participating in the chemical reactions. At the most fundamental level this is why chemical reactions occur. Electrons are always trying to achieve their lowest possible energy state and this requires that they find a means to release energy in the form of the emission of photons. Chemical reactions are one of the types of processes that allow this lowering of electron energy to occur through the emission of photons.

Work

Work is literally energy, but energy that is undergoing a transference process. Mechanical work can be done on an object by applying a net force to an object. The work (W) done on the object is the force (F) applied to the object multiplied by that distance (D) over which the force is applied to the object. This is given by the general equation:

$$W = FxD$$

An example is an object that is experiencing a constant force of 15 N. This force causes the object to accelerate. After the object travels a distance of 20 m, while experiencing the constant 15 N force, the work done on the object is equal to

$$W = (15 \ N) \ (20 \ m); \ W = 300 \ N\text{-}m.$$

The units N-m (Newton-meters) are equivalent to SI unit of energy, the joule (J). 1 N-m equals 1 joule. Also notice that units for the SI unit of force, the Newton, are equal to $kg \cdot m/sec^2$. Since a joule is 1 Newton times one meter, the units for the joule are also $kg \cdot m^2/sec^2$. The SI unit of work and the SI unit of energy are the same unit - the joule. This shows that work and energy are the same thing. As we will discuss later, heat is also equivalent to energy and to work

Gravitational Potential Energy

The gravitational potential energy of an object (PE) is calculated using the following equation

$$PE = mgh$$

For the above equation, m is the mass of the object, h is the height of the object above the surface of the earth and g is the acceleration that the object experiences due to the force of gravity. This acceleration (g) is a constant at or near the surface of the earth and is equal to 9.8 meters per second squared (9.8 m/s^2). As a specific example, consider an object with a mass of 10 kg that is resting motionless atop a ladder 5 meters above the surface of the earth. The gravitation potential energy of the object is

$$PE = (10 \text{ kg})(9.8 \text{ m/s}^2)(5 \text{ m}) = 490 \text{ kg·m}^2/\text{s}^2$$

The units kg·m^2/s^2 are the SI units for energy - the joule (J). The object therefore has a gravitational potential energy equal to 490 joules (490 J)

Kinetic Energy

Kinetic energy (KE) is the energy of motion for an object. An object with no velocity (at rest) has zero kinetic energy. The formula to calculate the kinetic energy of an object is

$$KE = \tfrac{1}{2} mv^2$$

In the equation above, m is the mass of the object and v is the velocity of the object. Notice that in the example above the object atop the ladder has no velocity and therefore no kinetic energy

The convertibility Between Kinetic and Potential Energy

If the object described above falls from the ladder, the earth's gravitational force begins to accelerate the object at 9.8 m/s^2. The object will experience the force of gravity over the entire vertical distance that it falls to the ground. This distance will be 10 meters. As we have previously discussed, the formula that gives the amount of work that is done on an object when the object is subjected to a constant force, such as the force of gravity, is:

Work=Force x Distance, or W=FxD

where distance is equal to the total distance over which the force is applied to the object. The object, when it began to fall, had a velocity of zero. The force acting on the object is the force of gravity and the distance is the object's height above the ground.

Since the general force equation is F=ma, the force of gravity experienced by our object can be written as

$$F_g = (m_o)(g)$$

where "m_o" is the object's mass and "a" is the acceleration due to "g" - the acceleration experienced by a mass at or close to the the surface of the earth. This gravitational acceleration is equal to 9.8 m/s^2.

Since work = force x distance, at the instant that the falling object strikes the ground, the object will have acquired an amount of energy equal to the work done on the object.

$$W = E \text{ and } W = mgh.$$

The work done on the object by the force of gravity over the distance of the object's fall to the ground is:

$$(10 \text{ kg})(9.8 \text{ m/s}^2)(5 \text{ m}) = 490 \text{ kg·m}^2/\text{s}^2.$$

Notice that, just as in the case of gravitational potential energy, the units kg·m^2/s^2 are the SI units of energy, the joule (J); 1 kg·m^2/s^2 is equal to 1 joule of energy.

This energy, 490 J, is equal to the object's kinetic energy at the instant before the object strikes the ground. Notice that this final kinetic energy is exactly equal to the object's initial gravitational potential energy. We can solve for the object's velocity the instant before it hits the ground by rearranging the equation kinetic energy equation

$$KE = \tfrac{1}{2} mv^2$$

$v = (2KE/m)^{1/2}$

Substitute the values for the object's mass, 10 kg, and the object's kinetic energy, 490 J, into the rearranged equation

$v = [(2)(490 J)/(10 kg)]^{1/2}$.

This reduces to $v = (98)^{1/2}$ or approximately the square root of 100 (since 98 is very close to 100). The velocity of the object the instant before it strikes the ground is approximately 10m/s.

The object's final kinetic energy, (the object's kinetic energy just before it strikes the ground), is equal to the object's initial potential energy (when the object was at rest 10 meters above the ground). This can be stated as:

PE = KE

This is equivalent to the equation:

$mgh = \frac{1}{2}(mv^2)$

This demonstrates that gravitational potential energy can be completely converted to kinetic energy. The reverse of this statement is equally true; kinetic energy can be completely converted to gravitational potential energy.

As a final example, consider an object with a mass of 20kg that has fallen from rest from an unknown height above the ground. The object strikes the ground with a kinetic energy of 980 J. The height of the object above the ground when the object began to fall can be calculated as shown below:

PE = mgh
h = PE/(mg)
KE = PE

h = KE/(mg)
KE = 980 J
h = 980 J/(9.8 m/s²)(20 kg)
h = 5 meters

Dimensional Analysis

One way to check that calculations are correct is by using dimensional analysis. The dimensions of a calculation are the units of measurement. In the equation above, h = 980 J/(9.8 m/s²)(20 kg). It is not obvious how the calculation results in an answer with units of meters. By substituting the units for a joule (J), $kg \cdot m^2/s^2$, into the equation, one can confirm that the answer will have units of meters.

h = 980 J/(9.8 m/s²)(20 kg)

h = (980 kg·m²/s²)/(9.8 m/s²)(20 kg)

The units of kg/s² are present in both the numerator and denominator of the equation, therefore these units cancel.

h = (980 m²)/(9.8 m)(20)

The units are now reduced to (m²/m), which simplifies to m (meters).

Chemical Potential Energy (Internal Energy)

We have seen how a large (macroscopic) object can acquire gravitational potential energy by moving from a lower height above the surface of the earth to a greater height above the surface of the earth. The work or energy required to lift an object against the force of gravity to a greater height is equivalent to the gravitational potential energy that the object acquires when it reaches the higher position above the surface of the earth. This energy can then be converted into kinetic energy of the object when the object begins to fall back to the surface of the earth.

At the microscopic scale, matter, in the form of molecules, can also acquire or release potential energy. This form of potential energy is acquired or released primarily by the formation of chemical bonds between the atoms of the molecules. This is called chemical potential energy. Chemical potential energy and several other quantities of a system of matter together comprise the **internal energy (U)** of a system of matter. In chemical reactions, the reactant molecules break existing chemical bonds and then form new chemical bonds resulting in the formation of new molecules (which are the products of the chemical reaction).

When a chemical bond is formed, energy is primarily released in the form of heat and heat energy is most commonly the energy that is utilized to break chemical bonds. If the amount of heat energy released by the formation of molecular bonds during a chemical reaction exceeds the amount of heat energy required to the break molecular bonds during the chemical reaction, then the overall reaction will produce heat and release this heat into the surrounding environment. This type of chemical reaction is called an exothermic (heat producing) reaction. The chemical potential energy of the reactant molecules has been converted into the heat energy produced by the reaction.

Heat

All forms of energy - kinetic energy and potential energy in particular - can be converted into work and that work can be converted back into any form of energy. Work and energy are therefore equivalent and the units of energy and work are the same. Heat ("H" or sometimes "Q")) is also equivalent to energy and to work and the units of heat are also given in joules. Heat can be converted to all forms of energy including kinetic and potential energy and all forms of energy including kinetic and potential energy can be converted to heat.

Exothermic and Endothermic Chemical Reactions

Heat is energy that is transferred between objects and this transfer occurs through radiation of electromagnetic energy and through transfer of kinetic energy of particles (conduction and convection). For the HESI, Heat is significant as it relates to the temperature of objects and as it relates to the physical properties of the solid, liquid and gas phases of matter, to phase transitions of matter and to the rates of chemical reactions. An example is the production of heat that occurs during an exothermic chemical reaction. As we discussed the potential chemical energy in such reactions is converted to heat. This is typically written in a general chemical reaction form as

$$A + B \rightarrow C + D, -\Delta H$$

The $-\Delta H$ is the amount of heat generated by the reaction. The negative sign shows that heat is removed from the reaction. If the reaction requires the addition of heat (an endothermic reaction) the ΔH is written as $+\Delta H$

The term **enthalpy** is often used in chemistry in place of the term heat. The heat of a chemical reaction, ΔH, if often called the enthalpy of the reaction.

Temperature

In most cases heat - on the atomic and molecular scale - is energy that ultimately is converted to kinetic energy. Although an object that is motionless has no net kinetic energy, every object has a temperature. **The temperature of an object is proportional to the average kinetic energy of the atoms that are contained in the object** (to be precise the temperature of a substance is directly proportional to the square root of the statistical mean of the kinetic energy of the particles - atoms or molecules - that comprise the substance). This is true not only for substances in the solid state, but for substances in the liquid and gas states as well. The higher the temperature of a substance the greater the average kinetic energy of the individual particles contained in the substance. The addition of heat to a substance usually increases the temperature of the object.

The Temperature Scales - Celsius, Kelvin and Fahrenheit

The Fahrenheit (F) temperature scale defines the freezing point of water as 32 °F and the boiling point of water as 212 °F

The Celsius (C) temperature scale defines the freezing point of water as 0°C and the boiling point of water as 100°C

The Kelvin (K) temperature scale is equivalent to the Celsius scale with the exception that the Kelvin scale defines absolute zero as 0 °K, and the triple point of water as exactly 273.16 degrees (we will discuss what a triple point is in the "phases of matter" discussion). Absolute zero on the Celsius scale is -273.15 °C.

Absolute zero is the theoretically lowest possible temperature of matter. It corresponds to a state where the atoms of matter have no kinetic energy at all - in other words, they are completely motionless. The laws of quantum mechanics show that this temperature can never occur in nature - it is physically impossible to cool anything down to a temperature of absolute zero.

The conversion formula for Celsius to Fahrenheit is
T (°C) = (T (°F) - 32) × 5/9
The Celsius to Kelvin conversion is
 T (°C) = T (°K) - 273.15

Entropy

Chemical energy also can be acquired or released by changes in the entropy of the atoms and molecules that participate in a chemical reaction. Entropy is a measure of how dispersed or spread out energy is within an object or system of objects. In any chemical reaction,

the change in entropy (ΔS) of the reaction can be calculated. When the change in entropy for the reaction is positive the reaction is progressing from a more highly concentrated overall energy state to a more dispersed or spread out energy state. The greater the positive change in entropy the greater the amount of chemical potential energy that is redistributed from a more concentrated to less concentrated (more "spread out") state by the reaction. This energy is equal to "$T\Delta S$" where T is the temperature at which the reaction occurs.

Gibbs Free Energy

Entropy may seem to be a very difficult concept to grasp but it is important for several reasons. The first is that whenever an isolated chemical reaction is occurring that reaction must be energetically favorable. In other words, the reaction must produce energy. We have seen that one source of energy production in a reaction is when there is heat energy produced by formation of new chemical bonds between atoms. This is the enthalpy (ΔH) of the reaction.

Recall that when ΔH is negative for a reaction this means heat is produced by the reaction and this is an exothermic reaction. This energetically favors the reaction, but if the reaction also produces a more well-ordered or lower entropy state compared to the reactants in the reaction, this requires the consumption of energy since the change in entropy is negative (entropy decreases).

To determine if a chemical reaction is energetically favorable both the change in enthalpy and the change in entropy of the reaction must be considered. The total chemical energy change for a chemical reaction is called the "Gibbs free energy" (ΔG). The formula to determine the Gibbs free energy for a reaction is
$\Delta G = \Delta H - T\Delta S$

For any chemical reaction, a negative ΔG corresponds to an energetically favorable reaction. Although exothermic reactions are usually energetically favorable is the change in entropy for the reaction is negative - in other words if the entropy decrease then the term "-TΔS" becomes a positive value (since -T times a negative number is a positive number). If the magnitude of a positive TΔS is greater than the magnitude of a negative ΔH. Then ΔG will be a positive value and the reaction will not be energetically favored.

The energy gained by the heat of the reaction ΔH is exceeded by the energy required to reduce the entropy of the products of the reaction. In fact, the reverse reaction will be energetically favored since the amount of Gibbs free energy produced by a given reaction is exactly the same amount of Gibbs free energy that will be consumed by the reverse of the given reaction (the same is true for the enthalpy change and entropy change of a given forward and reverse reaction).

To clarify this concept, consider a general chemical reaction

A+B→C+D

When the reaction is **exothermic** (-ΔH) and when the reaction results in an **increase in entropy**, then the Gibbs free energy change for the reaction is

ΔG = (-ΔH) - (TΔS)

Therefore:
ΔG is always negative

The ΔG in this case is always a negative value so the reaction liberates energy. The reaction is always energetically favored and the reaction is called an **exergonic** reaction. Exergonic reactions are by definition reactions with a negative ΔG and are always energetically favorable reactions.

ΔG = (+ΔH) - [(T)(-ΔS)]

Therefore:
ΔG is always positive

When the reaction is **endothermic** (+ΔH) and when the reaction results in a **decrease in entropy** (a negative ΔS), then the Gibbs free energy change for the reaction is always positive and this indicates that the reaction will absorb or consume energy. This is called an **endergonic** reaction. Endergonic reactions are always energetically unfavorable.

When the reaction is **exothermic** (-ΔH) and when the reaction results in a **decrease in entropy**, then the Gibbs free energy change for the reaction can be either positive or negative.

ΔG = (-ΔH) - [(T)(-ΔS)]

If ΔH is greater than TΔS, ΔG is negative and the reaction is exergonic.

If ΔH is less than TΔS, ΔG is positive and the reaction is endergonic.

When the reaction is **endothermic** (+ΔH) and when the reaction results in an **increase in entropy**, then the Gibbs free energy change for the reaction can be either positive or negative.

ΔG = (+ΔH) - (TΔS)

If ΔH is greater than TΔS, ΔG is positive and the reaction is endergonic.

If ΔH is less than TΔS, ΔG is negative and the reaction is exergonic.

There is no doubt that most students consider the topic of the entropy of chemical reactions among the most difficult to understand. The primary reason stems from confusion over the meaning of negative and positive values for ΔG, ΔH, and ΔS. In particular the term -TΔS becomes positive when ΔS is negative. This is just a mathematical fact that a negative times a negative is a positive. An increase in entropy is always energetically favorable, but this is a positive change in entropy.

To indicate that the reaction is producing energy by an increase in entropy (a positive value) this energy by convection must be indicated as a negative value. Just as a negative ΔH for a reaction indicates that the reaction produces heat and that a negative ΔG indicates that the reaction produces chemical energy when the combined contributions of enthalpy and entropy changes in the term "ΔH - TΔS" is negative.

The Four Phases of Matter

At the human or macroscopic scale, matter in the form of large collections of atoms and molecules can exist in four phases or "states". These phases are the solid phase, the liquid phase, the gas phase and the plasma phase. When we are discussing the phases of matter we are usually describing a macroscopic sample of a substance. That substance is usually a pure sample of huge numbers of a particular type of molecule.

A molecule is a particle that consists of more than one atom and those atoms are strongly bound together by electromagnetic forces either in the form of ionic bonds between oppositely charged atoms, or in the form of electrons in covalent bonds that form between the nuclei of two atoms. These binding forces are called intramolecular forces and except for the fourth state of matter - the plasma phase, the intramolecular covalent binding forces are not disrupted or broken during phase changes of the substance.

Ionic bonds are a different story - they are the forces that bind positive and negative ions together in an ionic crystalline solid. They are very strong and they must be

disrupted for the ionic compound to transition from a solid state to a liquid or gaseous state. Also, ionic solids are not composed of small molecules - instead they are composed of a three-dimensional lattice of alternating anions and cations. For the HESI discussions of the phases and phase changes of matter are almost certain to be referring to substances that are covalent molecular compounds and not ionic crystalline solid or liquid compounds.

Intermolecular Forces

The forces that are responsible for the unique properties of the solid and liquid phases are the attractive electrical forces that occur between molecules - intermolecular forces. These forces are weaker than the intramolecular forces of covalent bonds but can be surprisingly strong in the case of Hydrogen bonds.

Dipole-Dipole Interactions

Dipole-Dipole Interactions are the intermolecular forces that occur among molecules that have regions of permanent partial positive and negative charge. These molecules are called polar molecules, those with two poles - a positive and a negative pole - are called dipolar molecules. Molecules can have more than two partially charged regions.

These molecules with a spatial separation of charge are called multipolar molecules; an example is the water molecule H_2O which has four partially charged regions the positive and negative poles of adjacent molecules in a solid or liquid are attracted to each other. This is the permanent type of dipole-dipole intermolecular interaction These attractive forces are the forces that result in the specific properties of polar solids and liquids.

Hydrogen Bonds

Hydrogen bonds are the strongest type of dipole-dipole interactions. They occur between molecules that have hydrogen atoms that have a partial positive charge and also separate regions that have a partial negative charge. Important examples of molecules that experience intermolecular hydrogen bonding in the solid and liquid state are **water molecules** and ammonia (NH_3) molecules.

London Dispersion Forces

Collections of molecules that are non-polar can also exist in solid and liquid states. In these cases, the intermolecular forces are weaker than permanent dipole-dipole interactions. For very brief periods of time non-polar molecules will spontaneously develop random regions of partial positive or negative charge. These regions can induce opposing temporary regions of partial charge resulting in temporary attractions between nonpolar molecules. These types of temporary or instantaneous dipole attractions are called London dispersion forces. London dispersion forces are the weakest type of intermolecular forces.

Solids

In a solid, intermolecular forces are sufficiently strong to prevent individual particles from changing position relative to other particles in the solid. The kinetic energy of particles in a solid is manifested as vibrational motion. The particles in a solid have no translational velocity, but they are vibrating at a certain frequency. As the particles in the solid acquire more energy, they vibrate faster - and the temperature of the solid increases. Matter in the solid state maintains a constant 3-dimensional configuration (shape).

Liquids

As heat is continuously added to a solid, the temperature of the solid eventually rises to the solid's melting point. At the melting point, the individual particles' vibrational kinetic energy is sufficient to allow the particles to can begin to move or flow freely among the other particles in the solid. This process represents a phase change from the solid phase to the liquid phase.

In the liquid phase, the particles in the liquid still have little if any net translational motion. The continued addition of heat to a liquid increases the particles' kinetic energy by increasing the vibrational motion of the particles. At temperatures below the liquid's boiling point, the particles do not have sufficient energy to completely overcome the intermolecular force present within the liquid. The particles in a liquid remain in contact with one another.

The ability of particles in a liquid to move freely within the liquid results in one of the defining physical properties of a liquid - the ability to conform to the interior shape of the vessel that contains the liquid. Liquids will seek the lowest spaces available within a container and form a continuous horizontally level surface while occupying (filling) all of the accessible interior volume of the container that is below this liquid level surface.

As heat is continuously removed from a liquid, the liquid's temperature will eventually drop to the liquid's freezing point. At the freezing point, the reverse of the solid-to-liquid phase transition, the liquid to solid phase transition begins to occur. Notice that the freezing and boiling point temperatures of a substance are identical.

Gases

With the continuing addition of heat energy, the particles of a liquid move around faster and faster, both vibrationally and translationally. When the particles acquire enough kinetic energy, they can overcome their attraction to other particles. The particles in the liquid then begin to escape as individual particles into the surrounding environment. This corresponds to the temperature of the liquid's boiling point. At this temperature, the liquid particles begin to escape from the liquid and travel freely into the surrounding environment. This is the liquid to gas phase transition. the term for this process is evaporation.

The kinetic energy of gas particles is no longer due to vibrational motion, it is due to translational motion - the linear distance that an object travels per unit time - this kinetic energy is the form most of us are familiar with. The average speed (the magnitude of the velocity) of gas molecules can be calculated based on the temperature. The average speed of air molecules at 20 C is 500 m/s. This is equivalent to approximately 1100 miles per hour. Particles in the gas phase behave as if there are no intermolecular forces among the particles.

As gas molecules lose heat energy, the gas temperature eventually decreases to the condensation point (this is identical to the substance's boiling point) and the gas particles return to the liquid phase. This is the gas to liquid phase transition, the reverse of the liquid to gas phase transition; The term for this phase transition is condensation.

Plasmas

The plasma phase of matter occurs when matter reaches extremely high temperatures. At sufficiently high temperature the kinetic energy of individual molecules overcomes the strength of intramolecular bonds and molecules are torn apart into individual atoms. The atom's electrons absorb additional energy and eventually are energetic enough to overcome the attractive electromagnetic force that binds electrons to atoms.

As electrons are stripped away from atomic nuclei, a collection of naked positively charged atomic nuclei and intermingling negatively charged free electrons form. This represents the plasma phase of matter. The plasma phase seldom occurs on earth except when artificially generated by highly specialized and sophisticated technological processes. Elsewhere in the universe, the plasma phase of matter is the most common phase since it is the phase of matter that exists within stars and interstellar dust. It is unlikely that HESI questions will involve any more detailed

knowledge regarding the plasma phase of matter.

Sublimation and Deposition

Under certain conditions substances in the solid phase may transition directly to the gas phase. This is called sublimation. Similarly, substances in the gas phase may transition directly to the solid phase. This phase transition is called deposition. The temperature at which this occurs is the sublimation/deposition point for the substance. An example of this is carbon dioxide, which transitions directly from a solid to a gas at atmospheric pressure with a sublimation/deposition point of -78.5°C

Specific Heat Capacity

The amount of heat energy that is required to increase the temperature of a given amount of a substance by a given number of degrees Celsius depends on the physical nature of the substance. Several factors determine the magnitude of this heat value but the actual value must be determined experimentally for each particular substance.

This measured quantity is designated as the specific heat of a substance, it is given in units of energy per unit mass per degree Celsius usually either Joules/g-degree Celsius or calories/g-degree Celsius.

An example, the specific heat capacity of liquid water is 4.18 J/g·°C. This means that it requires 4.18 joules of heat energy to raise the temperature of 1 gram of water by 1 degree Celsius. The specific heat capacity of water is one of the highest values for any substance, for instance the heat capacity of solid iron is 0.45 J/g·°C, This means it requires approximately ten times more heat energy to raise the temperature of one gram of liquid water by one degree Celsius than is required to raise the temperature of one gram of solid iron by one degree Celsius.

An example of a specific calculation is to calculate the amount of energy required to raise the temperature of 20 grams of liquid water by 15°C. The calculation is shown below.
$$(4.18 \text{ J/g·°C})(10g)(15°C) = 1254 \text{ J}$$

Heats of Phase Transitions

There are circumstances when the addition of heat to a substance does not increase the temperature of the substance. In particular this occurs during phase transitions. Once a substance reaches the temperature of a phase transition, any subsequent heat energy added to the substance is utilized by specific physical processes that are required for the phase transition to occur.

During the phase transition, the temperature of the substance remains at the phase transition temperature point. For instance, at a pressure of 1 atm, a pan of boiling water positioned over an active heating element - a gas flame or hot electric burner - remains at a temperature of 100℃ until all of the liquid water has completely evaporated. The amount of heat energy required to convert a given amount of a substance from the liquid phase to the gas phase is called the **latent heat of vaporization**. For a solid to liquid phase transition, this is called the **latent heat of fusion**.

An example of a calculation involving latent heats of transitions is, given that the latent heat of vaporization for liquid water is approximately 2200 J/g, to determine how many grams of water will be converted from liquid to gas if 6600 Joules of heat are added to a volume of boiling water. The calculation for this question is shown below.

$(2200J/g)(x \text{ grams}) = 6600 \text{ J}$

$x \text{ grams} = 6600 \text{ J}/2200 \text{ J/g}$

$x = 3 \text{ grams of water}$

Phase Equilibriums

At the highest level of difficulty, the HESI may test one's understanding of phase equilibrium. A certain percentage of substance particles continually pass from one phase to the other regardless of the temperature and pressure conditions. For instance, water molecules

in are always in an equilibrium with water molecules in the gas phase as long as there is a volume (or space) above the water surfaces available for the gas phase to exist. This is significant because the cooling effect of sweat evaporating from the skin occurs at temperature ranges well below the boiling point of water. The boiling point is the temperature where all of the water molecules are at or very near the kinetic energy required to escape into the gas phase.

Evaporation at equilibrium at any lower temperature reflects the statistical fact that a few water molecules in the liquid state at the surface randomly acquire enough kinetic energy to escape into the gas phase. These energetic water molecules carry heat from the body.

Physical Properties of Gases

Matter in the gas phase has several properties that are independent of the atomic or molecular structure of individual gas particle. These properties of gases are described by the **kinetic theory of gases**. The theory is almost certainly beyond the scope of the HESI but several assumptions of the theory are used to describe an ideal gas.

An ideal gas is a theoretical gas composed of gas particles that behave as if they have **no interactive forces** acting among other gas particles. They also behave as if they always travel in straight line trajectories unless they collide with other gas particle or other solid surfaces or objects. When ideal gas particles do collide, these **collisions are perfectly elastic** - meaning the gas particles rebound in a geometrically predictable manner and the kinetic energy of the collisions is conserved (not converted into other forms of energy).

The Ideal Gas Law

The ideal gas law can be used to describe a sample of gas that is confined in a container with a given internal volume (V) an absolute temperature (T) given in degrees kelvin and a given number of gas particles given in molar units (moles). The equation for the ideal gas law is

$$PV = nRT$$

P is the pressure of the gas within a container with a volume of V. The term n is the number of moles of gas present within the container volume and the term R is the universal gas constant. The value of the gas constant 'R" depends on the choice of units used to express the pressure and volume of the system. A common value for the gas constant is R=0.082 L atm mol^{-1} K^{-1}. An example of an application of the ideal gas law is to calculate what volume one mole of gas would occupy at standard temperature and pressure (STP).

For ideal gases, standard pressure is defined as one atm and standard temperature as 273.15 K (0 degrees Celsius). The ideal gas law can be used to calculate theoretical values for the ideal gas law variables - volume, temperature, pressure and number of moles of gas particles present in an enclosed sample gas system. As an example, the volume of a sample gas system that contains one mole of gas particles at standard temperature and pressure can be determined by rearranging the ideal gas law to solve for volume:

$$V = (nRT)/P$$

When the actual values of R=0.082 L atm mol^{-1} K^{-1}, one mole for n, 273.15 K for T, 1 atm for P are used to carry out the above equation the result is that **1 mole of any ideal gas will occupy a volume of 22.4 liters when the gas is at a STP** (a pressure of 1 atm and a temperature of 273.15 K).

The notable feature of this relationship - that one mole of a molecular substance will - as a gas at STP - occupy a volume 22.4 liters is the remarkable difference in volume of the molecular substance in the liquid or solid phase compared to the gas phase. Consider that the molecular substance (or molecular compound) methane has a chemical formula of CH_4. One mole of methane has a mass of 12 grams (the atomic mass of one carbon atom is 12 AMU) + 4 (the atomic mass of four hydrogen atoms is 4 AMU). The Molecular weight of methane is therefore equal to 16 and therefore one mole of methane has a mass of 16 grams.

The density of liquid methane is 0.42 g/cm^3 therefore the volume of 1 mole of liquid methane is (16 g)/(0.42 g/cm^3) = 38.1 cm^3. One cubic centimeter is equal to 0.001 liters (there are 1000 cm^3 in one liter). The volume of one mole of liquid methane in liters is therefore (0.001)(38.1)= 0.038 liters. In the gas phase at STP, one mole of methane will occupy a volume of 22.4 liters. The ratio of these two volumes is 22.4/0.038 = 589 to 1. This shows that one mole of methane in the gas phase occupies a volume almost 590 times as large as the volume of one mole of methane in the liquid phase. This ratio is of comparable magnitude for the volumes of most molecular compounds in the gas phase compared to the liquid phase.

Initial and Final States of a Sample Gas System

The most useful application of the ideal gas law to be aware of is the calculations of an initial and final state of an ideal gas. To illustrate this, we can rearrange the ideal gas law as follows

$$PV = nRT$$
therefore,
$$(PV)/(nT) = R$$

Since R is a constant, we can write an equation for the initial and final states of a gas where P_i, V_i, T_i and n_i are the initial pressure, volume, temperature and number of moles of a gas and where P_f, V_f, T_f and n_f are the final pressure, volume, temperature and number of moles of a gas

Equation 1: $(P_iV_i)/(n_iT_i) = R = (P_fV_f)/(n_fT_f)$
Therefore
Equation 2: $(P_iV_i)/(n_iT_i) = (P_fV_f)/(n_fT_f)$

Equation 2: $(P_iV_i)/(n_iT_i) = (P_fV_f)/(n_fT_f)$, is the general equation for the initial and final states of a gas and it can be used to make several types of calculations. One of the most frequent is to consider initial and final states where the number of moles of gas remains constant (no gas molecules enter or escape from the system). Since the number of moles of gas does not change the general equation (equation 2) can be written as:

Equation 3: $(P_iV_i)/T_i = (P_fV_f)/T_f$

Consider the initial and final states of the gas to represent two different systems. The initial system consists of a certain amount of gas molecules confined in a container with initial volume temperature and pressure. Assume that the container in the system is a cylindrical piston and that the top or head of the piston can move up or away from the floor of the piston. This will increase the volume of the interior of the piston.

We can also move the piston head downward or toward the floor of the piston. This will decrease the volume of the piston. Assume that we may directly change the temperature of the initial system by heating the container (adding energy to the system) or by cooling the container (removing energy from the system). For our initial system assume that the volume of the piston is 5 liters the pressure of the system is 760 torr (1 atm) and the temperature of the system is 300 Kelvins. Substituting these values as the initial values in equation three we get:

$(760 \text{ torr})(5 \text{ liters})/(300K) = (P_fV_f)/T_f$

Assume we lock the piston so that the volume cannot change and then add heat to the system until the temperature of the gas rises to 600K. Now we substitute the new temperature value of 600K for the final temperature. The final volume is unchanged (5 liters). The unknown final value is the final pressure of the system. We can rearrange the equation above to solve for the final pressure

$(600K)(760 \text{ torr})(5 \text{ liters})/(300K)(5 \text{ liters}) = P_f$
This simplifies to
$(2)(760 \text{ torr}) = 1520 \text{ torr}$

We see now that if the volume of the system remains constant and the temperature of the gas doubles, the pressure of the gas doubles. Since the volume of the system does not change, the general equation for this is

$P_i/T_i = P_f/T_f$

Boyle's Law
Boyle's Law is a special case of the general relationship between the initial and final states of a gas given in Equation 3: $(P_iV_i)/T_i = (P_fV_f)/T_f$, where the temperature of the initial and final states is unchanged (notice that there is also no change in the amount of gas) but the volume and pressure of the system may change. Since the temperature of the initial and final states is unchanged, equation 3 simplifies to:

Equation 4: $(P_iV_i) = (P_fV_f)$

Assume the initial pressure and volume of the system are 760 torr and 5 liters respectively. Substituting these values into equation 4 gives:

$(760 \text{ torr})(5 \text{ liters}) = (P_fV_f)$

If we decrease the volume of the system by a factor of two the final volume will be 2.5 liters. We rearrange the equation above to solve for the final pressure

$(760 \text{ torr})(5 \text{ liters})/(2.5 \text{ liters}) = P_f$

$P_f = 1520 \text{ torr}$

In this case the temperature increases by a factor of 2 (doubles). Recall that this is an inversely proportional relationship. Boyle's law therefore can be stated as **"when the amount (number) of gas particles and temperature on a sample of an ideal gas are kept constant, the pressure and volume of the ideal gas are inversely proportional."**

Scientific Methods and Reasoning

In the laboratory, we could use our system of gas contained in a piston to reduce the volume of the piston from 5 liters to 2.5 liters, but to do this we would need to apply an external force on the piston head sufficient to generate a downward pressure that is greater than the pressure of the gas. As the piston head moves down the force is being applied over the distance that the piston head moves. Recall that work is force times distance and that work is energy. Therefore, we must do work on the gas and therefore we are transferring energy into the system. This energy will be converted into increased kinetic energy of the gas molecules and therefore the temperature of the gas will increase. We would then need to remove energy from the system to decrease the final temperature of the gas to the initial temperature.

To do this we must draw some of the energy out of the gas perhaps by immersing the piston in cold water. Heat would flow out of the system by conduction through the walls of the cylinder into the cold water. If the temperature of the gas were higher than the external temperature we could also draw heat out of the system by using the gas as a heat source in a heat engine to perform work on the external environment.

Charles' Law

Charles' Law is also a special case of the ideal gas law that pertains to initial and final states of a gas when the pressure of the gas does not change from the initial compared to the final state. Since pressure does not change the general ideal gas relationship of equation 3: $(P_iV_i)/T_i = (P_fV_f)/T_f)$ simplifies to the following:

$$V_i/T_i = V_f/T_f$$

Assume the initial volume and temperature of the system are 5 liters and 300K respectively. Substituting these values into equation 4 gives:

$$(5 \text{ liters})/(300k) = V_f/T_f$$

If we heat the gas to increase the temperature to 450K we have increased the temperature by a factor of 1.5 We rearrange the equation above to solve for the final volume.

$(5 \text{ liters})(450K)/(300K) = V_f$

$V_f = 7.5 \text{ liters}$

Notice that when the temperature of the system increased by a factor of 1.5 the volume of the system increased by a factor of 1.5. Recall that this is a directly proportional relationship, so Charles Law may be stated as: **"When the amount (number) of gas particles the pressure on a sample of a gas is held constant, the temperature (in degrees kelvin) and the volume will be directly proportional."**

Fundamental Concepts of Chemical Reactions

Many of the concepts that we have discussed affect chemical reactions. We will discuss the nature of chemical reaction in greater detail shortly but this is a good stage to preview several important concepts that relate to chemical reactions. Consider the general form of a chemical reaction as follows

$$aA + bB \rightarrow cC + dD$$

Stoichiometric Coefficients

In most cases this chemical reaction involves molecules on the right side "A" and "B" whose atoms "react" to rearrange themselves into new types of molecules "C" and "D". The molecules A and B on the left side of the equation are called reactants and the the molecules C and D on the right side of the equation are the products of the reaction. the reactant molecules rearrange into the product molecules by breaking existing chemical bonds and forming new chemical bonds. The lower case letters, a,b,c and d are called stoichiometric coefficients. They are integer numbers that indicate the proportional numbers of the molecules A, B, C and D that participate in the reaction. For instance, this could be

$$2A + 3B \rightarrow C + 4D$$

This indicates a reaction where two molecules of A and three molecules of B react to produce one molecule of C and four molecules of D. Notice that when the stoichiometric coefficient is "1" that the number 1 is not used, in this case for the product molecule C. When reactant or product molecules are not preceded by a coefficient it is understood that the coefficient is "1".

As we have discussed the coefficients may be thought of as numbers of individual molecules, but more often they are considered to be very large collections of molecules as given by moles - for the example above this would be interpreted as "two moles of A and three moles of B react to produce one mole of C and four moles of D". The key concept is that the stoichiometric coefficient describes the relative amounts of reactants and products participating in the chemical reaction.

Phases of Chemical Reactions

Chemical participants in a reaction can be in the solid, liquid or gas phases. This is indicated in the example below

$$aA(s) + bB(g) \rightarrow cC(l) + dD(l)$$

The parenthetical terms (s) (g) and (l) identify the phase of the molecule participating in the reaction: (s) indicates a solid phase, (g) a gas phase and (l) a liquid phase. In the example above, A is in the solid phase, B is in the gas phase and both C and D are in the liquid phase. A good example of these concepts is shown in the chemical reaction of photosynthesis where carbon dioxide (CO_2) and water (H_2O) react to form glucose ($C_6H_{12}O_6$) and molecular oxygen (O_2):

$$6CO_2(g) + 6H_2O(l) \rightarrow C_6H_{12}O_6(s) + 6O_2(g)$$

Most chemical reactions do not involve reactants purely in the solid state such as is shown below.

$$A(s) + B(s) \rightarrow C(s) + D(s)$$

This is because it is difficult for the molecules in solids in one reactant to intermingle with the molecules of solids in the other reactant. It is also uncommon to encounter pure liquids in a chemical reaction.

$$A(l) + B(l) \rightarrow C(l) + D(l)$$

In most cases reactions will occur where the reactants are either in the gas phase or are dissolved in a liquid solvent (resulting in a solution). We will limit this discussion to solutions where the solvent is liquid water. This type of solution is called an aqueous (aq) solution. Nearly all biochemical reactions are reactions where the chemical participants are in an aqueous solution (dissolved in water). A general example is

$$A(aq) + B(aq) \rightarrow C(aq) + D(aq)$$

Reversible Reactions

Recall that most reactions are reversible reactions where the reactants on the left can become products and the products on the right become reactants:

$$C(aq) + D(aq) \rightarrow A(aq) + B(aq)$$

Reversible chemical reactions are indicated by the double arrow symbol ⇌ as in the example below

$$A(aq) + B(aq) \rightleftharpoons C(aq) + D(aq)$$

Recall that spontaneous reactions (as written from left to right) are reactions that liberate Gibbs free energy (G) and that this is indicated when the change in Gibbs free energy (ΔG) is a negative value. For example

$$A(aq) + B(aq) \rightleftharpoons C(aq) + D(aq); \Delta G \text{ is negative}$$

In this case the forward reaction is energetically favored and will proceed spontaneously.

The critical concept to understand when we indicate that **the ΔG for a reaction is a specific value is that depends on the conditions under which the reaction is occurring at the precise moment in time that it is occurring.** The critical conditions of the reaction are the concentrations of the reactants and products if they are in an aqueous phase, the partial pressures of the reactants and products if they are in the gas phase and products and the absolute temperature (degrees kelvin) at which the reaction is occurring.

When a reaction is proceeding in the forward direction, the concentrations or partial pressures of the reactants are decreasing and the concentrations or partial pressures of the products are increasing. This means that the **during any ongoing chemical reaction the ΔG of the reaction is constantly changing** (in fact it is constantly becoming less negative). When a specific ΔG value is assigned to a reaction it represents the ΔG at the exact moment in time when reactants and products have specific precise concentrations or partial pressures.

ΔG^0

Standard conditions for a reaction are defined when the reaction begins with reactants and products at **concentrations equal to 1 mole/liter** or one atmosphere partial pressure, and a reaction temperature of **25 degrees Celsius**. The ΔG for a reaction that is under

standard conditions is the symbol ΔG^0. For example, consider the reaction:

$$A(aq) + B(aq) \rightleftharpoons C(aq) + D(aq); \Delta G^0 \text{ is negative}$$

A negative ΔG^0 indicates that when the reaction begins with all reactants and products, a concentration of 1 mole per liter and at a reaction temperature of 25 degrees Celsius, the forward reaction is energetically favorable and will proceed spontaneously. As the reaction proceeds the concentrations of the reactants decrease and the concentrations of the products increase and the ΔG of the reaction is becomes less negative.

Chemical Reaction Equilibrium and the Equilibrium Constant "Keq"

At some point the ΔG becomes zero and the reaction appears to stop. At this point the concentrations of the reactants and products remain constant. The reaction has reached equilibrium. There is no longer any free energy difference between reactants and products and therefore no energy available to drive the reaction further in either the forward or reverse direction. This equilibrium occurs for all reversible reactions and a constant, Keq (the equilibrium constant) can be calculated for any reversible reaction as is shown for the general reversible reaction below:

$$aA(aq) + bB(aq) \rightleftharpoons cC(aq) + dD(aq)$$

$$Keq = [C]^c[D]^d \div [A]^a[B]^b$$

The equation shows that the Keq for a reversible reaction is obtained by multiplying the concentrations of the products raised to the power of their stoichiometric coefficients and dividing this value by the product of the concentrations of the reactants raised to the power of their stoichiometric coefficients

Scientific Methods and Reasoning

This explanation of the concept of equilibrium and equilibrium constants for a reaction is probably spectacularly confusing because as often happens these types of processes are awkward to explain in word. It is much easier to understand using a specific example as follows:

Imagine we are in the laboratory and are investigating a general reaction that is

A(aq) + B(aq) ⇌ C(aq) + 2D(aq)

We measure out one mole of the chemical compounds A, B, C and D solutions and dissolve them in one liter of water. We now have a reaction vessel that contains A, B, C and D each in concentrations of 1 mole per liter. We measure the concentrations of the participants of the reaction and observe that the concentrations of A and B are decreasing over time and the concentrations of C and D are increasing over time. After several hours, we are no longer able to detect any changes in the concentrations of A, B, C or D. We conclude the reaction has reached equilibrium.

We measure the actual concentrations and find that the concentration of A is 0.02 mol/L, the concentration of B is 0.02 mol/L, the concentration of C is 0.98 mol/L and the concentration of D is 1.96 mol/L. Obviously the reaction began with a large negative ΔG since the forward reaction proceeded until almost all of the reactants were consumed.

Since the reaction is now at equilibrium we can calculate the Keq of the reaction by using the general formula $Keq = [C]^c[D]^d \div [A]^a[B]^b$ and substitute the actual concentrations of A, B, C and D into the equation. Notice that since the product D in the chemical reaction has a coefficient of 2, the concentration of D must be raised to the power of two (A, B, and C have coefficients of 1).

(0.98 mol/L)(1.96 mol/L)²/(0.02 mol/L)(0.02 mol/L) = 3.76/(1x10⁻⁴) = 9,400 or 9.4x10³

The Keq of 9.4x10³ indicates that the forward reaction is so energetically favorable it does not reach equilibrium until the concentration of products exceeds the concentration of reactants by a factor of several thousand times. In fact, the reaction almost goes to completion, completion meaning there are no reactants remaining.

Factors that Influence Chemical Reactions

The equilibrium constant (Keq) is the most important value to know for any chemical reaction and it reveals many interesting features of chemical reactions. One is that reactions that are generally thought to be very energetically favorable (typically very exothermic reactions such as combustion reactions) under certain circumstances can become energetically unfavorable.

Initial Concentrations of Reactants and Products - The Reaction Quotient "Q"

One of the ways to determine how far away a reaction is from equilibrium and to determine in which direction a reversible reaction will proceed is to calculate a **reaction quotient (Q).**

Scientific Methods and Reasoning

Consider our experiment where we determined that the Keq for the reaction A(aq) + B(aq) ⇌ C(aq) + 2D(aq) was 9.4x10³. If we had begun the experiment with different concentrations for the reactants and products, the reverse reaction could have been the reaction that occurred. For instance, if the concentrations of A and B had been 0.1 mol/L each rather than 1 mol/L and the concentrations of C and D had been 10 mol/L rather than 1 mol/l each then **the reaction quotient (Q) which is calculated in the same manner as the equilibrium constant** would be:

(10 mol/L)(10 mol/L)²/(0.1 mol/L)(0.1 mol/L) = 1000/0.01 = 100,000 or 1x10⁵.

This value for the reaction quotient "Q" is roughly 10 times greater than the equilibrium constant of 9.4x10³. Since every reversible reaction moves toward its equilibrium constant concentrations, the products of the forward reaction (as written) C and D must decrease in concentration and the reactants of the forward reaction (as written) must increase in concentration in order to reach the equilibrium constant concentrations.

By changing the initial concentrations of the reaction, we have converted the for forward reaction into an energetically unfavorable reaction (a reaction with a positive ΔG). This means we have also converted the reverse reaction into an energetically favorable reaction (a reaction with a negative ΔG).

Gas Phase Chemical Reactions

Chemical equilibrium also occurs in reversible reactions where some or all of the chemical participants in the reaction are in the gas phase. Consider the following general reaction:

$$A(g) + B(g) \rightleftharpoons C(g) + 2D(g)$$

Partial Pressures of Gases

The participants in the reaction above are all in the gas phase. The reaction is occurring in a sealed flask and there are no other gases present in the flask. The total gas pressure inside the flask is equal to the sum of the partial pressures (p) of the individual participants in the reaction (assuming no other gases have contaminated the system).

The individual partial pressures for each participant can be calculated using the ideal gas law $PV = nRT$. Since n is the number of moles of gas we can begin the reaction with one mole of each participant and will get equal partial pressures for each participant. In this case the partial pressures of each participant will add together to give the total pressure of gas within the reaction flask. Since there are four participants, each with identical partial pressures, the total pressure within the flask will be four times the partial pressure of any one of the participants. The Keq and reaction quotients for gas phase reactions is the same as that for solution reaction except that concentrations are given in partial pressures rather than in units of moles per liter

We can write a reaction quotient Q for the beginning of the reaction as follows $(pC)(pD)^2/(pA)(pD)$.

The actual partial pressures of the participant will depend on the reaction temperature and the volume of the flask. Since we have ensured that all of the partial pressures are equal at the start of the reaction we can arbitrarily assign a partial pressure since this is a hypothetical situation. Let's say the partial pressure that occurs for each participant under our laboratory conditions is 0.5 atm.

$$(0.5 \text{ atm})(0.5 \text{ atm})^2/(0.5 \text{ atm})(0.5 \text{ atm}) = 0.5 \text{ atm}$$

If the forward reaction proceeds the partial pressures of A and B will decrease and the partial pressures of C and D will decrease since the forward chemical reaction shows that one molecule of A reacts with one molecule of B to produce one molecule of C and two molecules of D. If the Keq for this reaction is larger than 0.5 atm then the forward reaction will proceed since the partial pressures of C and D must increase and the partial pressures of A and B decrease for the value of the overall equation to become larger. If the Keq for the reaction is less than 0.5 atm then the reverse reaction will proceed by the same reasoning.

Pressure Change Effects on Reactions

Another way to drive reactions in a desired direction is to take advantage of the effects that changes in the partial pressures of chemical participants can have on chemical reactions. In the example of a pure gas phase reaction $A(g) + B(g) \rightleftharpoons C(g) + 2D(g)$, the forward reaction produces 3 moles of product (1 mole of C and 2 moles of D from 2 moles of reactant (one mole of A and one mole of B). The forward reaction therefore produces a larger amount of gas molecules from a smaller amount of gas molecules.

In a sealed reaction vessel, the forward reaction tends to increase the partial pressures of the reaction participants within the reaction vessel. If the reaction vessel is a piston, external force can be exerted by the piston head on the gas in the reaction vessel. As the partial pressures increase, the reaction moves farther away from the equilibrium partial pressures the reverse reaction becomes more favorable since this causes lowering of the partial pressures of participants within the vessel by converting a larger number of gas molecules into a smaller number of gas molecules via the reverse reaction.

By increasing the volume of the reaction vessel, the forward reaction is favored by the same reasoning. It is important to realize that this effect is actually due to increasing the concentration of the participant gases. Other methods of increasing the pressure of the reaction vessel - such as pumping additional non-reactive gas into the vessel - will not have any effect on the reaction.

Temperature Effects on Reactions

We have seen how changes in concentrations and in partial pressures of participants in a chemical reaction can tend to drive reactions in the forward or reverse direction. This is because both methods move the reaction quotient of the reaction farther away from the Keq of the reaction. Temperature changes to the environment in which reactions are occurring actually change the Keq of reactions.

For exothermic reactions increases in temperature drive the reverse reaction, which removes heat from the system. Lowering the temperature increases the forward reaction, which adds heat to the reaction environment. The reverse is true for endothermic reactions. Increasing the temperature of the reaction environment

will favor the forward reaction since this removes heat from the reaction environment and decreasing the temperature will favor the reverse reaction by the same reasoning.

Scientific Methods and Reasoning - Other Methods to Control Chemical Reactions

In the laboratory or in industry chemical reactions that are energetically unfavorable or that are only marginally favorable can be converted into highly favorable reactions. Consider the reaction

$$aA(aq) + bB(aq) \rightleftharpoons cC(aq) + dD(aq)$$

where the Keq under standard condition is very large. This favors the forward reaction. If the objective is to produce chemical A and from the reaction.

The laboratory process can begin with C and D as starting materials and allow the reaction to proceed. Since there are no amounts of A and B present when the reaction begins, the reaction quotient is technically infinite but practically huge compared to the Keq for the reaction, so some amount of A and B will be produced as the reaction attempts to lower the reaction quotient to the Keq value. If as the reaction proceeds and either A and or B can be removed from the reaction as it or they are produce, the concentrations of A and or B will never reach levels high enough to allow the reaction to reach the lower Keq value.

In this manner, a very unfavorable reverse reaction can be driven to completion. There are several methods to accomplish the removal of a participant in a reaction from the reaction process. Two of these are based on the fact that solids and pure liquids are not included in Keq constants.

Precipitation of Desired Products

Pure solids and pure liquids do not change concentrations during reactions so they are assigned an unchanging concentration value of 1. If the solution where our reaction occurs has properties where the participant chemical A immediately forms a solid that precipitates out of the solution the the concentration of A in the solution will never reach levels that will allow the reaction to reach equilibrium and theoretically the highly unfavorable reverse reaction can produce a nearly 100% yield of the desired substance A.

One common method to achieve this effect is by selecting a reaction solution that has a specific pH or level of acidity that favors the precipitation of the desired product but that does not favor the precipitation of the reactant that produce the product.

Evaporation and Condensation

Reaction participants can also be removed by heating the reaction solution so that the participant becomes a gas, thereby escaping from the reaction solution. In the gas phase, reaction participants can be removed from the reaction environment by cooling the reaction vessel to the condensation point of the participant so that a specific participant becomes a liquid that can be drained away from the reaction vessel.

Each method can also result in preventing reaches from reaching equilibrium and drive reactions to completion in the desired direction. These methods can be combined using various laboratory techniques. In general, these separation methods are termed "**distillations**".

Sequential or Chain Reactions

When the production a desired product of a reaction is energetically unfavorable - i.e. the ΔG of the forward reaction is positive and therefore the K_{eq} of the forward reaction is very small - the reaction can be driven forward by creating conditions in the reaction system so that the products of the reaction immediately undergo a second chemical reaction that is very energetically favorable. If the second reaction involves another

product of the first reaction the desired product will accumulate in the reaction system.

Step 1: $A + B \rightleftharpoons C + D$
Step 2: $D + E \rightleftharpoons G + H$

More importantly for human biology, this process can drive energetically unfavorable early reactions toward more energetically favorable stages of a sequence of reactions (chain reactions). This is very common in many important biological processes that involve the synthesis of complex molecules from simpler molecules (anabolic metabolism).

Coupled Reactions

A very common method that the human body uses to drive energetically unfavorable reaction is to couple the unfavorable reaction with a very energetically favorable reaction. When this is done the overall reaction becomes very energetically favorable. In particular this is frequently accomplished by coupling unfavorable reaction with the hydrolysis of ATP. ATP (adenosine triphosphate) is a molecule that is often described as the energy molecule or energy currency of the body. The Hydrolysis of ATP is a reaction that converts ATP into ADP (adenosine diphosphate) and a phosphate group (PO_4).

$ATP + H2O \rightleftharpoons ADP + PO_4 + H^+$; $\Delta G = -34$ kJ/mol

The ΔG for ATP hydrolysis can actually be much higher depending on the local chemical environment in which the hydrolysis occurs. The coupling of ATP hydrolysis with an energetically unfavorable reaction is shown with the example below

Desired reaction:

$A + B \rightleftharpoons C$; $\Delta G = +24$ kJ/mol (very energetically unfavored).

Coupled reaction:

$A + B + ATP + H_2O \rightleftharpoons C + ADP + PO_4 + H^+$; $\Delta G = -14$ kJ/mol (very energetically favored).

Keq in Dissociation Reactions

We will discuss the types of chemical reactions that may be encountered in HESI questions in general shortly, but one type or reaction, the dissociation reaction is closely related to our discussion of equilibrium in chemical reactions and in particular the Keq for chemical reactions. A dissociation reaction involves the breakdown of one molecule (often generalized as "AB") into two or more molecules. A general formula for a dissociation reaction is

$AB \rightleftharpoons A + B$

Solubility Products - Ksp

Since most reactions in the human body occur as aqueous solutions, an important type of dissociation reaction is the dissolving of a solid substance into water.

$AB(s) + H2O \rightleftharpoons A(aq) + B(aq) + H2O$

This general reaction actually represents the formation of an aqueous solution by dissolving a solute (AB) into a solvent (in this case H_2O) to create a solution. Notice that H_2O is involved in the process where a solid is undergoing conversion to aqueous decomposition products, but that H_2O is not actually being chemically converted by the process. Typically, this is shown as H_2O written above the double arrow symbol. Indicating that water is required, but does not participate in the chemical reaction.

$$AB(s) + \overset{H_2O}{\rightleftharpoons} A(aq) + B(aq)$$

There is a limit to how much solute can be dissolved into a solution and this is indicated as the equilibrium concentration for a solution. There is of course an equilibrium constant, called "Ksp" that can be calculated for this reaction that is derived using the same formula as is used for any chemical reaction equilibrium. Recall that this general calculation for the general reaction

$aA(aq) + bB(aq) \rightleftharpoons cC(aq) + dD(aq)$ is:

$Keq = [C]^c[D]^d \div [A]^a[B]^b$

For our reaction of a dissociation reaction of a solid into aqueous breakdown products, we can write a version of Keq, The Ksp which is the equilibrium solubility product of the reaction

$$AB(s) + \overset{H_2O}{\rightleftharpoons} A(aq) + B(aq) ;$$
$$Ksp = [A][B]$$

Notice that The solid "AB" and the solvent H2O are not included in the Ksp, because, among other reasons, the concentrations of solids and solvents do not change during chemical reactions.

A specific example is the solubility of sodium chloride (NaCl) - common table salt - in water to form an aqueous solution of sodium and chloride ions (Na^+ and Cl^-)

$$NaCl(s) \overset{H_2O}{\rightleftharpoons} Na^+(aq) + Cl^-(aq), Ksp = 36$$

Since one mole of NaCl gives one mole of Na^+(aq) and one mole of Cl^-(aq), the concentrations of the two ions is equal when they ions are derived from solid sodium chloride dissolved into pure water. We can use the unknown value "x" for each concentration value and solve the Ksp equation as follows:

$Ksp = [Na^+][Cl^-] = [x][x] = [x]^2$
$[x]^2 = 36; x = 6$

The units of concentration are "moles per liter" unless otherwise specified. The value for x is therefore 6 moles per liter. This indicates that a maximum of 6 moles of solid NaCl will dissolve in one liter of water resulting in an aqueous solution containing Na+ and Cl- ions that are each in concentrations of 6 moles per liter.

This is referred to as the equilibrium concentration for Na+ and Cl- ions in an aqueous solution. This value is also temperature dependent. The Ksp for decomposition reactions changes depending on the temperature of the reaction environment. Usually Ksp values are given for temperatures of 20 degrees Celsius.

Notice that the units for Ksp depends on the stoichiometric coefficients of the reaction participants that are included in the equilibrium calculation. In the above reaction the Ksp equation units are $(Mol/L) x (Mol/L) = (Mol/L)^2$ or Mol^2/L^2. Often the dissolution of a solid is not a simple bimolecular breakdown but more complex, such as

$$AB_2(s) \overset{H_2O}{\rightleftharpoons} A(aq) + 2B(aq)$$

Since the equilibrium equation is $Keq = [C]^c[D]^d \div [A]^a[B]^b$, to calculate the Ksp for this reaction the concentration of B must be raised to the power of its stoichiometric coefficient, which is 2.

$$Ksp = [A][B]^2$$

In this case the units for the Ksp equation are $(Mol/L) x (Mol/L)^2$ which gives $(Mol/L)^3$ or Mol^3/L^3. An example of a specific reaction of this type is the decomposition of lead chloride ($PbCl_2$) in water to form Pb^{2+} and Cl^- ions in an aqueous solution. The Ksp for this reaction is $2.0 x 10^{-5}$ (the units will be Mol^3/L^3)

$$PbCl_2(s) \rightleftharpoons Pb^{2+}(aq) + 2Cl^-(aq)$$
$$Ksp = [Pb^{2+}][Cl^-]^2$$

Since one mole of $PbCl_2$ gives one mole of $Pb^{2+}(aq)$ and two moles of $Cl^-(aq)$, the concentration of $Cl^-(aq)$ is twice the concentration of $Pb^{2+}(aq)$ when they ions are derived from solid lead chloride when dissolved into pure water. We can use the unknown value "x" for each concentration value and solve the Ksp equation as follows:

$Ksp = Ksp = [Pb^{2+}][Cl^-]^2 = [x][2x]^2 = [4x]^3$
$[4x]^3 = 2.0 x 10^{-5}$; $x = 0.27$ Mol/L

Of course, this calculation requires a calculator and would not appear on the HESI, but the concentration of one of the ions could be given and the question could ask for the concentration of the other ion that would be required to begin to precipitate the ions out of solution as solid $PbCL_2$. For example, if the concentration of Cl^- is $1.0 x 10^{-2}$ Mol/L, then the concentration of Pb^{2+} that will be required to begin precipitating solid $PbCL_2$ from the solution will be

$[Pb^{2+}][Cl^-]^2 = 2.0 x 10^{-5}$
$[Pb^{2+}][1.0 x 10^{-2}]^2 = 2.0 x 10^{-5}$
$[Pb^{2+}][1.0 x 10^{-4}] = 2.0 x 10^{-5}$
$[Pb^{2+}] = 2.0 x 10^{-5}/[1.0 x 10^{-4}] = 2.0 x 10^{-1}$

The solution to the equation shows when the concentration of Cl^- is $1.0 x 10^{-2}$, solid $PbCL_2$ will begin to precipitate out of the solution when the concentration of Pb^{2+} reaches a value of $2.0 x 10^{-1}$ Mol/L.

The relevance of solubility and Ksp for the HESI relates to several physiological processes. First there are critical dissolved ions in body fluids and within cells called electrolytes. These are most importantly the sodium (Na^+), potassium (K^+), chloride (Cl^-), phosphate ($PO4^-$) and magnesium (mg^{2+}) ions. In certain circumstances, such as in the renal tubules, for instance, the solubility of calcium ion can exceed the solubility product for calcium containing solids. When this occurs a kidney stone, consisting of calcium and other substances can for and obstruct the excretory system.

The gases oxygen (O_2) and carbon dioxide (CO_2) also have a solubility in blood, body fluids and fluids within cell. The respiratory and other systems are designed so that oxygen can move as a gas into fluid and carbon dioxide in fluids can move out of the fluid and into the gas phase in the lungs.

Another important physiological function is the regulation of the pH of body fluids; pH is a measure of the hydrogen ion (H^+) content of fluids and is closely related to the concept of solubility products and Ksp.

Finally, water (H_2O) has a dissociation constant that is very important in terms of the pH levels of the human body. We will discuss acid-base reactions and the dissociation of water in greater detail later in this review, but we will also preview these topics now due to their close relationships to solubility products and Ksp.

The Dissociation Constant of Water - K_w

Pure water is in equilibrium with the hydrogen ion (H+) and the hydroxide ion (OH-) as shown below

$$H_2O \rightleftharpoons H^+(aq) + OH^-(aq)$$

This is also frequently alternatively described as pure water is in equilibrium with the hydronium ion (H_3O^+) and the hydroxide ion (OH-) as shown below

$$2H_2O \rightleftharpoons H_3O^+(aq) + OH^-(aq)$$

It makes little difference what the definition is because the hydronium ion (H_3O^+) behaves exactly the same as a free hydrogen ion (H^+) in chemical reactions and the dissociation constant is exactly the same. For our purposes, we will use the hydrogen ion version (H^+) since this is how acid base reactions are usually described and nearly all acid base reactions occur in water.

The dissociation constant is similar to a Ksp since water is a pure liquid and similar to a solid, is not included in the calculation of the dissociation constant of water. The dissociation constant for water is written as the K_w for water. For the reaction:

$$H_2O \rightleftharpoons H^+(aq) + OH^-(aq)$$
$$K_w = [H^+][OH^-] = 1 \times 10^{-14} \text{ Mol/L}$$

The pH and pOH of Pure Water

The concentrations of $H^+(aq)$ and $OH^-(aq)$ are important quantities in nearly all chemical reactions in the human body and are commonly referred to by their "p" values. The value "pH" refers to the concentration of hydrogen ion (H+) in a solution and "pOH" refers to the concentration of hydroxide ion (OH-)in a solution. **The pH and pOH values are the negative log values of the hydrogen and hydroxide ion concentrations respectively.** In the case of pure water as

shown in the above equation, we see that H_2O is in equilibrium with $H^+(aq)$ and $OH^-(aq)$ and that the Keq for this equilibrium is called the K_w. Specifically, for pure water, $K_w = [H^+][OH^-] = 1 \times 10^{-14}$ Mol/L. Since one molecule of H_2o dissociates into one molecule each of $H^+(aq)$ and $OH^-(aq)$, at equilibrium the concentrations of $H^+(aq)$ and $OH^-(aq)$ must be equal. We can therefore calculate the equilibrium pH and pOH values for pure water as shown below

$$K_w = [H^+][OH^-] = 1 \times 10^{-14} \text{ Mol/L}$$
$$K_w = [x][x] = 1 \times 10^{-14} \text{ Mol/L}$$
$$[x]^2 = 1 \times 10^{-14} \text{ Mol/L}$$
$$[x] = 1 \times 10^{-7} \text{ Mol/L}$$

This calculation shows that the equilibrium concentrations of $H^+(aq)$ and $OH^-(aq)$ are both equal to 1×10^{-7} Mol/L. **The negative log of 1×10^{-7} is 7. Therefore, the pH of pure water is 7** and the pOH of pure water is also 7. One of the most significant facts about the pH of water is that the pH value of 7 is used to define whether a solution is acidic or basic. A solution with a **pH value of 7 is defined as a neutral pH solution.** Solutions with **pH values less than 7 are defined as "acidic" solutions** and solutions with **pH values greater than 7 are defined as "basic" solutions.** Notice that pure liquid water is - by definition - a pH neutral liquid.

Acids, Bases and pH

An important category of chemical reactions for the HESI is acid-base reactions. Acids are - according to the Bronsted-Lowry definition **proton donors** or more specifically - substances or compounds that in a solvent (almost always water) dissociate, and one of the dissociation products is H^+ (the +1 hydrogen ion - which is actually a single naked proton). The general formula for the dissociation of an acid is

$$HA \rightleftharpoons H^+(aq) + A^-(aq)$$

Strong Acids

Strong acids will completely dissociate in water. The classic example of a strong acid is hydrochloric acid (HCl). To determine the pH of a strong acid, consider an aqueous solution of HCL that has a concentration of 1×10^{-2} Mol/L.

HCl $\rightarrow$ H$^+$(aq) + Cl$^-$(aq)

Notice there is a single arrow in this equation, indicating the dissociation of HCL is complete. There is actually no concentration of HCL in solution. The HCl molecules have completely dissociated into H$^+$(aq) and Cl$^-$(aq) ions. Since one molecule of HCl dissociates into one H$^+$(aq) ion (and one Cl$^-$(aq) ion), 1×10^{-2} Mol/L of HCl will dissociate into 1×10^{-2} Mol/L of H$^+$(aq) ion. The negative log of 1×10^{-2} is 2, therefore the pH of the HCl solution is 2.

Weak Acids

Weak acids do not dissociate completely in aqueous solutions. The pH of weak acid solutions depends on the equilibrium concentrations of the weak acid "HA" and its dissociation components "H$^+$(aq)" and "A$^-$(aq)". For weak acids, " A$^-$(aq)" is referred to as the **conjugate base** of the acid "HA".

HA $\rightleftharpoons$ H$^+$(aq) + A$^-$(aq)

The equilibrium constant for acids is called the K$_A$ and is given by the formula

K$_A$ = [H$^+$(aq)] [A$^-$(aq)]/[HA]

In chemistry K$_A$ values are converted to pK$_A$ values. pK$_A$ values are the negative log of the K$_A$ value, just as pH and pOH values are the negative logs of the H$^+$ and OH$^-$ concentration values of a solution.

The K$_A$ equation can be rearranged to solve for the H$^+$ concentration as shown below (the "aq" notation has been eliminated to simplify the equation)

[H$^+$) =K$_A$ [HA] /[A$^-$]

If we convert this equation to negative log values, the equation becomes the **Henderson-Hasselbalch equation**

pH = pK$_A$ + log ([A$^-$] /[HA])

Scientific Methods and Reasoning

The primary importance of the Henderson-Hasselbalch equation is that it identifies the **isoelectric point** for a weak acid. This is the the pH level of the weak acid

solution where [A$^-$] = [HA]. this means that log [A$^-$] /[HA] =1 and since the log (negative or positive) of 1 is equal to zero, log ([A$^-$] /[HA]) = 0. Therefore, at the isoelectric point, the weak acid solution pH is equal to the pK$_A$

pH = pK$_A$; the isoelectric point of a weak acid "HA" solution.

This isoelectric pH value is important in chemistry because it is **the optimum pH for a buffered solution -** a solution that is resistant to changes in pH when additional acids or bases are added to the solution. In the human body the **bicarbonate buffering system** plays a crucial role in maintaining fluid pH values between a range 0f 7.35 and 7.45

A classic weak acid is acetic acid (the acid found in vinegar). The chemical formula for acetic acid is CH$_3$CO$_2$H. The partial dissociation of acetic acid in water is

CH$_3$CO$_2$H $\rightleftharpoons$ H$^+$(aq) + CH$_3$CO$_2^-$(aq)

The pK$_A$ of acetic acid is 4.76, and 1 molar aqueous solution (1 Mol/L) of acetic acid has a pH of 2.4, meaning the equilibrium H$^+$(aq) ion concentration of the solution is between 1×10^{-2} Mol/L (a pH of 2) and 1×10^{-3} Mol/L (a pH of 3).

We will not describe the mathematics required to determine the precise concentration of acetic acid in solution that would result in a solution pH that is equal to the pK$_A$ of acetic acid, but this is a common calculation in chemistry used to prepare an optimally buffered solution with a pH of 4.76. The choice of which weak acid to use to prepare buffered solutions depends on the pH level that one wishes to maintain and then to select a weak acid with a pK$_A$ that is as close to possible to the desired pH level.

Bases

Bases are substances that according to the Bronsted-Lowry definition are **proton acceptors** or more specifically - substances or compounds that in a solvent (almost always water) dissociate, and one of the dissociation products is (usually) the OH$^-$ ion. The general formula for the dissociation of a base is

$$BOH \rightleftharpoons B^+(aq) + OH^-(aq)$$

The concepts discussed for acids are nearly exactly analogous for bases. Strong bases completely dissociate in aqueous solutions and weak bases partially dissociate in aqueous solutions. There are K$_b$, pK$_b$ and pOH values for base dissociations and. The B$^+$ in the above equation is called the conjugate acid of the base (analogous to the conjugate base, A$^-$ of an acid dissociation reaction).

We will revisit acid-base reactions in greater detail in our later discussion of specific types of chemical reactions. The relationship of acid and base dissociations to equilibrium concentrations and associated equilibrium constants as we have discussed in this section are key concepts to understanding of chemical equilibriums and future discussions of acid-base reactions.

Colligative Properties of Solutions

Colligative properties of solutions are properties that are independent of the type of solute particles (molecules or ions) in a solution. Instead they **depend only upon the concentrations of solute** particles in a solution. Colligative properties include freezing point depression, boiling point elevation, vapor pressure lowering, and osmotic pressure. In our discussion, we will use the example of water as the solvent liquid, but the explanations that follow are generally true for any solvent liquid.

Freezing point depression, boiling point elevation and vapor pressure lowering, are best understood in comparison to the freezing and boiling points and vapor pressures of pure solvents. Pure liquid water at standard pressure of 1 atm has a freezing point of 0 degrees Celsius and a boiling point of 100 degrees Celsius. Any amount of material that is dissolved in water will decrease the vapor pressure and the freezing point of water and increase the boiling point of water.

The magnitude of these temperature changes depends on the concentration of the dissolved particles in the water. We are of course now describing an aqueous solution where water is the solvent and the dissolved particles are the solutes. An additional qualification for the colligative property effects is that the solutes are non-volatile, meaning they do not tend to evaporate out of the liquid phase and into the gas phase, but remain in solution regardless of temperature changes.

Vapor Pressure Lowering

For vapor pressure changes recall that liquid water is in equilibrium with water in the gas phase and this equilibrium depends on the temperature of the liquid water at 25 degrees Celsius the vapor pressure of water is 23.8 torr. This is the equilibrium partial pressure of water vapor above the surface of liquid water.

At equilibrium, the number of water molecules in the gas phase that are entering the liquid phase at the water surface are equal to the number of water molecules that are leaving the liquid phase by leaving the water surface as gas molecules. When solute particles are present in liquid water some of them are taking the place of liquid water molecules at the liquid surface. This means fewer water molecules are available at the surface to enter the gas phase, but these surface solute particles do not prevent gas phase water molecules from entering the liquid phase at the water surface.

A gas phase water molecule can displace a surface solute molecule as easily as it can a surface water molecule. This phenomenon shifts the vapor pressure equilibrium, favoring the movement of gas phase water molecules into the liquid phase over the movement of liquid phase water molecules into the gas phase. The consequence is that the solutes lower the vapor pressure of water at any temperature. The higher the concentration of the solute particles, the greater the reduction in the vapor pressure of water

Freezing Point Depression and Boiling Point Elevation

The exact same phenomenon is responsible for the lowering of the freezing point and the raising of the boiling point of water by dissolved solutes in the liquid phase of water. Fewer water molecules are present at the surface to escape into the gas phase during the phase transition of a solid to a liquid but there is no reduction in the rate of gas molecules re-entering the liquid phase.

This shifts the temperature of the phase transition of water at (a pressure of 1 atm) from liquid to gas (the boiling point) from 100 degrees Celsius to a higher temperature.

The magnitude of the increase in the boiling point temperature increases as the concentration of solute particles increases. This effect occurs at any point on the pressure-temperature phase transition boundary for water. The same shifts in liquid water leaving the solid state to the liquid state vs. liquid water molecules entering the solid-state account for the decrease in the freezing point of water at all pressure values for the phase transition between the solid and liquid state.

The actual numerical values for the changes in vapor pressure, boiling points and freezing points of water due to the concentration of solutes in liquid water are given by the same general type of equation. It is very unlikely that the HESI will expect one to perform a direct calculation of the magnitude of changes in vapor pressure, boiling points and freezing points based on the specific concentrations of solutes contained in a solution.

In general, one should be aware of the direction of the changes - vapor pressures decrease, boiling points increase and freezing points decrease. Also, one should be aware that the magnitude of these changes becomes larger as the concentration of solutes increases.

Osmotic Pressure

Osmotic pressure is a colligative property that is present in solutions when there is a semipermeable barrier between two solutions with different solute concentrations. To explain the phenomena of osmotic pressure we first need to describe what a semipermeable membrane is and second to describe the process that drives fluid and solutes across a semipermeable membrane. This process is called diffusion.

Semipermeable Membranes

Semipermeable membranes are typically thin sheets of material that separate (at least) two fluid compartments. The barrier is generally permeable to the solvent liquid within the compartments. Permeable means "able to pass through". The semipermeable membrane is impermeable to some or all of the solutes in the solutions within the compartments. Impermeable means "unable to pass through".

Semipermeable membranes are critical in biology because the membrane of a cell - which separates the interior contents of the cell from the external environment of the cell is a semipermeable membrane. The cell's semipermeable membrane is permeable to water (which is the solvent in biological solutions). The membrane is impermeable to most other substances that are dissolved in biological solutions.

Diffusion

Diffusion is the passive (non-energy requiring) process that occurs when solvents and solutes are moving from one local region to another local region due to differences in the concentrations of solutes between the two regions. When a concentration gradient exists between two regions, the solute particle in the region of higher concentration will move or flow to the region of lower concentration. The greater the difference in concentration between the two regions, the greater the driving force for the movement of solutes from higher to lower concentrations.

The other consideration in determining how strong the driving force of diffusion is the distance that the separates the highest and lowest concentration regions. The shorter the distance between the high and low concentration regions, the stronger the driving force of diffusion. Diffusion will continue until the concentrations of the two regions are equal.

If a semipermeable barrier exists between the high and low concentration regions, where the barrier is permeable to the solvent but not to the solutes. The solutes will be unable to diffuse between high and low concentration regions. In this case the solvent liquid will diffuse through the semipermeable barrier in an attempt to dilute the higher concentration region and thereby equalize the concentration of the solution between the two regions.

The phenomena of osmotic pressure can be best described by example. Imagine we have a U-shaped tube standing upright on a table with the ends of the tube pointing upward. Next there is a semipermeable membrane separating the right and left interior space of the tube located at the midpoint of the bend of the U at the lowest point of the tube - where it rests on the table.

The membrane is permeable to water, but not to either sodium or chloride ions. If we fill the tube with water from the top so that the water fills half of the tube, we will have equal water levels within the right and left sides of the tube. (If NaCl crystals are added to one side of the tube, lets choose the right side - the crystals will dissolve into Na+ and Cl - ions and an aqueous solution of Na+ and Cl - ions will be formed.)

Let's assume the resulting concentration of the solution is 1 Mol/L. The concentration of solute on the left side is zero so water will begin to diffuse from the left side of the tube, through the semipermeable membrane and into the right side of the tube in an attempt to equalize the solute concentrations between the right and left fluid compartments. As water moves from left to right, the volume of the left compartment decrease and the volume of fluid in the right compartment increases. Since there are no solutes in the left compartment the two compartments can never reach a point where the solute concentrations are equal.

The difference in height between the fluid column on the right vs the fluid compartment on the left represents a difference in pressure between the left and right fluid compartments. The weight of the fluid on the right, that is above the level of the fluid on the left compartment, creates a pressure that is acting to drive fluid back through the semipermeable membrane and restore the fluid between the two compartments to an equal level. This pressure is created by the differences in concentrations of solutes between the two compartments.

Eventually this increasing pressure due to the increasingly higher level of water on the right side becomes equal to the concentration gradient pressure that is driving the diffusion of water from the left to the right sides. We can then measure the difference in height between the two columns and use the density of the fluid and the volume of the fluid in the higher

volume to determine the mass of the fluid in the higher volume.

We can then use the formula for gravitational potential energy PE = mgh, to calculate the exact amount of pressure that the higher-level volume of fluid is exerting on the fluid beneath the higher-level fluid column. This pressure is the osmotic pressure that is generated due to the differences in concentration of non-permeable solutes between the two fluid compartments that are separated by the semipermeable membrane.

There are several key concepts that are demonstrated by this discussion of osmotic pressure. The first is that concentration gradients represent a form of potential energy. The concentration gradient in the u-shaped tube was able to lift a column of water by a certain height. The process of lifting this mass of solution requires energy. The source of that energy is the differences in concentration between the two fluid compartments. In this case the potential energy generated a mechanical force that was capable of driving the right-side fluid column upward.

The second concept is that this potential energy is a component of the internal energy of a chemical system - it can drive chemical reactions. In the mitochondria of cells a concentration gradient of hydrogen ions is built up between spaces separated by a membrane. The potential energy of this concentration gradient is used to drive hydrogen ions across the membrane through a membrane gate that is designed to generate ATP molecules from the energy of hydrogen ions as they pass through the gate. This is the final step in the aerobic cellular respiration cycles that extract energy from the conversion of glucose and oxygen to carbon dioxide and water.

Cells also use energy to pump solute particles across cell membranes to create concentration gradients. This is how an electrical potential is created across cell membranes. These transmembrane electrical potentials are critical features that allow nerve cells to generate electrical impulses and that allow muscle cells to contract.

Finally, the distribution of fluids between fluid

compartments within the human body - the intracellular compartments, the extracellular compartments and the intravascular compartments - is carefully regulated. The regulation process is based to a large extent on the regulation of concentrations of fluids within these compartments.

An example is the concentration of sodium ions (Na+) within the body. If sodium concentrations within a cell are too low compared to levels in the fluids surrounding the cell, water will move into the cell and the cell will begin to swell. If the cell is a brain cell this swelling can cause the cell to dysfunction or even die. Even slight disruptions in the balance of sodium levels within the body can cause this result in the human brain and the effects are often fatal.

The process of diffusion and the phenomena of osmotic pressure are fundamental processes that underlie a vast number of physiological processes at all levels of complexity in the human body from the cellular level to the organ and organ system level and to the overall level of the human body as a functional whole.

The Atom

The atom is the smallest unit of matter that can retain the physical and chemical properties of a specific substance. Atoms are composed of three subatomic particles; electrons - which are fundamental (not composed of smaller subatomic particles), and protons and neutrons which are each composed of quarks. Quarks are fundamental subatomic particles.

Atomic Radius

The electrons of an atom orbit the atom's nucleus. The outermost orbiting electrons define the surface boundary of the atom and define the size of the atom. Usually this size is given in terms of atomic radius or atomic diameter.

The Atomic Nucleus

The central region of an atom - the nucleus - is composed of protons and the neutrons. The only exception to this statement is that one isotope of the element hydrogen - hydrogen 1 - consists of atoms that have a nucleus that contains one single proton and no neutrons. Protons and neutrons are more generally classified as "nucleons". The nucleons of an atomic nucleus are held together by the strong nuclear force.

Atomic Mass

By definition, the mass of a proton is equal to exactly one atomic mass unit (1 AMU). The mass of a neutron is nearly equal to but slightly higher than that of the proton. For the HESI the mass of the neutron is also 1 AMU. The mass of an electron is several thousand times less than 1 AMU and for the HESI the mass of the electron is so small that it will irrelevant in comparison to proton and neutron masses. The mass of a single atom therefore is almost entirely due to the sum of the masses of the nucleons (protons and neutrons) in the atom's nucleus. For example, an atom whose nucleus contains six protons and seven neutrons has an atomic mass of 6 AMU + 7 AMU = 13 AMU.

Nuclear Radius

The radius of an atom's nucleus is thousands of times smaller the atomic radius. Nearly all of the mass of an atom and almost none of the volume of an atom are contributed by the atomic nucleus. This means that the atom is almost entirely empty space and that the nucleus is incredibly dense.

Electrons and Atomic Charge

The nucleus is surrounded by electrons. Electrons have an electric charge of -1, protons have an electric charge of +1 and neutrons have zero charge. Particles with opposite electric charges are attracted to one another by the electromagnetic force (particles with the same electric charge repel each other). It is the electromagnetic force that attracts electrons to an atom's positively charged nucleus. When an atom contains the same number of electrons and protons, the positive charge due to the protons in the nucleus and the negative charge of the electrons surrounding the nucleus cancel out. As a result, the atom has a net electric charge of zero. When this is the case, the atom is called a neutral atom.

Ions

Atoms can have fewer or more electrons than protons. When the number of electrons exceeds the number of protons, the atom has a net negative charge. When the number of protons exceeds the number of electrons, the atom has a net positive charge. The net charge is equal to the sum of the positive charges due to protons and negative charges due to electrons. For instance, if an atom has eight electrons and six protons, then the net charge of the atom is (-8)+(6)= -2.

Atoms (and molecules) with net charges are called ions. Negative ions are called anions and positive ions are called cations.

The Elements
A specific element is defined as the group of all atoms that individually contain the same number of protons within their nuclei. Atoms with nuclei that contain different numbers of protons are different elements. The atoms of every individual element have a unique set of physical and chemical properties. Isotopes of an element have virtually identical chemical properties but can have different physical properties due to the difference in mass among the isotopes.

Isotopes
The simplest atom is the hydrogen atom. Any atom that has one and only one proton in its nucleus is an atom of the element hydrogen. Hydrogen atoms may also have one or two neutrons in their atomic nucleus. These three types of hydrogen nuclei - one with one proton only, one with one proton and one neutron and one with one proton and two neutrons - all have one proton in their nucleus, but the nuclei have different numbers of neutrons. Elemental atoms with different numbers of neutrons in their nucleus are designated as isotopes of the element. Therefore, there are three isotopes of the element hydrogen. The other elements have varying numbers of isotopes.

Atomic Weight
The atomic weight of an element is defined as the average atomic mass of atoms of an element. Since almost every element has at least two isotopes, the average mass of the elemental atoms depends on the masses of the isotopes and the fractional percentage (relative abundance) of the isotopes that occur in nature.

Hypothetically, imagine that hydrogen's three isotopes occur naturally in percentages of 50% H-1 (one proton or 1 AMU), 20% H-2 (1 proton and 1 neutron or 2 AMU) and 30% H-3 (one proton and 2 neutrons or 3AMU). The average atomic weight of hydrogen atoms in general would be

$$(0.5)(1 \text{ AMU}) + (0.2)(2 \text{ AMU}) + (0.3)(3 \text{ AMU}) = 0.5 + 0.4 + 0.9 = 1.8$$

If these were the actual percentages of hydrogen's three isotopes, the average mass of hydrogen atoms would be 1.8 AMU and the atomic mass of the element hydrogen would be 1.8. In reality, nearly all hydrogen (99.99%) is the isotope H-1, therefore the tiny fractions of heavier isotopes are too small to change the mass except at several digits to the right of the decimal point. Therefore, the atomic mass of the element hydrogen is very nearly equal to that of the hydrogen-1 isotope, which is 1.008.

For the lighter elements, usually the most common isotope by far is the isotope that has equal numbers of protons and neutrons, so most atomic weights are close to twice the element's atomic number (the number of protons in the elemental atom nucleus). This is not always true. For instance, the element chlorine has an atomic number of 17 and an atomic weight of 35.45. This indicates that the element chlorine contains a relatively large percentage of the heavier chlorine isotopes.

The Periodic Table
The periodic table arranges all of the elements in a modified grid-like chart. Each element occupies a unique position in the table. The position correlates with the element's atomic number (as we have mentioned, the atomic number of an element is equal to the number of protons contained in the nucleus of atoms of the element). The first element - hydrogen- occupies the upper left corner position in the table. Elements of sequentially increasing atomic number are added to the next available position in the same row of the chart immediately to the right until the row of the table is complete. The element with the next higher atomic number is assigned to the first position on the left of the row immediately below the completed

HESI A^2 - Spire Study System

upper-row of the table.

Groups and Periods

The rows of the periodic table are called periods; the columns of the table are called groups. The first two columns on the left side of the table, beginning with the first column on the left, are the group I elements and - for the adjacent column on the right - the group II elements. The last column on the right side of the table is designated as the group XIII elements. The columns that are located to the immediate left of the group VIII column, beginning with the adjacent column, are the group VII, VI, V, IV and III elements,

The first period (top row) of the table has only a group 1 position - hydrogen - and a group VIII position - helium. They are separated by a wide gap in the periodic row. The second period has eight positions that include all of the groups I-VIII. The group I and group II positions are separated by another large gap from the group III-VIII positions. The third period has eighteen positions. Between the group II and the group III positions are ten new positions. The elements corresponding to these ten new positions are designated as transition metal elements.

The gaps in the periods ultimately reflect differences and similarities in properties of the elements that emerge as electrons arrange themselves in various configurations. We will describe the manner in which electrons are arranged around an atomic nucleus shortly.

Atomic Energy States

All atoms strive to attain their lowest possible energy states. First this is favored by achieving charge neutrality for the atom. The nuclei of atoms have a positive charge equal to the number of protons in the atom's nucleus. All protons have a charge of +1. The most energetically favorable state for an atom in terms of charge is the neutral state. An electron has charge of -1 the exact opposite charge of proton. When an atom contains equal numbers of protons and electrons the proton and electron charges cancel out and the atom's net charge is zero. By definition, neutral atoms have a net charge of zero. Neutral atoms however can lower their overall energy state even further if they can achieve a particular arrangement of electrons.

Electron Shells - the N levels

Electrons that are electromagnetically bound to an atom arrange themselves in concentric electron shells around the nucleus. In an atom, the innermost electron shell is the "n=1" electron shell. The "n=1" electron shell contains the lowest energy level positions available to electrons. For this reason, the n=1 shell is the first to be filled by electrons. The n level can be any positive integer n=1,2,3... the larger the integer value for n, the higher the energy of the n electron shell.

Electron Subshells (Orbitals)

The regions within an electron shell that electrons may occupy are called subshells or electron orbitals. The n=1 level shell has only one type of subshell/orbital. This is a spherical orbital called an "s" orbital. Since this s orbital is located at the n=1 shell, it is designated as the "1s" orbital. Individual subshell orbitals can accommodate no more than 2 electrons. There is only one s orbital at any n shell level. Therefore, only two electrons can be accommodated at the n=1 level.

An atom achieves a significant lowering of its energy state when it fills its n=1 shell. Atoms of the element helium have two protons and therefore will achieve charge neutrality by acquiring 2 electrons. Additionally, these two electrons will fill the 1s orbital. This also simultaneously completes the n=1 electron shell. There is no additional electron configuration that will further lower the energy state of helium atoms. Helium is therefore chemically inert - it will almost never participate in any chemical reactions with other elements.

Period 2 Elements and p Orbitals

For elements with atomic numbers higher than 2 (by definition, atoms that have nuclei containing more than 2 protons), additional electrons must be acquired for the atoms to achieve charge neutrality. Beginning with helium, the n=1 electron shell is filled. For all elements with atomic numbers greater than 2, additional electrons must occupy higher energy positions within orbitals beginning at the n=2 electron shell.

At the n=2 level, there are two types of orbitals - the s orbital and a new type of orbital, the "p" orbital. At the n=2 shell level, and at all subsequently higher shell levels (n= 3, 4 ...) There are one "s" orbital and three "p" orbitals. Within any n level electron shell, this new type of orbital - the p orbital - is at a higher energy level in comparison to the s orbital.

Since the maximum electron capacity of any single orbital is always 2 electrons, the n=2 shell can accommodate a total of eight electrons; 2 in the single s orbital and 2 electrons in each of the three p orbitals. These orbitals at the n=2 level are designated as the 2s orbital and the $2p_x$, $2p_y$ and $2p_z$ orbitals.

Elements in the second period (row) of the periodic table have electrons that occupy positions within the orbitals of the n=2 electron shell. There are eight elements in the second period of the table, beginning with lithium on the left in the group I column directly beneath hydrogen. The elements to the right of lithium sequentially add one additional electron to the n=2 level orbitals. At the final position on the right (and the 8th position of the period) is the element neon (atomic number 10). Notice that neon has completed the n=2 electron shell and that neon is in the group VIII column directly below helium.

Electron Configuration Notation

The electron configuration (positions) of an atom can be specified by listing the electron shells and orbitals that contain electrons. The electron positions are specified beginning with the lowest energy orbital on the left and then to progressively higher energy orbitals. For hydrogen, this would be indicated by the following notation:

$1s^1$

For helium (atomic number 2) this would be:
$1s^2$

For neon (atomic number 10) this would be
$1s^2\ 2s^2\ 2p^6$

Since at any given n electron shell level, the s orbitals are lower energy than the p orbitals, the s orbitals fill

before electrons begin to occupy positions in p orbitals. For example, the electron configuration for boron (atomic number 5) is

$1s^2\ 2s^2\ 2p^1$

NOT

$1s^2\ 2s^1\ 2p^2$

AND NOT

$1s^2\ 2p3$

NOTE: The electron energy level notation indicates the lowest possible electron energy state for an atom. This is called the **ground state** for electrons in an atom. Electrons can acquire energy by absorbing photons and consequently jump to higher energy level orbitals. This is termed an **excited energy state**. If an electron absorbs sufficient energy it can escape from the parent atom entirely. The energy required for this is equal to the parent atom's elemental ionization energy.

Valence Electrons

At this point we can begin to explain and even predict the chemical properties of the elements as well as many physical properties of the elements. For the ten period 2 elements, the n=2 electron shell is the outermost electron shell. Recall that all ten of the period 2 elements have an innermost n=1 electron shell that is filled by 2 electrons. These electrons are very tightly bound to their atomic nuclei and under normal circumstances never participate in chemical reactions. It is the electrons in the outermost or highest energy shells of an atom that participate in chemical reactions. These outermost shell electrons are usually called valence electrons.

The Octet Rule

The energy of an atom is lowered by a large amount when the n=1 electron shell is completed by the acquisition of 2 electrons that occupy the 1s orbital. Beginning at the n=2 energy level, an additional large reduction of energy occurs when the 2s orbital and the three 2p orbitals of the shell are filled by electrons. This is an underlying explanation for the octet rule. The octet rule states that there is a fundamental reason that atoms engage in chemical reactions. The reason is atoms strongly desire to acquire exactly eight valence electrons in their valence s and p orbitals. The reason for this desire is that this eight-electron configuration in the valence s and p orbitals results in a large reduction in an atom's electron energy level. Atoms that do not have a filled valence octet can "fill" the octet by taking electrons from other atoms (and consequently becoming an anion). Alternatively, **atoms may achieve a valence octet by sharing additional electrons with other atoms through the formation of covalent chemical bonds with those other atoms.**

Lewis Dot Structures

The s orbital and three p orbital valence electron configuration of an atom can be represented by Lewis dot structures. The Lewis dot structures are useful because they provide additional information about the valence electron configurations of an atom. To illustrate this, consider **the Lewis dot structure for nitrogen** (atomic number 7)

$$\cdot \overset{\cdot\cdot}{N} \cdot$$

Notice that there are four positions to place dots on the Lewis dot structure. These are the top, bottom and left and right sides of the atomic symbol (in this case N for nitrogen). These four locations represent the s and each of the three p valence shell orbitals of the atom. Nitrogen has 5 valence electrons; two in the 2s orbital and one each in each of the three 2p orbitals.

Electrons in an electron shell will not pair up in a p orbital until there is at least 1 electron in the other p orbitals. The two dots on the left side of the nitrogen symbol indicate there are 2 electrons in the 2s orbital of the nitrogen atom. This is an arbitrary position; the s orbital may be represented at any of the four positions surrounding the atomic symbol. The Lewis dot structure for nitrogen has single dots above, below and to the right of the nitrogen symbol. This indicates that there is one electron in each of nitrogen's three 2p orbitals.

Another example is **the Lewis dot structure for oxygen**

$$H : \overset{\cdot\cdot}{\underset{\cdot\cdot}{O}} : H$$

Oxygen (atomic number 8) has six valence electrons; 2 in the 2s orbital and four distributed among the three 2p orbitals. Notice that the Lewis dot structure indicates that each 2p orbital has at least one electron and that the final valence electron has been forced to pair with another electron in one of the 2p orbitals. Valence electrons that are paired in an orbital are called "lone pair" electrons.

The Lewis dot structure for neon is shown below. Notice that this is a structure that represents a completion of the octet rule. Neon, like all of the group VIII elements after helium, has a complete valence octet. All of the group XIII elements (the noble gases) have an identical Lewis dot structure. We see that this structure indicates that there are two electrons in the s and two electrons in each of the three p valence orbitals.

$$: \overset{\cdot\cdot}{\underset{\cdot\cdot}{Ne}} :$$

Periodic Properties of the Elements

The term "periodic" in the periodic table reflects the fact that the chemical and many physical properties of the elemental atoms tend to periodically repeat. This is because elemental atoms with the same number of s and p orbital valence electrons attempt to satisfy the octet rule in the same manner. Atoms of the elements that are in the same column of groups I through VIII have the same number of s and p valence electrons.

With the exception of helium, all of the elements in group VIII (the noble gases) have satisfied the octet rule as neutral atoms. They have no energetic advantage to gain by participating in chemical reactions with other elemental atoms. Consequently, the noble gases are chemically inert.

The Trends in the Periodic Table - From Left to Right Electronegativity

The ability of an elemental atom to draw electrons from other atoms to share in a covalent bond or, in extreme cases, to take an electron away from an atom is determined by the electronegativity of the atom. The electronegativity of elemental atoms is primarily determined by how near the atom is to completing a valence octet. The group VII element atoms (the halogens) are one electron short of completing their valence octets and are therefore the most electronegative of the group I through VII elemental atoms.

The group I elemental atoms (the alkali metals) are 7 electrons short of completing their valence octets. They are the farthest away from completing their valence octet and have little to gain by attempting to acquire additional electrons. The group I elemental atoms therefore have the lowest electronegativity of the groups I through VII elemental atoms.

The trend in the electronegativities of elements in the periodic table is that electronegativities increase from left to right across a period. This trend is broken at the last element on the right of a period. This is the group VIII element. The noble gases (group VIII) have no desire for additional electrons and therefore have almost zero electronegativity.

Ionization Energies

The ionization energy for an atom is the amount of energy required to overcome the electrons attraction to its nucleus. The extraction of the first electron from an atom requires the lowest amount of energy. This is called the first ionization energy. This process results in a +1 charged atomic ion. Extracting a second electron requires a larger amount of energy. This process results in a 2+ atomic ion. Each subsequent ionization requires progressively higher amounts of energy.

An elemental atom's ionization energies are usually correlated to the elemental atoms electronegativity. Elements with the lowest first ionization energies are the Group I elements and those with the highest first ionization energies are the group VIII elements. The

exception to this correlation is the noble gases. The noble gases have the lowest electronegativities of the all of the periodic groups but have the highest ionization energies of all of the periodic groups.

The trend in the ionization energies of elements in the periodic table is that ionization energies increase from left to right across a period.

Atomic Radius

The trend from left to right in the periodic table for the atomic radii of the elemental atoms is that the atomic radius decreases from left to right. The reason for this is that in the periodic table the progression from left to right correlates with an increasing number of protons contained in the nucleus and therefore an increasing positive nuclear charge of the elemental atoms. This increasing positive nuclear charge exerts a stronger electromagnetic force on the electrons orbiting the nucleus. As a result, the electrons are physically drawn closer to the nucleus, including the electrons located in the outermost electron shell. Since the outermost electron shell determines to outer boundary surface of an atom, increasing nuclear charge will decrease the atom's atomic radius.

The Trends in the Periodic Table - from Top to Bottom

Electronegativities and ionization energies decrease from top to bottom in the periodic table and atomic radii increase from top to bottom in the periodic table. There is a common phenomenon that explains all three trends. This is the phenomenon of electron shell shielding of the atomic nucleus.

Electron Shell Shielding of Nuclear Charge

When an electron shell is filled, it partially shields higher energy shell electrons from the positive electric charge of the atomic nucleus. This reduces the electromagnetic force that the positive charge of the nucleus is able to exert on electrons that occupy positions outside of the lower filled electron shell or shells. As a result, the outer electrons move farther away from the nucleus. Of course, they must be farther away simply because they must be located outside of the lower electron shells, but the shielding phenomenon results in a larger actual radius of the outer shell electrons than is required by the geometry of the concentric shell arrangement.

Since electronegativity and ionization energies are a result of the strength of the electromagnetic attraction of the positively charged nucleus for electrons, the reduction in the charge due to shielding reduces the energy required to ionize an atom (ionization energy) and also reduces the ability of the atom to attract additional electrons (electronegativity). Shielding does not occur among electrons in unfilled shells. Adding electrons in a given shell does not result in any shielding of other electrons in the shell.

Chemical Bonding

With the exception of the group VIII elements, all elemental atoms to varying degrees will engage in chemical reactions with other atoms. The groups I through VII elemental atoms attempt to satisfy the octet rule either by taking one or more electrons away from other atoms (ionization) or by sharing electrons with other atoms through the formation of interatomic bonds.

Ionic Bonds

When an atom succeeds in taking one or more electrons from another atom, the atom that takes the electrons becomes a negatively charged ion (an anion). The atom that loses the electron(s) becomes a positively charged atom (a cation). Usually the electron donor and the electron acceptor atoms become strongly bonded due to the electromagnetic force between the negative and positive charges of the two atoms. This type of interatomic or molecular bond is called an ionic bond.

Atoms with very high electronegativities are able to take electrons away from atoms with very low electronegativities. Ionic bonds therefore occur between atoms of very high electronegativity and those with very low electronegativity. The tendency to form ionic bonds is highest for elements located on the left and right of the periodic table -groups I and II as cations and groups VI and VII as anions - and progressively lower towards the middle of the table. The formation of the cation in an ionic bond requires less energy and is therefore more likely progressing from top to bottom, but the formation of an anion is less energetically favorable and therefore less likely progressing from top to bottom in the periodic table.

Ionic Solids

When two different types of atoms form ionic bonds the atoms arrange themselves in crystal - **a three-dimensional lattice of alternating anions and cations**. There is no sharing of electrons in a pure ionic bond. The force that holds the ionized atoms in place is the attractive electromagnetic force between positively and negatively charged atomic ions. This is a very strong type of bonding and ionic crystalline solids have very high melting and boiling points since all of the ionic bonds in the solid and liquid phase must be weakened in the solid to liquid transition (melting) and completely broken in the liquid to gas transition (boiling).

An example of an ionic crystalline solid is common table salt, sodium chloride (NaCl). Solid sodium chloride consists of sodium cations ($Na+$) and chloride anions ($Cl-$) arranged in an alternating three-dimensional crystalline structure that is typical of ionic compounds.

An important characteristic of many ionic solids is that they are easily dissolved in polar liquids such as water. The partial positive and negative charges on polar molecules are able to weaken the ionic attractions between the ionic solid ions and stabilize them as individual atomic ions within the dissolving polar liquid.

Covalent Bonds

In most cases, the difference in electronegativity between bonding atoms is insufficient for one atom to take an electron away from the other bonding atom. The two atoms instead share one electron each through a covalent bond. Atoms can share additional electrons through the formation of additional covalent bonds with other atoms or by forming additional covalent bonds with the same atom resulting in double or triple covalent bonds.

The number of covalent bonds that an atom forms depends on how many electrons the atom requires to complete its valence octet. For instance, oxygen, with 6 valence electrons, is 2 electrons short of completing its valence octet. Therefore, oxygen typically forms two covalent bonds with other atoms. This results in the sharing of two additional electrons by the oxygen atom through the two covalent bonds with other atoms. In this manner, the oxygen atom has completed its valence octet.

Polar Bonds

In covalent bonds, electrons are not equally shared when there is a significant difference in electronegativity between the bonding atoms. For example, in the molecule hydrogen fluoride (HF), fluorine is much more electronegative than hydrogen and the hydrogen fluoride molecule has a partially negative pole near to the fluorine atom and a partially positive pole near to the hydrogen atom. The covalent bond between hydrogen and fluorine is said to have a partial ionic character.

Ionic bonds also have some covalent character, more so as the difference in electronegativities between the bonding atoms decreases.

Some covalent bonds are pure covalent bonds; in particular when the molecule consists of atoms of the same element such as O_2 or N_2. Importantly, the carbon-hydrogen bonds in hydrocarbon atoms have almost no ionic character, and hydrocarbon molecules are **nonpolar molecules**. This is significant because **nonpolar molecules will not dissolve in polar liquids such as water.** Water molecules are very polar and liquid water is a powerful polar solvent. Hydrocarbons and molecules composed in large part of hydrocarbons (fats and other lipid molecules) or insoluble in water but will dissolve in nonpolar liquids such as benzene or other hydrocarbon liquids.

Properties of the Group I-VII Elements

The Group VIII elements - the noble gases - are chemically inert and therefore are not included in this discussion of the chemical properties of the groups of the periodic table.

Group VII Elements - The Halogens

All Halogens are represented by the same Lewis dot structure shown as shown below for the halogen fluorine.

$$:\!\ddot{F}\!:$$

As we have discussed, the halogen atoms are one electron short of completing their valence octet. They are therefore the most electronegative of the periodic table groups. They are sufficiently electronegative to take electrons away from atoms with weak electronegativity, usually the group I and group II elemental atoms. This results in the formation of ionic bonds between the halogen anions and the group I or group II cations. Halogens form -1 anions in ionic compounds because they require only one additional electron to complete their valence octet.

When halogens form covalent bonds, they almost always form only one covalent bond, since this results in the gain of one additional electron through sharing of electrons in the covalent bond. This additional electron completes the halogen atoms' valence octets.

Typical halogen-containing molecules that are likely to appear in questions on the HESI are the crystalline-ionic-solids sodium chloride, NaCL, potassium chloride, KCl, Calcium chloride $CaCl_2$ and magnesium chloride $MgCl_2$. Chlorine may also appear on the HESI as the chloride ion Cl^- in solutions.

Group VI Elements - The Oxygen Family

For the HESI, oxygen and sulfur are the only likely elements in group VII whose properties will be expected knowledge. Oxygen is two electrons short of completion of a valence octet. Oxygen is very electronegative and can form ionic bonds with group I and group II atoms. Oxygen atoms form -2 anions in ionic compounds because they require two additional electrons to complete their valence octets. Oxygen atoms will form two covalent bonds with other atoms in order to gain two additional electrons through sharing of electrons in the two covalent bonds. Sulfur is not well represented by Lewis dot structure because sulfur very often forms six covalent bonds with other atoms

Typical oxygen containing molecules that are likely to appear in questions on the HESI are molecular oxygen O_2, water, H_2O, carbon dioxide CO_2, carbohydrates such as glucose, and in solutions as the hydroxide ion OH^- and as the bicarbonate ion $HCO3-$

Group V Elements - The Nitrogen Family

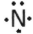

For the HESI, nitrogen and phosphorus are the only likely elements in the group VI elements whose properties will be expected knowledge. Nitrogen is

three electrons short of completion of a valence octet. Nitrogen is moderately electronegative but does not commonly form ionic bonds. Nitrogen will typically form three covalent bonds with other atoms to gain 3 additional electrons through sharing of electrons in the three covalent bonds. Phosphorus, like sulfur, is not well represented by Lewis dot structure because phosphorus very often forms six covalent bonds with other atoms

Typical nitrogen containing molecules that are likely to appear in questions on the HESI are molecular oxygen nitrogen N_2, ammonia NH_3, amino acids, nitrogenous bases of nucleic acids and urea $CO(NH2)_2$. On notable fact regarding ammonia is that it is a moderately strong base with a pH of 11.6

Phosphorous will likely appear as an important mineral element in bones and as a phosphate group, PO_4^- in ATP molecules and in the sugar phosphate polymer chain that forms the structural long axis of DNA and RNA molecules.

Group IV Elements - The Carbon Family

The chemical properties of carbon are perhaps the most important chemical properties to be familiar with for the HESI. Carbon - with four valence electrons - nearly always forms four covalent bonds with other atoms. This allows carbon to form the carbon skeletons of the tens of thousands of very large and complex molecules that are required to create a living organism. Carbon does not participate in ionic bonding.

The element silicon is the carbon family element directly below carbon. Silicon has very different chemical and physical properties than those of carbon. Silicon is a metalloid - an element with properties that are somewhere between those of metals and of nonmetals. Silicon is a critical element in the semiconductor industry and is the major element that is used to form the circuitry in most modern electronic devices.

Typical carbon containing molecules that are likely to appear in questions on the HESI are carbon dioxide CO_2 and almost every organic molecule including the three types of hydrocarbons; the alkanes (C_nH_{2n+2}), the alkenes (C_nH_{2n}), and the alkynes (C_nH_{2n-2}); carbohydrates, fats and other lipid molecules, amino acids, and in solution, carbonic acid H_2CO_3 and the bicarbonate ion HCO_3^-.

Group III Elements

Boron and the other group III elemental atoms have unpredictable and complex chemical properties and bonding characteristic which are not expected knowledge for the HESI.

Group II Elements - The Alkali Earths

:Be

All of the group II elements have very similar chemical and physical properties and the HESI expects that these properties be recognized for any element in group II. Group II elements are very weakly electronegative. They have only two valence octet electrons and these are easily extracted by the strongly electronegative halogens and oxygen. The result is that group II elemental atoms tend to form 2+ charged cations that are ionically bonded to 1- charged halogen anions in a 2 to 1 ratio or to 2+ charged oxygen anions in a 1 to1 ratio.

Typical group II containing molecules that are likely to appear in questions on the HESI are the crystalline ionic solids calcium chloride ($CaCl_2$) and magnesium chloride $MgCl_2$. They may also appear on the HESI as the magnesium and calcium ions Mg^{2-} and Ca^{2-} in solutions.

Group I Elements -- The Alkali Metals

•Li

All of the group I elements have very similar chemical and physical properties and the HESI expects that these properties be recognized for any element in group I. Group I elements have the lowest electronegativity among the groups I through VII. They have only one valence octet electron which is very easily extracted by the strongly electronegative halogens and oxygen. As a result, the group I elemental atoms tend to form 1+ charged cations that are ionically bonded to 1- charge halogen anions in a 1 to 1 ratio or to 2+ charged oxygen anions in a 1 to 2 ratio.

Typical group I containing molecules that are likely to appear in questions on the HESI are the crystalline ionic-solids sodium chloride, NaCL and potassium chloride, KCl, Sodium and potassium may also appear on the HESI as the sodium and potassium ions Na^- and K^- in solutions.

The Period 3 Elements -The 3s and 3p Orbitals

The third period (third row) of the periodic table represents elements whose atoms have already completed their n=1 and n=2 electron shells. The electrons contained in these two completed electron shells (10 electrons total) are now so strongly bound to their atomic nuclei that they never participate in chemical reactions.

At the n=3 electron shell level, atoms are able to place electrons into not only a 3s orbital and three 3p orbitals, but also into a new type of orbital. This new orbital is the "d" orbital. At electron shell levels where n is equal to three or higher, each shell has five d orbitals. Two electrons may be placed into each of these five d orbitals. Therefore, a total of ten electrons can be placed into d orbitals at any n=3 or higher electron shell.

The third period consists only of the group I through VIII elements. This is due to the fact that the 3s and 3p orbitals are preferentially filled before any electrons are placed in 3d orbitals. Notice that in the third period these eight positions in the periodic table correspond to the groups I through VIII just as occurs in the period two elements.

The Transition Metal Elements - The d orbitals

In the fourth period (row) of the periodic table there are 18 elements. The fourth period begins with the group I and group II elements. The group II element is followed by ten elements in new rows of the periodic table. These ten new element positions are followed by the group III through VIII elements. The ten elements between the group II element and the group III element are transition metal elements.

These ten transition metal elements, beginning in the fourth period, are elements that have electrons in their d orbitals. In the fourth period, **the 3d orbitals are higher energy orbitals than the 3s, 3p and 4s orbital but are lower energy orbitals than the 4p orbitals.** Therefore, elemental atoms in the fourth period first place electrons into the 4s orbitals. After filling the 3s orbitals, elemental atoms begin to place electrons into the 3d orbitals. Notice that the n=3 energy shell is not completed until the elements zinc places the tenth electron into the final available position for electrons in the n=3 shell. The six elements to the right of zinc are the groups III through VIII elements. These elements have completed their 4s and 3d electron orbitals and now begin to place electrons into the 4p orbitals.

The Electron Conduction Band in Transition Metals

The d orbital electrons, in pure samples of a transition element or in combinations (alloys) of transition metal elements merge to form **a delocalized conduction band of electrons.** Electrons move freely within the conduction band, acting as a fluid that surrounds all of the transition metal nuclei. The result is that, in transition metal solids, the individual atomic nuclei are not confined to rigid positions as occurs in ionic and other crystalline solids. The atoms are relatively easily rearranged within the transition metal mass.

Physical Properties of Transition Metals

Malleability and Ductility

The ability of transition metal nuclei to move relatively easily in relation to other transition metal nuclei within the solid state of a transition metal sample explains the physical properties of transition metals of ductility and malleability. The metals can be shaped (malleability) and stretched (ductility) and yet the atoms within a transition metal object are still strongly attracted to one another. Although the metal objects can be forged or stretched into different shapes, including very thin wires, it is extremely difficult to actually separate a metal object into two or more separate objects. These properties of ductility, malleability and tensile strength make the transition metals ideal elements for use as structural materials. They are strong yet can be machined into a wide variety of useful shapes - tools, weapons and parts of complex machinery.

Electrical and Thermal Conductivity

The mobile electrons in the conduction bands of transition metal also make the transition metals excellent conductors of electricity. Transition metals have very high specific heats of fusion and vaporization. It requires very large amounts of heat to melt or vaporize transition metal objects, but the specific heats of transition metals are very low, so they are excellent conductors of heat (and extremely poor insulators).

Nonmetals

The HESI expects that one understands several chemical and physical properties of the group of elements that are classified as nonmetals. These properties should be appreciated in contrast to the same properties of the elements of the transition metal category and the Group I category - the alkali metals. Further discussion of the underlying physical principles that distinguish these categories becomes too technical and counterproductive for preparation for the HESI. It is best to simply memorize that the most significant nonmetal elements are carbon (C), nitrogen (N), oxygen (O) phosphorus (P), sulfur (S) and all of the group VII elements - the halides.

These properties of nonmetals are generally the opposite of the transition metals. The nonmetals - in their elemental form and as molecular compounds with other elemental atoms - tend to form small molecules that are strongly covalently bonded but with weak intermolecular attractions. These compounds in the solid state tend to be brittle or powdery. The nonmetals are extremely poor electrical and thermal conductors and therefore excellent electrical and thermal insulators.

Metalloids

There are one or two elements that are located at the positions in each period, beginning with Boron at group III in period two and then advancing to group IV, V and VI in a descending stair step fashion moving from top to bottom of the periodic table that have properties that are partially metallic and partially those of the nonmetal elements. The second period group IV through VI elements - carbon, nitrogen and oxygen are all nonmetals. Several other of the group IV through VI elements including phosphorus and sulfur are nonmetals and all of the group VII (halogens) and group VIII (noble gases) are nonmetals. The metalloids most notably have intermediate electrical conductivity and are often classified as semiconductors. Semiconductors are critical materials used in the electronics industry. The most familiar metalloids are the elements silicon and germanium.

The Fifth and Higher Periods of the Periodic Table

At the 5th and higher periods of the periodic table, additional electrons begin to be added to new types of orbitals. At the fourth period, the "f" orbital becomes available and at the fifth period a "g" class orbital becomes available. Elements that are adding electrons to these new orbitals are the lanthanide and actinide elements. Once these f and g orbitals are filled then d orbitals begin to fill. The chemistry of the lanthanide and actinide orbitals are beyond the scope of the HESI. The group I (alkali metals) the group II (alkali earths), group VII (halogens) and the group VIII (noble gases) at all higher periods of the periodic table retain their specific group properties - and this is expected knowledge for the HESI.

Transition Metal-Nonmetal Chemistry

The chemistry of transition metal-nonmetal interactions is indirectly addressed in the HESI as a class of chemical reactions called reduction-oxidation (redox) reactions. There are many redox reactions that do not involve transition metals, but nearly all of the chemical reactions involving transition metals with nonmetals are redox reactions. Transition metals - due to their d orbital electron capacities - can easily exist in a wide range of oxidation states within various chemical compounds. It is these wide range of oxidation states that cause bright and highly variable coloration characteristic of solutions that contain transition metal compounds.

Quantum Mechanics and Chemistry

The discussion above of the nature of atomic elements, electron orbitals and the periodic table provides a descriptive understanding of processes that govern chemical behavior. There is a much deeper level of understanding of these topics that can be gained by understanding the quantum mechanical principles that underlie these processes.

At the atomic level the nature of matter and the physical interactions of matter are entirely different from the apparent properties of matter and the physical interactions of matter that we see at a macroscopic scale. Recall that we discussed that photons, the subatomic particles that are electromagnetic energy, Usually, behave not as if they were point particles like tiny billiard balls but rather they appear to behave as if they were waves of energy.

In some circumstances photons do behave as if they were tiny billiard balls. It is really not correct to say that photons are either a particle or a wave, but rather that they have some particle-like character and some wave-like character. This **wave-particle duality** is true not only for photons, but also for electrons and particularly so for electrons that are electromagnetically bound within an atom and for electrons that are bound within a molecule.

The first principle to understand about quantum mechanics is that energy **exists as individual packets or quanta**. When energy is absorbed or emitted by matter it must be absorbed or emitted as an exact amount or quantum of energy. This is an all or none process; either the entire quantum of energy is absorbed or emitted or none is absorbed or emitted, and no fractionally less or greater amount of energy can be absorbed or emitted.

The next principle, for chemistry, is that **atoms and**

molecules form a quantum system. Within this quantum system, **electrons behave as if they are waves.** All of the properties of these electron waves can be described by exactly **four quantum numbers** (which are not really numbers, but letters). These letters are **n, l, m and s.** The quantum number **n is the principal quantum number** and it is the exact same number as the n for electron energy shells in an atom. In a quantum system such as an atom electrons can have any n value that is positive integer value beginning with **n=1 (n=1, 2, 3,...).** The reason that there are these energy levels is that they represent the allowed quantum energy value differences for electrons within an atom. **Electrons are forbidden to have fractional energy levels between the principal energy levels n.**

The quantum number ℓ is the **azimuthal quantum number.** The electron with a principal quantum number of n, can have any single azimuthal quantum number ℓ with integer values of **(0, 1, 2,...n-1).** For instance, if an electron has a principal quantum number n=4, then it can have any single quantum number ℓ value 0 to 3 (n-1 =3 where n=4). These possible ℓ values would be 0, 1, 2 or 3. **The specific ℓ values correspond to the subshells or orbitals of the n levels.** An ℓ=0 value corresponds to an **s orbital,** an ℓ=1 value corresponds to a **p orbital,** an ℓ=2 value corresponds to a **d orbital** and an ℓ=3 value corresponds to an **f orbital,** an ℓ=4 value corresponds to a **g orbital.**

Notice that for the n=1 level, there is only one possible value for ℓ and therefore only one allowed type of orbital, the l=0 orbital which is the s orbital. The same reasoning explains why at the n=2 level there are only s and p orbitals allowed and at the n=3 level there are only s, p and d orbitals allowed.

The quantum number m is the **magnetic quantum number.** An electron with an azimuthal quantum number of ℓ can have any single magnetic quantum number m with **integer values of (-ℓ...0...+ℓ).** For instance, if an electron has an azimuthal quantum number ℓ=2, then it can have any single magnetic quantum number m value from -2 to +2. These possible m values would be -2, -1, 0, +1 and +2.

The magnetic number m specifies **the different**

orientations that an orbital can have within an n level. The m number explains why at any given n level there is only **one s orbital,** only **three p orbitals** and only **five d orbitals.** An s orbital has an ℓ=0 value. This means it can have only an m= 0 value. Therefore, there is only one possible orientation of an s orbital at any n level. For p orbitals, ℓ=1, therefore the possible m values are -1, 0, +1. This means there are three possible orientations of p orbitals at any n level. Therefore, there are three available p orbitals at any n level.

For the d orbitals, ℓ=2 and the possible m values are -2, -1, 0, +1, and +2. This means there are five possible orientations of d orbitals at any n level. Therefore, there are **five available d orbitals** at any allowed n level. Using the formula for m values, we can see that there will be **7 possible f orbitals** (beginning at the n=4 energy shell) and **9 possible g orbitals** (beginning at the n=5 energy shell).

The final quantum number, s, is the spin quantum number. For electrons the allowed s or spin values are **either +½ or -½ .** The Pauli exclusion principle state that **no two electrons within a quantum system can have the exact same quantum numbers n, l, m and s.** When we bring all of the quantum information of electrons in atoms together, all of the details of how electrons arrange themselves within an atom becomes apparent.

First, any electrons in a specific orbital must have the same n, l and m quantum numbers. For instance, electrons in the 2s orbital have the quantum numbers n=2, l=0 (a s orbital) and m=0. since no two electrons can have the same set of quantum numbers there are **only two electrons that can simultaneously occupy any single orbital,** one electron must have a spin of +½ and the other electron must have a spin of -½ .

The limitation of two electrons per orbital explains the electron capacities of the various orbitals and of the n levels. For instance, at n=2 there is one s orbital and three p orbitals. At 2 electrons per orbital this gives 8 electrons as the capacity of the n=2 level. At the n=3 level, there are one s orbital and three p orbitals and five d orbitals. Therefore, there are a total of nine orbitals at the n=3 level and at 2 electrons per orbital,

18 electrons that can be accommodated at the n=3 level.

Electron Density and Bonding Orbitals

The wave-like nature of electrons in quantum systems such as atoms and molecules also explains how intermolecular bonding orbitals are formed and **predicts the geometry of molecules** as well as many other characteristics of individual molecules.

Rather than imagine that electrons are point particles orbiting atomic nuclei, it is more accurate to think of an electron as **a cloud of electron density** that is spread out over the entire orbital that an electron occupies around a nucleus. When a covalent bond is formed between two atoms, the bond occurs because valence electrons reconfigure themselves into a new type of orbital - **a bonding orbital**. To accomplish this, the electron orbital that contains the electrons that will form a bonding orbital must overlap. When they overlap, the two orbitals can transform into one bonding orbital (actually two new orbitals - a bonding orbital and an antibonding orbital).

For instance, the 1s orbitals of two hydrogen atoms can overlap and create a bonding orbital where the majority of the electron cloud resides between the two hydrogen nuclei. As a result, the hydrogen nuclei are drawn toward the electron cloud between them, thus forming a covalent bond.

Considering a covalent bond to represent a cloud of electron density between two atomic nuclei also explains how covalent bonds can become polar and how molecules can be polar. The more electronegative atom in a covalent bond will draw a larger percentage of the electron cloud density toward the more electronegative nucleus and away from the less electronegative nucleus.

The more electronegative nucleus thereby acquires a partially negative charge and the other nucleus develops a partially positive charge. The result is that a **dipole** is formed and the molecule containing this **polar bond** becomes a **polar molecule.**

Sigma Bonds

Two hydrogen molecules sharing two electrons in a bonding orbital fills the N=1 energy shell of both atoms and this is the reason that hydrogen molecules are H_2 or "diatomic" molecules. They form a single bond by overlapping their 1s orbitals. **Single bond orbitals are called "sigma" bonds.** Sigma bonds are called covalent bonds because they are formed from valence orbitals between two atoms. In a covalently bonded molecule, every atom forms one sigma bond with at least one other adjacent atom.

Pi Bonds

Once a sigma bond is formed between two atoms, it may be possible for the two atoms to form one or two additional covalent bonds between the two atoms. This occurs when the adjacent atoms have valence p orbitals available that can overlap.

The p bond is bi-lobed or dumbbell-shaped and can overlap top-lobe to top-lobe and bottom lobe to bottom-lobe with an adjacent p orbital on another atom to create a new bonding orbital called a **pi orbital**. Pi orbitals are also called **pi bonds**. If two valence p orbitals are available on adjacent atom Then a pi bond can form between the two atoms.

Since the adjacent atoms already have formed a sigma bond, formation of an additional pi bond results in a **double bond** between the two atoms. Formation of a second pi bond results in a **triple bond** between the two atoms. For example, the oxygen molecule, O2, forms a sigma bond and one pi bond between two oxygen atoms, resulting in a double bond between the two oxygen atoms, the nitrogen molecule, N2, forms a sigma bond and two pi bonds between two nitrogen atoms, resulting in a triple bond between the two nitrogen atoms.

Hybrid Orbitals

Another consequence of the ability of electrons in orbitals to recombine into new types of orbitals is that valence orbitals can recombine within a single atom. For instance, a carbon atom has two electrons in the 2s orbital and one electron each in two of the three available 2p orbitals. These four valence electrons have four valence orbitals that can recombine to form hybrid orbitals. A valence s orbital can combine with one valence p orbital to form **two sp hybrid valence orbitals**. A valence s orbital can combine with two valence p orbitals to form **three sp₂ hybrid valence orbitals** and a valence s orbital can combine with three valence p orbitals to form **four sp₃ hybrid valence orbitals**. All atoms are capable of forming hybrid valence orbitals and will do so if the formation of these orbitals allow the atom to lower the electron energy state of the atom by using the orbitals to form intramolecular bonds with other atoms.

With the exception of hydrogen atoms, nearly all atoms form hybrid orbitals to use as the orbitals that participate to form covalent sigma bonds (hydrogen forms sigma bonds with a 1s orbital; the second bond in double bonds and the second and third bonds in triple bonds are always formed by adjacent p orbitals of two atoms). The sp, sp2 and sp3 hybrid orbitals are teardrop-shaped with the apex of the tear pointing toward the atomic nucleus. **Any type of hybrid orbital can overlap with any other type of hybrid orbital to form a sigma bonding orbital.**

VSEPR - Valence Shell Electron Pair Repulsion Theory

The hybrid orbitals that atoms generate to participate in covalent bonding consist of negatively charged electron density clouds. Since these hybrid orbitals have the same charge (negative) they are repelled from one another and will arrange themselves geometrically in three dimensions so that they are as far apart as possible. This principle is the basis for **valence shell electron pair repulsion theory (VSEPR)**. The theory explains and predicts of the three-dimensional geometries of molecules and a wide variety of other properties of molecules

Hybrid Orbital Geometries

For **sp orbitals**, of which there are two, the optimum geometry to reduce the repulsive force between the two orbitals is to orient them **linearly** so that they are on opposite sides of the nuclei with an angle between the two orbitals of **180 degrees**. For **sp2 orbitals** the three orbitals arrange themselves on a **trigonal** (triangular) **plane** with each orbital separate from the other two by an angle of **120 degrees**. For **sp3 orbitals**, the four orbitals are directed towards the four apices of a regular

tetrahedron with the angle between the four bonds being about **109 degrees**.

This information allows chemists to predict the **geometry of atoms around a central bonding atom**. For small molecules, such as CH4 this is the geometry of the entire molecule and for larger molecules it is the geometry of one or more region of the molecule oriented around a central atom or atoms.

For molecules that are covalently bonded the individual atoms within the molecule will form bonds in an attempt to satisfy the octet rule. If the atom desires to form one or more covalent bonds it will usually form at least two hybrid orbitals. If the atom seeks to form two single covalent bonds often this would be accomplished by first forming the sp hybrid orbital since two sp orbitals are formed by the combination of an s and a p orbital.

If the atom desires to form three single bonds then it will form at least three hybrid orbitals, this would often be the sp2 hybrid orbital (3 sp2 orbitals form from one s orbital and two p orbitals). If the atom desires to form four single bonds then it will form four hybrid orbitals, this would be the sp3 hybrid orbital (four sp3 orbitals from one s orbital and three p orbitals).

Lone Pair Electrons

Often an atom will form more hybrid orbitals than are required for bonding because the atom will have valence electrons that do not participate in bonding. Usually these are pairs of nonbonding electrons that are deposited in a single orbital. These valence electrons in a single orbital are called **lone pair electrons**. An example of lone pairs are those that exist in the atom oxygen when oxygen is covalently bonded within a molecules.

Due to the octet rules, an oxygen atom desires to form two covalent bonds. Oxygen could form two sp orbitals to participate in formation of sigma bonds with other atoms to satisfy its octet rule, but oxygen - when it forms two covalent bonds - has four valence electrons that do not participate in bonding.

These lone pairs have strong negative charges and it is

more energetically favorable for oxygen to minimize the repulsive forces generated by the lone pair electrons by forming four sp3 bonds. Two of the sp3 bonds will participate in forming sigma bonds and the other two sp3 orbitals will contain two of the four remaining valence electrons apiece. The result is that the bonded oxygen atom has two lone pairs of electrons in sp3 hybrid bonds. This is significant because it explains many of the **unique properties of the water molecule H_2O.**

This quantum mechanical picture of electrons within atoms and the VSEPR theory of bonding orbitals within molecules may seem confusing, but it is extremely helpful in understanding a vast amount of chemical information that would otherwise require rote memorization. As an illustration, let us consider four small molecules, methane (CH_4), ammonia (NH_3) carbon dioxide (CO_2) and water (H_2O).

Methane - CH_4

Hydrogen desires to form one covalent bond to complete the n=1 energy shell and carbon, with four valence electrons desires to form four covalent bonds in order to acquire four additional electrons to complete its s-p orbital valence octet. Both types of atoms fulfil their objectives by forming the molecule CH4 where each of the four hydrogens have formed one covalent bond and simultaneously the central carbon of CH$ has formed four covalent bonds.

The most energetically favorable means to achieve this is for carbon to combine the 2s orbital and the three 2p orbitals to form four sp3 hybrid orbitals. Each of the orbitals then overlaps with a hydrogen 1s orbital to form four equivalent covalent sigma bonding orbitals. The hydrogens will be located at the apices of a regular tetrahedron and the CH4 molecule will have a three-sided-pyramid shape. All of the bonds in CH4 are single bonds.

Although methane is highly combustible with oxygen, it usually requires a very high initial heat source such as an open flame to induce combustion. This is because single bonds are difficult to attack chemically because They are in between and thus shielded by the bulk of two the bonding atoms. CH4 is the simplest of the hydrocarbon class of molecules.

All hydrocarbons consist of carbon chains with the carbon-chain carbons also bonded to hydrogens. Hydrocarbon molecules with only single carbon bonds are called alkanes. Those with at least one carbon-carbon double bond are called alkenes and those with at least one carbon-carbon triple bond are called alkynes. The carbon-hydrogen bonds in hydrocarbons are nonpolar and hydrocarbons as a class of molecules are nonpolar. Consequently, hydrocarbons and molecules that are predominantly composed of hydrocarbons are not soluble in water.

Ammonia - NH_3

Ammonia has five valence electrons and desires another three electrons to complete its valence octet. Therefore, ammonia can achieve this by forming three covalent bonds. This could be accomplished by forming three sp2 orbitals, but notice that this leaves two unbonded valence electrons on the nitrogen atom. To minimize electron repulsion from the lone pair of electrons, as predicted by the VSEPR theory, nitrogen forms four sp3 hybrid orbitals. Three of the sp2 orbitals overlap with hydrogen 1s orbitals and form three sigma bonds. This predicts a different geometry than if nitrogen had used sp2 orbitals to form sigma bonds with three hydrogens.

The sp2 hybridized ammonia molecule would have been a planar molecule with 120 degrees between any two of the three sigma bonds. Instead the ammonia molecule has three hydrogens located at three of the four apices of a tetrahedron and a lone pair of electrons at the remaining apex of the tetrahedron.

The angle between nitrogen hydrogen bonds is 109 degrees and the molecule has the geometry of a three-sided pyramid. The lone pair electrons that occupy the fourth sp3 orbital are negatively charged (of course) but are also very exposed to chemical attack. For this reason, **ammonia is a weak base. The lone pair electrons will readily bind to hydrogen ions** (the definition of a base) and form the ionic molecule NH4+.

Many other important chemical reactions involve interactions with the lone pair electrons of ammonia.

The lone pair electrons also give the ammonia molecule a polarity and allow ammonia to participate in **hydrogen bonding**. This makes ammonia one of the few small molecules that are **liquid at room temperature** and also make ammonia an **excellent polar solvent.**

Carbon Dioxide - CO_2

The carbon dioxide molecule illustrates how atoms will hybridize orbitals in whatever fashion is required to achieve an optimal lowering of electron energy. In carbon dioxide, both oxygen atoms form two covalent bonds - which we know they desire to do - and a central carbon atom forms four covalent bonds - also as we know carbon desires to do.

To achieve this carbon must form two sets of double bonds and each oxygen one set of double bonds with the central carbon atom. Since only p orbitals can form the second bond in a double bond, carbon requires two of its three p orbital to remain as p orbitals and each oxygen requires one of its p orbitals to remain as a p orbital.

One oxygen and one carbon p orbital overlap between the central carbon and each of the two oxygen atoms. This generates a pi orbital forms between each of the oxygen atoms and the central carbon atom. Carbon must also form two sigma bonds, one with each of the two oxygen atoms. Carbon combines the remaining p orbital and the 2s orbital to form two sp orbitals.

The oxygen atoms have two sets of lone pair electrons to deal with so each oxygen atom forms three sp2 orbitals from their 2 remaining p orbitals and their 2s orbital. The sp2 orbitals off the carbon atom overlap one of the sp3 orbitals of the oxygen atoms to form sigma bonds (single bonds) between the oxygen atoms and the central carbon atom.

The result of these orbital hybridizations and formations of sigma and pi bonds produces double bonds between each of the two oxygen atoms and the central carbon atoms. The two sets of lone pair electrons on each oxygen atom are place in the remaining two sp2 hybrid orbitals of each oxygen atom.

Since the central atom of CO_2 is the carbon atom and since the carbon sigma bonds are sp bonds, the angle between the two oxygen atoms is 180 degrees and CO_2 is therefore a linear molecule. With overlaps of combinations of p orbitals. sp orbitals and sp2 orbitals to form bonding orbitals, the molecule CO_2 illustrates how versatile atoms can be in manipulating electron orbitals even within very small molecules in order to achieve an optimum lowering of electron energy.

Water - H_2O

The molecular structure of H_2O reflects the desire of oxygen to form two covalent bonds to satisfy its valence octet and of hydrogen atoms to form one covalent bond to complete the n=1 electron energy shell. This is accomplished in the water molecule by one oxygen atom forming single sigma bonds with two hydrogen atoms. To accomplish this the oxygen atom hybridizes it's one 2s orbital and its three 2p orbitals to form four sp3 hybrid orbitals.

Oxygen places one pair of electrons in each of two of the sp3 hybrid orbitals and overlaps the remaining two sp3 orbitals (each containing one electron) with the 1s orbital of each of the two hydrogen atoms creating sigma bonding orbitals between the central oxygen atom and the two hydrogen atoms.

The result is an H_2O molecule with the hydrogen atoms at the two of the apices of a tetrahedron and with a lone pair of electrons in an sp3 hybrid orbital at each of the other two apices of a tetrahedron. This results in a "bent" or angular geometry of an H_2O molecule where the bond angle between the two oxygen - hydrogen bonds is almost 109 degrees.

Oxygen is much more electronegative than hydrogen so both hydrogen-oxygen bonds are strongly polar with large partial negative charges located at regions near the hydrogen atoms. The two lone pair electron regions acquire a strong partially negative charge.

The result is that an H_2O molecule is a quadrupole, with two partially negative regions and two partially positive regions. Furthermore, the geometry of these polar sites corresponds to the sp3 hybrid bond angles of 109 degrees. This is important because the 109-degree three-dimensional arrangement of the polar regions is ideal to allow for the simultaneous formation by an H_2O molecule of as many as four hydrogen bonds with other H_2O molecules.

Hydrogen bonds are up to 10% as strong as a covalent single bond. Raising the temperature or changing the phase of liquid water to gas or solid water to liquid requires disruption of up to four hydrogen bonds per water molecule.

No other small molecule has this hydrogen bonding capacity and as a result liquid water has **extraordinarily high heat capacity, heats of fusion and heats of vaporization**. The hydrogen bonding that occurs in water also results in a **very high surface tension** for liquid water. The surface molecules of liquid water are strongly attracted to each other and this attraction resists forces that attempt to penetrate the water surface.

The bond angle of the positive and negative regions of the water molecule, combined with the small size of water molecules allows water molecules to penetrate and wedge into solid substances and to surround ions within solids. The partial polar regions of the water molecule can surround ions and polar molecules, disrupting the charge attractions that hold liquid and solid ionic or polar compounds together. This polar geometry of water molecules is what makes liquid water by far **the most efficient and versatile of all polar solvents**.

Chemical Reactions

Throughout or previous discussions we have described general features of chemical reactions and the fundamental physical processes that drive chemical reactions. We have addressed in considerable detail major features of several types of one major form of chemical reaction - the decomposition reaction. In particular we described the concept of chemical equilibrium - where chemical reactions will proceed from initial conditions to reach an equilibrium state.

This equilibrium state refers to the concentration of chemical participants that exist when a chemical reaction appears to have stopped - with no further changes in the concentrations of chemical participants occurring over time.

This chemical equilibrium state can be defined by an equilibrium constant - Keq for chemical reactions in general; Ksp for one type of decomposition reaction the dissolving of solids or liquids in a liquid solvent to form solutions and, Ka and Kb in acid and base decompositions respectively in a solvent; and Kw for the decomposition of pure liquid water in hydrogen and hydroxide ions. In the next section, we will review several of these basic principles of chemical reactions and discuss several types of reactions in greater detail.

General Form of a Chemical Reaction

The convention for writing chemical reactions is to place the reactants on the left followed by a rightward pointing arrow followed by the products of the reaction.

$$aA + bB \rightarrow cC + dD$$

The small letters, a, b, c, d are the relative amounts in number of particles for each participant A, B, C, D in the reaction (These are called the stoichiometric coefficients of the reaction). Of course, there may be more or less than two individual reactants and/or products of a specific chemical reaction.

The General Types of Chemical Reactions

Simple chemical reactions can be categorized as one of four types of reactions. These are the synthesis reaction, decomposition reaction, single-replacement reaction and double -replacement reaction. The general formula for each of these types of reactions are shown below

Synthesis
$$A + B \rightarrow AB$$

Decomposition
$$AB \rightarrow + A + B$$

Single Replacement
$$AB + C \rightarrow + A + BC$$

Double Replacement
$$AB + CD \rightarrow + AD + BC$$

The general formulas for these four types of reactions should be self-explanatory in terms of what occurs during the reactions. There are more complex reactions where combinations of these four basic reactions occur simultaneously. This categorization of reactions actually provides very little useful information, other classifications of reaction types are much more important to recognize, in particular whether the reaction is an acid-base reaction, a reduction- oxidation reaction a hydrolysis or dehydration reaction, a polymerization reaction or phosphorylation or dephosphorylation reaction.

Balancing Reactions

Balancing chemical reactions is a process that begins with the elements and elements of molecules that constitute the reactants and products of a chemical reaction but with no ratios of the elements that compose molecules nor stoichiometric ratios of elements and/or molecules that participate in the reaction.

To balance a chemical reaction the total numbers of each type of atom on the left must equal the total numbers of each type of atom on right. When the ratios of elements are unknown for the molecules that participate in chemical reactions, the information provided in the periodic table and in particular the octet or equivalent rule for individual elements can be used to predict what the ratios of elements should be.

Once this information is known, the stoichiometric coefficients can be reasoned out using common sense or simple algebra. To illustrate this balancing process, several examples are provided below.

Reaction 1: Synthesis of liquid water from molecular hydrogen gas and molecular oxygen gas

Perhaps the most basic chemical reaction is the reaction of hydrogen molecules (H_2) and oxygen molecules (O_2) to form a hydrogen-oxygen molecule

$$H_2(g) + O_2(g) \rightarrow HO\ (l)$$

The reaction shown above is a **unbalanced chemical reaction** where hydrogen and oxygen combine to form a molecule consisting of hydrogen and oxygen The (g) for H_2 and O_2 indicate that, in this reaction, both O_2 and H_2 react as gasses. The (l) for HO indicates the product "HO" is a liquid.

There are two atoms of hydrogen and two atoms of oxygen on the right and one atom each of hydrogen and oxygen contained on the molecule HO on the left. One could write a balanced reaction 1 as

$$H_2(g) + O_2(g) \rightarrow 2HO\ (l)$$

This is a balanced reaction - there are the same number of hydrogen and oxygen atoms on the left and right sides of the reaction, but **it is incompatible with what we know atoms are attempting to do in chemical reactions** - namely to satisfy the octet rule. Recall that oxygen requires two additional electrons to satisfy the octet rule. Hydrogen is unique in that it does not have an octet rule, but does have the equivalent.

When hydrogen has 2 electrons it achieves a substantial lowering of energy by filling the n=1 electron shell. Oxygen therefore wishes to share 2 electrons by creating two covalent bonds and hydrogen wishes to share one electron by creating one covalent bond. Therefore, we can predict that one oxygen atom will form 2 covalent bonds, one with each of 2 hydrogen atoms. The Lewis dot structure for this is as follows

$$H\!:\!\overset{\displaystyle ..}{\underset{\displaystyle ..}{O}}\!:$$
$$H$$

The two dots between the hydrogen and oxygen atoms represent covalent bonds between hydrogen and oxygen atoms. Each atom is sharing one of its valence electrons in each covalent bond.

This structure demonstrates that both hydrogen and the oxygen atoms have all attained a desired electron configuration; each hydrogen has 2 electrons that are shared in a covalent bond with oxygen and oxygen has eight octet valence electrons, an additional two which are acquired through sharing of electrons in single covalent bonds with the two hydrogen atoms. This indicates the correct chemical reaction for reaction 1 is

$$2H_2(g) + O_2(g) \rightarrow 2H_2O\ (l)$$

Synthesis of Carbon Dioxide from Carbon and Hydrogen

Another important example of predicting the composition of molecules based on the octet rule is the formation of a carbon-oxygen molecule from carbon and oxygen atoms

$$C+O \rightarrow CO$$

Using Lewis dot structures, we can create a molecule where carbon and oxygen have satisfied their octet rules.

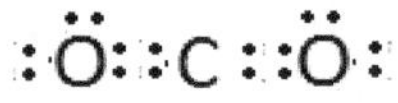

:Ö::C::Ö:

In the structure above the four dots between carbon and oxygen represent two covalent bonds. This is a double bond and can be represented as

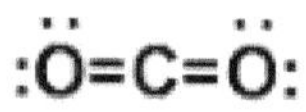

:Ö=C=Ö:

Each horizontal line between carbon and oxygen atoms represents a single covalent bond. All four of carbon's valence electrons are participating in covalent bonds with oxygen atoms and again each oxygen atom is donating two electrons apiece to the formation of two covalent bonds with carbon. The result is that both of the oxygen atoms and the carbon atom now have complete valence octets. This predicts that the carbon-oxygen molecule formula will be

$$CO_2$$

The balanced chemical reaction for the synthesis of carbon dioxide as a gas from solid elemental carbon and oxygen molecules as a gas is shown below

$$C(s)+O_2(g) \rightarrow CO_2(g)$$

Hydrocarbons

Lewis dot structures and the octet rule can be used to predict the molecular formula for almost all classes of molecules. An important example is the prediction of the molecular structures of hydrocarbons. The hydrocarbons are molecules that consist exclusively of carbon and hydrogen atoms. The simplest of these are the alkanes.

Alkanes

Alkane molecules contain only single bonds between carbon and hydrogen and between any two carbon atoms. The simplest alkane is the molecule methane

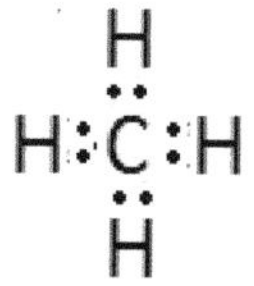

H
..
H:C:H
..
H

Notice that when carbon forms four single covalent bonds with four hydrogen atoms the resulting molecule - methane - results is 2 valence electrons apiece for all four hydrogens and a valence octet for carbon. This predicts the methane molecule has a formula of CH_4.

In hydrocarbons with more than 1 carbon atom, carbon atoms form carbon-carbon covalent bonds as illustrated by the 2 carbon alkane – ethane that is shown below.

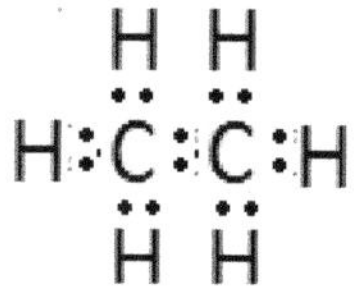

H H
.. ..
H:C:C:H
.. ..
H H

Ethane can be extended to larger hydrocarbons with larger numbers of carbon atoms forming additional carbon-carbon covalent bonds. Since each carbon-carbon bond leaves two fewer carbon-hydrogen bonds that can form, the general formula for an alkane is

$$C_nH_{2n+2}$$

Naming Hydrocarbons

Three carbon alkanes are propanes and four carbon alkanes are butanes. Larger alkanes are named by the prefix for the number of carbons contained in the alkane, for 5 carbon alkanes this is pentane, for 6 this is hexane, and so on. For alkenes "ene" is substituted for the corresponding specific carbon number "ane". For example, a five-carbon alkene is a pentene. For alkynes, "yne" is substituted for "ane" as in" butyne", which is the four-carbon alkyne.

Alkenes

$$H:C:C::C$$

with H atoms arranged around the carbon chain.

The Alkenes have at least one carbon-carbon double bond. The example above is the 3-carbon alkene - propene. The general formula for all alkenes with one carbon-carbon double bond is

$$C_nH_{2n}$$

Alkynes

$$H:C:C:::C:H$$

with H atoms arranged around the carbon chain.

The Alkynes have at least one carbon-carbon triple bond. The example above is the 3-carbon alkyne - propyne. The general formula for all alkenes with one carbon-carbon triple bond is

$$C_nH_{2n-2}$$

Notice that for all hydrocarbons carbon always forms four covalent bonds either with single bonds to hydrogen or with combinations of single, double or triple bonds with other carbon atoms.

Reduction-Oxidation (Redox) Reactions

A major alternative classification of reactions is the reduction-oxidation or "redox" class of chemical reactions. Any of the four categories of general chemical reactions - synthesis, dissociation (or decomposition), single replacement and double replacement can be redox reactions. The critical element in determining whether or not a reaction is a redox reaction is to determine whether during the reaction, any atom participating in the reaction has changed its oxidation number.

Oxidation States (Numbers)

Oxidation numbers or oxidation states for elements are closely related to the charge of the elemental atom. Elemental atoms in a pure state, such as a sample of a pure metal or as elemental molecules such as H_2 and O_2 or as non-metallic crystals - for instance pure carbon as the 2-dimensional crystalline form known a graphene or in a three-dimensional crystal (a diamond) have a neutral electrical charge and are defined as having an oxidation state of zero (0). When elemental atoms become ions, the oxidation state of the atoms is equal to the ionic charge. For instance, a magnesium ion; Mg^{2+} ion has an oxidation number of +2 and a chloride ion Cl^- has an oxidation number of -1.

Molecules also have an overall oxidation state the is the arithmetic sum of the oxidation states of atoms that constitute the molecule. Molecules always have an overall oxidation state of zero unless the molecule is an ion with a net positive or negative charge. The overall oxidation state of molecular ions is equal to the charge of the molecule. For instance, the bicarbonate ion, HCO_3^- has an oxidation state of -1 and hydronium ion H_3O^+ has an oxidation state of +1.

Changes in Oxidation States

When atoms are covalently bonded in molecules they usually do not have oxidation numbers of zero. Instead, their oxidation numbers are determined by which atoms they are covalently bonded with. The more electronegative atom in a covalent bond - for purposes of determining its oxidation number - is treated as if it had actually ionized the less electronegative atom in the covalent bond. Rather than sharing two electrons in the bond, it is as if the more electronegative atom had extracted the electron contributed to the covalent bond by the less electronegative atom and an ionic bond rather than a covalent bond existed between the two atoms. The more electronegative atom then is considered to be a -1 ion and the less electronegative atom is considered to be a +1 ion. In this example, the more electronegative atom is assigned an oxidation number of -1 and the less electronegative atom is assigned an oxidation number of +1.

To clarify this explanation, consider the reaction where hydrogen molecules and oxygen molecules react to form H_2O molecules

$$2H_2 + O_2 \rightarrow 2H_2O$$

On the left side of the reaction hydrogen and oxygen are both in their elemental states as hydrogen molecules and oxygen molecules. The hydrogen and oxygen atoms of the respective molecules by definition have oxidation states (numbers) equal to zero. On the right side of the reaction, the molecule H_2O consists of a single central oxygen atom which is very electronegative relative to the two covalently bonded hydrogen atoms.

This reaction is a redox reaction because atoms in the reaction have changed their oxidation states. In the H_2O molecule, oxygen is treated as though it had acquired one electron from each hydrogen atom and therefore the oxygen atom has changed its oxidation state from zero to -2. **Since this represents a decrease or more negative change in the oxidation state of the oxygen atom has undergone a reduction** (its oxidation number has become smaller or more negative).

The hydrogen atoms are treated as if they have each lost their single electron to the oxygen atom and their oxidation states have changed from zero to +1. **Since this represents an increase in the oxidation states of the hydrogen atoms, the hydrogen atoms have been oxidized (the opposite of being reduced).**

This example demonstrates several additional rules for redox reactions. The first is that **the total oxidation state for the left side of a redox reaction must equal the total oxidation state for the right side of the reaction.** In our example, the left side of the reaction consists of six atoms - four hydrogens and two oxygens - all with oxidation states of zero.

The total oxidation state of the left side of the reaction is therefore equal to zero. On the right side of the reaction there are two oxygen atoms with oxidation states of -2 and four hydrogen atoms each with oxidation states of +1. Arithmetically the oxidation state are equivalent to $2(-2)=-4$ for the oxygen atoms and $4(+1)=+4$ for the hydrogen atoms.

The oxidation states overall cancelled out since $(-4) + (+4) = 0$. This demonstrates that the overall oxidation state of the left and right side of the reaction are equal, which is consistent with the rule that the overall oxidation state of the left and right halves of a reaction

do not change. A Close corollary with this rule is that **whenever an oxidation or reduction occurs in a reaction there must be a corresponding reduction or oxidation of equal magnitude that occurs simultaneously during the reaction.**

"Rules" for Assigning Oxidation Numbers

The rules for assigning oxidation numbers to atoms within a molecule are essentially rules of thumb based on the valence electrons that neutral atoms contain, the octet rule and the relative electronegativities of elemental atom. **The most useful rules for assigning oxidation numbers to atoms bonded in a molecule are:**

- the group 1 (alkali metals) and the group ii (alkali earths) elements have oxidation numbers of +1 and +2 respectively.
- The group VII (halogen) elements have oxidation numbers of -1
- Oxygen (usually) has an oxidation number of -2. When bonded to a halogen - then oxygens oxidation number is increased by +1 for every bonded halogen. When oxygen is bonded to another oxygen atom, both oxygen atom's oxidation state is increased by +1.
- Hydrogen has an oxidation number of +1 when bonded with nonmetal atoms and -1 when bonded with metal atoms.
- Transition metals can exist in multiple oxidation states. The actual oxidation state for a transition metal compound or molecule depends on the atoms that are bonded to the transition metal atom within the molecule

Advisory Regarding Redox Reactions

In chemistry, an analysis of complex chemical reactions as redox reactions is a useful means of balancing complex reactions and sequences of reactions. The reduction and oxidation steps can be separated into **half-cell reactions** that have voltage potential values that have been determined experimentally and can be used to predict how much energy reactions will produce or require and also allow for the calculation of equilibrium values for reactions.

Example of half-cell reactions

H2 + F2 → 2HF

The oxidation reduction reaction shown above can be separated into two half-cell reactions

Reaction 1: $H_2 \rightarrow 2H+ + 2e-$
Reaction 2: $F_2 + 2e- \rightarrow 2F-$

The two half-cell reactions can be "added" together. The two electrons on the left in reaction 1 cancel out the two electrons on the right in reaction 2. The hydrogen ion H+ on the right in reaction 1 and the fluorine ion F- on the right in reaction combine to give the molecule HF and the overall reaction $H_2 + F_2 \rightarrow 2HF$ is the result.

A comprehensive understanding of redox chemistry requires a large amount of additional discussion and this includes the participation of hydrogen ion or hydroxide ions that are present in the reaction solutions. These reactions often involve **transition metal compounds that undergo multiple oxidations and reductions.** An example is the unbalanced redox reaction shown below

$$HNO_3 + CuS \rightarrow NO + CuSO_4 + H_2O$$

There are several additional rules for balancing this reaction. When these rules are applied to this reaction - with the understanding that the solution is acidic - the overall balanced reaction including all ions that participate is

$$8NO_3^- + 3CuS^{2+} + 3S^{2-} + 8H^+ \rightarrow 8NO + 3Cu^{2+} + 3SO_4^{2-} + 4H_2O$$

The rules for balancing this equation provide the means to determine the correct stoichiometric coefficients for the reaction. When the ions in the equation are combined the overall balanced reaction is

$$8NO_3 + 3CuS \rightarrow 8NO + 3CuSO_4 + 4H_2O$$

Notice that the stoichiometric ratios for this balanced reaction is not obvious from the initial unbalanced reaction. We provide this example to illustrate the complexity of redox reaction chemistry - **It is almost certain that the HESI will not expect an understanding of redox chemistry at this level.** It is therefore counterproductive to attempt to master the intricacies of redox chemistry. Rather it is sufficient to be able to determine what the oxidation states of atoms are in a molecule and to identifying which atoms have changed their oxidation states from the left to right sides of a chemical reaction. This allows one to identify which atoms or molecules have been oxidized and which have been reduced.

Transition Metal Redox Reactions in Biology

While the precise details of complex redox reactions involving multiple oxidation states of participating transition metal atoms is beyond the scope of the HESI it is useful to note two critical chemical processes that involve these types of redox reactions. One is the binding of O_2 to the hemoglobin molecule in red blood cells and the other is the electron transport chain that generates large amounts of ATP molecules in the mitochondria of human cells.

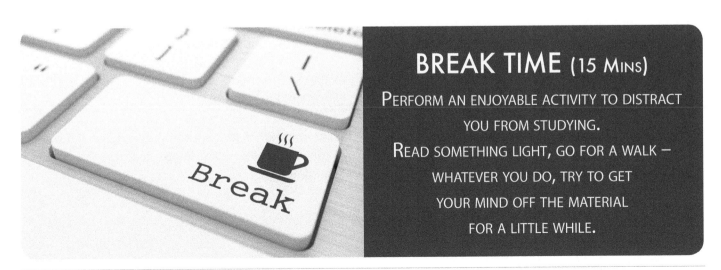

VOCABULARY

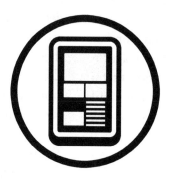

WORDS IN CONTEXT

When reading through a chapter in a book or a passage on a test, you will sometimes encounter a word you've never seen before. You may not know what it means, but don't worry! You can still figure out a basic definition of the word, even if you don't have a dictionary in hand (or if you don't want to get off the sofa and get one).

In every sentence, any given word is surrounded by clauses, phrases and other words. When you find a word you don't recognize, you can learn more about it by studying the context surrounding it. These surrounding words, phrases and clauses are called context clues. Using these, you can determine the definition for almost every unfamiliar word you encounter. This is a skill that will become especially helpful when you start reading higher-level texts with fancy words or training manuals with lots of jargon.

TYPES OF CONTEXT CLUES

As you read, you can use several different types of context clues to help you discover the meaning of unknown words. Some important and common types of context clues are outlined below. Try to use the specific context clue to determine the meaning of the bolded word.

ROOT WORD & AFFIX
This is a context clue that uses your existing knowledge of common root words.

EXAMPLE: SCIENTISTS WHO DIG UP DINOSAUR BONES ARE EXPERTS IN **PALEONTOLOGY.**

This context clue assumes you have knowledge of dinosaurs and can relate that to the study of "paleontology."

Compare/Contrast

This is a context clue that signals a similarity or difference by using words or phrases that denote a comparison or contrast. Words that imply similarity (or comparison) include *like*, *also*, *just as*, *too*, etc. Words that imply difference (or contrast) include *whereas*, *opposed to*, *unlike*, *versus*, etc.

EXAMPLE: A COMET, LIKE AN **ASTEROID**, IS MADE FROM LEFTOVER MATTER IN THE UNIVERSE.

This context clue compares an "asteroid" with a comet to imply a similarity to the given definition of a comet.

Logic

This is a context clue wherein you must infer the definition of the unknown word by using the relationships within the sentence.

EXAMPLE: BUILDERS ROUTINELY USE **FASTENERS** THAT WILL HELP HOLD THEIR STRUCTURES AND BUILDINGS IN PLACE.
This context clue describes the job that "fasteners" do.

Definition

This is a context clue that includes a basic definition of the unknown word.

EXAMPLE: NEW BIOLOGICAL SPECIES CAN BE FORMED THROUGH A PROCESS CALLED **SPECIATION**.
This context clue defines "speciation" outright.

Example or Illustration

This is a context clue that uses an example or illustration of the unknown word.

EXAMPLE: ANIMALS CLASSIFIED IN THE PHYLUM PORIFERA LIVE IN A **MARINE** HABITAT LIKE THE ATLANTIC AND PACIFIC OCEANS.

This context clue uses Atlantic and Pacific Oceans as examples of "marine" habitats.

HOMOGRAPHS

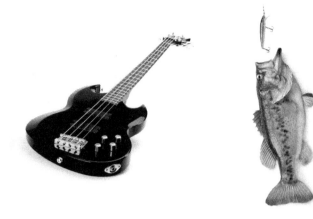

Now that you've had a refresher on context clues, let's talk about homographs. A homograph is a word that is spelled exactly like another word, but has a different meaning. For example, "bass" can mean "a low, deep sound" or "a type of fish." Here's a more complex homograph: "minute" can mean "a unit of time" or "something very small."

Although questions with homographs aren't necessarily difficult, you'll need to pay extra attention to the context clues. If you're rushing or don't read the entire sentence, you can accidentally mark an incorrect answer by mistaking the homograph for the wrong meaning. As long as you take your time and use the context clues, you'll most likely have no problem.

Here's something to consider when you take the exam. Within the question, replace the vocabulary term with your selected answer choice. Read the sentence and check whether or not it makes sense. This won't guarantee a correct answer, but it will help identify an incorrect one.

Another point to keep in mind is that sometimes there will not be an answer choice that exactly fits into the sentence. Don't panic! You probably did not misread the context clues or come up with an incorrect meaning. Many times, questions will ask you to select the *best* word from the given answer choices, even though that correct answer choice may not be the best *possible* answer overall. These types of questions want you to choose the *most* correct answer choice. These can be tricky to tackle, but expect to see questions like this on the exam. Just remember the

CRITICAL READING

DETAIL QUESTIONS

Reading passages and identifying important details is an important part of the critical reading process. Detail questions ask the reader to recall specific information about the main idea. These details are often found in the examples given in the passage and can contain anecdotes, data or descriptions, among other details. For example, if you are reading a passage about certain types of dogs, you may be asked to remember details about breeds, sizes and coat color and patterns. As you read through the passage, make sure you take note of numbers, figures and the details given about the topic. Chances are you will need to remember some of these.

There is a wealth of information, facts, pieces of data and several details that can be presented within any passage you read. The key to uncovering the main idea and understanding the details presented is to take your time and read through everything contained in the passage. Consider each example and figure presented. Think about how they relate to the main idea, how they support the focus, and how those details add to the information and value of the passage.

Strategies for Answering Detail Questions:

- Identify key words in the question that help you find details and examples to answer the question.

- Take note of how words are used and if phrases are repeated. Look for the overall meaning of each paragraph and passage.

- Some questions will pull words or phrases from the passage and quote them in the question. In this case, find those quotes and make sure they are being used the same way in the passage and the question. Many questions will change the meaning of these to make the question wrong or confuse the reader.

- Some questions will ask you to determine if a particular statement or topic is true. In this case, look over the paragraphs and find the overall theme or idea of the passage. Compare your theme or idea to the statement in the question.

UNDERSTANDING QUESTION STEMS

In addition to careful reading of the passages (including marking up the text for topic and concluding sentences, transitional words and key terms), you must also be able to identify what is being asked of you in each of the questions. Recognition of the task in each question can be easily accomplished if you are familiar with the question stems, or the most commonly phrased wording that will be associated with each type of question on the test. Keep reading for an explanation of each question type, along with sample stems, and suggested approaches for tackling them.

Supporting Details

Supporting details are those that back up the main ideas presented in the passage. These can include examples, clarifying explanations, or elaborations of basic ideas presented earlier in the reading. Supporting details are directly stated in the passage, so you must rely on your careful reading to guide you to the correct answer. Answers may not be stated in the original language of the passage, but the basic ideas will be the same.

Here are some common ways this type of question is asked:
· The passage states...
· The author says...
· According to what you read...

Main Idea

Questions asking you to identify the main idea expect that you will be able to determine the overall point of the passage (often called the thesis), NOT secondary details or supporting points. Attempting to put the main idea into your own words after reading WITHOUT looking at the text again is a very helpful strategy in answering this type of question. If you can sum up the author's main point in your own words, then you will find it very easy to find the right "match" amongst the answers provided for you. Alternately, the main idea may often be found in the opening or concluding paragraphs, two common places where an author may introduce a topic and his perspective about said topic, or he summarize the main points.

Here are some common ways this type of question is asked:
· The main idea for this paragraph...
· The central point of the passage...
· A possible title for the passage...
· The author's primary point...

Inference

Inferences are those ideas which can be gleaned from the suggestions that may be implied in other statements made by the author. They are never explicitly stated, but we understand that they are true from "reading between the lines". The answers to inferences questions, therefore, are assumptions, and cannot be found from direct statements in the text. You will have to rely on your ability to logically deduce conclusions from your careful reading. More than one answer may sound correct, but only one is. Make sure that, whichever answer you choose, you can find statements in the text which would support that idea. If you cannot do that, then that choice is likely not the right answer.

Here are some common ways this type of question is asked:
· The passage implies...
· The author suggests... ·
The reader could logically conclude that...
· The reader would be correct in assuming that...

Tone/Attitude

Some questions will ask you about the author's tone or attitude. A good place to start with this type of question is to consider whether the passage is positive, negative or neutral. Does the author seem angry? Maybe sad? Or torn between two points of view? The language that an author uses can be very telling about his tone and attitude. Is the author critical? Praiseworthy? Disappointed? Even if you find some finer details of passage difficult to understand, the tone and attitude are often fairly easy to identify. Look for adjectives and statements that reveal the author's opinion, rather than facts, and this will help you know his tone or attitude.

Here are some common ways this type of question is asked:
· The tone of the passage is...
· The attitude of the author is...
· The writer's overall feeling...

Style

Style refers to a writer's "way with words". Most seasoned writers have a well-developed and easily recognizable style, but often the topic of a written work can dictate style. If the topic is serious the language will likely be more formal. Works for academic settings may be heavy with the jargon of that discipline. Personal reflections can be rife with imagery, while instructional manuals will use simple and straightforward language. Identifying style is not difficult; simply pay attention to the words used (simple or fancy?), the sentence structure (simple or compound-complex?), as well as the overall structure of the piece (stream of consciousness or 5-paragraph essay?). You must answer these questions in order to determine the style of the passage.

Here are some common ways this type of question is asked:
· The overall writing style used in the passage...
· The author's style is...
· The organizational style of the passage is...

Pattern of Organization

Pattern of organization questions want you to consider how the writing of a piece was developed. What features did the writer utilize to make his point? Did he include personal anecdotes? Data or statistics? Quotes from authorities on the topic? These are all modes of organizing a passage that help the writer support his claims and provide a logical focus for the work.

Here are some common ways this type of question is asked:
· The author proves a point through...
· In the passage, the author uses...
· Throughout the passage, the author seems to rely on...

Purpose and Attitude

Questions asking about purpose and attitude require you to consider why the author took the time to write. The authors motivations are directly behind the purpose of the piece. What question did he wish to answer? What cause did he want to show support for? What action did he wish to persuade you to take? Identifying these reasons for writing will reveal the purpose and attitude of the passage.

Here are some common ways this type of question is asked:
· The purpose of the passage is...
· The author's intent for writing the passage is...
· The attitude the author displays is...

Fact/Opinion

There will be some questions on the test that will ask you whether a statement is a fact or an opinion. Without being able to fact-check, how will you do this? A rule of thumb would be that opinions reflect only the thoughts, feelings or ideas of the writer, whereas facts are verifiable as true or false, regardless of one's feelings. If a writer cites a statistic about the environmental effects of oil drilling on migratory mammals in the Pacific Northwest, then that is verifiable and can be considered factual. If, however, the writer claims that oil drilling in the Pacific Northwest United States is bad and should be stopped, then that is his opinion. He may at some point provide examples of why this is so, but that viewpoint is based on his thoughts and feelings about oil drilling, and can only be considered opinion.

Here are some common ways this type of question is asked:
· Which statement is a fact rather than an opinion?
· This statement is meant to be...
· An example of fact is when the author says...
· An example of opinion is when the author states that...

ELIMINATING WRONG ANSWERS

An author often writes with an intended purpose in mind, and they will support their main idea with examples, facts, data and stories that help the overall meaning of their written text to be clear. You may be asked a question regarding one of these details or examples, or you may be asked something about the overall theme or main idea of the passage. These types of questions require you to read the passage carefully for meaning and to look at all the supporting details used. However it's also important to learn how to identify incorrect answer choices and eliminate them right away. This will help you narrow down the answer choices that are likely to be correct.

ARITHMETIC REASONING

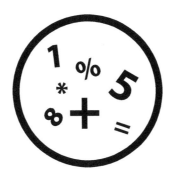

Addition, Subtraction, Multiplication, Division Operations with Decimals

The sign conventions for positive and negative decimal arithmetic operations are the same as those for whole number operations outlined in Module 1. But, there are special details to recall when performing arithmetic operations with decimal values to ensure correct answers.

When adding and subtracting decimal values, it is important to make sure that the decimal points are aligned vertically. This is the simplest method to ensure a reliable result. For example adding 0.522 and 0.035 should be performed as follows:

$$
\begin{array}{r}
0.522 \\
+0.035 \\
\hline
0.557
\end{array}
$$

Subtraction operations should be aligned similarly.

$$
\begin{array}{r}
0.522 \\
-0.035 \\
\hline
0.487
\end{array}
$$

It is important to note that multiplication requires a different convention to be followed. When multiplying decimals, the operations are NOT aligned necessarily the same way as addition and subtraction. For example, multiplying 0.7 and 2.15 is performed as follows:

$$\begin{array}{r} 2.15 \\ \times\, 0.7 \\ \hline 1.505 \end{array}$$

When multiplying decimal values, the decimal point placement in the answer is determined by counting the total number of digits to the right of the decimal point in the multiplied numbers. This detail is often overlooked in testing choices where the same numbers may appear in several multiple-choice answers, but with different decimal point placements.

Division of decimal values is simplified by first visualizing fractions that are equivalent. The mathematics terminology is that a dividend / divisor = quotient. For example:

7.35 / 1.05 is the same as 73.5 / 10.5, which is the same operation as 735 / 105.

The last fraction, in the example above, means that to solve 7.35 / 1.05 we can divide 735 / 105 and find the correct whole number answer. This method just requires that when dividing by a decimal number, the divisor must be corrected to be a whole number. This requirement is achieved by moving the decimal points in both the dividend and divisor the same number of decimal places. If the dividend still contains a decimal point, the place is maintained in the long division operation, and the correct quotient is still achieved. The quotient remains in the form of a decimal number.

ADDITION, SUBTRACTION, MULTIPLICATION, DIVISION OPERATIONS WITH FRACTIONS

The sign conventions for positive and negative fractional arithmetic operations are the same as those for whole number operations outlined in Module 1. However, there are special details to recall when performing arithmetic operations with fractional values to ensure correct answers.

Remember that fractions are made up of a numerator and a denominator. The top number of the fraction, called the numerator, tells how many of the fractional parts are being represented. The bottom number, called the denominator, tells how many equal parts the whole is divided into. For this reason, fractions with different denominators cannot be added together because different denominators are as different as "apples and oranges." So, when adding or subtracting fractions with different denominators, a common denominator must be found. In this case, simple geometric models will be used to explain the common denominator principle. Usually, this principle is illustrated with circles divided into "pie slices." A simpler and more effective example involves the use of squares or rectangles divided into fractional parts.

Representing fraction parts, $1/_3$ and $1/_4$ will be demonstrated with the following square diagrams. In this case a whole square is the number "1" and the fractional parts will be the slices of the square as follows:

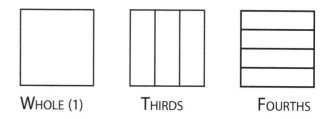

WHOLE (1) THIRDS FOURTHS

If we superimpose the four horizontal slices over the three vertical slices, there are twelve separate parts of the whole as follows:

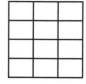

In the last diagram, any column representing a third, has four of the twelve small rectangles from the diagram, or $4/_{12}$ as the equivalent fraction. Similarly, any row of the last diagram, representing a fourth, has three of the twelve small rectangles from the diagram, or $3/_{12}$ as the equivalent fraction. With this modification of the two fractions, both are now in the form of a common denominator, and the addition of the two fractions can be completed:

$$1/_3 + 1/_4 = 3/_{12} + 4/_{12} = 7/_{12}$$

Notice that this result is exactly analogous to the simple diagram above. Common denominator fractions need not be simplified with this type of diagram, but

HESI A^2 - Spire Study System

it is a valuable example to explain the principle. The common denominator is required whenever adding or subtracting fractions with different denominators. If the denominators are the same, then the addition or subtraction of numerators is all that is required. If more assistance is needed on how to find common denominators, the Arithmetic Reasoning chapter in Module 1 will provide information on finding the Least Common Multiple, or the lowest common denominator, required for addition and subtraction. Remember that the individual fractions will retain the same value only if the numerator and denominator are multiplied by the same value.

Multiplication of fractions is a simple operation because fractions multiply as follows:

$$\frac{7}{8} * \frac{3}{4} = \frac{(7*3)}{(8*4)} = \frac{21}{32}$$

This fraction is in its simplest form because there are no common factors. If common factors exist in the numerator and denominator of a fraction, then that fraction must be simplified.

Division of fractions should never be attempted in the form of a ratio. The method is confusing, elaborate and unreliable in a testing situation. Instead, every fraction division problem is a simple operation because the division operation can be rewritten as a multiplication operation. To begin, as stated previously:

dividend / divisor = quotient
This can be rewritten as:
dividend * ($\frac{1}{divisor}$) = quotient

This yields exactly the same outcome as division. The quantity ($\frac{1}{divisor}$) is called a reciprocal, and for a fraction, it's as simple as flipping the fraction upside down. Therefore:

$$(\tfrac{5}{8}) / (\tfrac{1}{4}) = \tfrac{5}{8} * \tfrac{4}{1} = \tfrac{20}{32} = \tfrac{5}{8} \text{ (in simplified form)}$$

FRACTION TO DECIMAL CONVERSIONS

Every fraction represents a division problem. The decimal value of any fraction is represented by the numerator, (top value), divided by the denominator (bottom value). Certain combinations, such as $\frac{1}{3}$, will result in repeating decimals that will always be rounded in a multiple-choice testing situation.

The fraction $\frac{1}{2}$ has a decimal value of 0.5, which is the value of 1 divided by 2. The values of improper fractions such as $\frac{3}{2}$, $\frac{5}{2}$, or $\frac{7}{2}$ (larger numerator than denominator) are determined by dividing as previously stated or more easily by multiplying the numerator by 0.5. So the improper fraction of $\frac{7}{2}$ is 7 * 0.5, or 3.5. Often, the determination of the unit fraction (1 divided by the denominator) followed by the decimal multiplication is simpler in a testing situation.

The fraction $\frac{3}{5}$ has a decimal value of 0.6, which is the value of 3 divided by 5. Alternately, the value of the unit fraction of $\frac{1}{5}$ is 0.2, and that unit fraction multiplied by 3 is 0.6. If you know the unit fractions for common fraction values, the answer selection process may be simplified.

When a fraction such as $\frac{5}{7}$ is evaluated, the quotient of 5 divided by 7 results in a lengthy decimal value of 0.71428.... That extended value will never appear as a multiple-choice test answer selection. Typically, that value will be rounded to either 0.71 or 0.714. Remember that testing instructions say to choose the best answer. Your best choice may be a rounded number.

DECIMAL TO FRACTION CONVERSIONS
All decimals are also fractions and can be written in that form. The fractions that result all have powers of 10 in the denominator and usually need to be simplified in order to be compared to multiple-choice answers in a testing situation.

For example, simple decimal values, such as 0.25, can be written as the fraction $\frac{25}{100}$. This fraction must be simplified to be correct. $\frac{25}{100}$ can be rewritten as a product:

$$\frac{(25 * 1)}{(25 * 4)}$$
or
$$\frac{25}{25} * \frac{1}{4}$$

The fraction can be expressed correctly as $\frac{1}{4}$ since the fraction $\frac{25}{25}$ is simplified to 1. Recognizing the common factors in the numerator and denominator is the essential element in making these conversions.

For testing purposes, decimal conversions will often be based on common fraction values. For example, $1/16$, if divided with long division, is 0.0625. Any integer multiple of this value results in a fraction with 16 in the denominator.

The value 0.0625 is first rewritten as the fraction:

625/10000

Simplifying with factors of 5 in the numerator and denominator gives the fraction:

125/2000

Simplifying with factors of 25 in the numerator and denominator gives the fraction:

5/80

Simplifying with factors of 5 in the numerator and denominator one more time gives the simplified fraction:

1/16

While either of these methods may require an extra amount of time to complete, usually the answer choices may be logically reduced to two of the four examples. Testing the answer choices is simply a matter of multiplying the decimal value by the denominator to determine if the numerator is correct.

Another solution method, logical deduction, can be used as a simple, reliable and time saving approach to finding the fractional value of 0.435. In this example, the following is a list of possible multiple-choice answers:

A   3/16

B   5/16

C   7/16

D   9/16

Logically, any fraction greater than $1/2$ is immediately eliminated since:

0.435 < 0.5

So, first eliminate answer D. Incorrect answer choices will be eliminated with this type of logical deduction. Second, notice that in the answer choice:

3/16 < 1/4

and in decimal form

3/16 < 0.25

So, choice A can logically be eliminated since our answer comparison is with 0.435.

Third, notice that in the answer choices:

5/16 > 1/4

and in decimal form

5/16 > 0.25

Since $5/16$ is just slightly more than $1/4$, choice B can be eliminated since our comparison is with 0.435.

Finally, C is chosen as the most likely answer choice. It is the logical choice since:

7/16 < 1/2

and

0.435 < 0.5

PERCENTAGES

Percentages is a concept you are most likely familiar with from real-world applications, so these are some of the less scary math problems that appear on tests. However, test writers take that confidence into account and can use it against you, so it's important to be careful on problems with percentages. Let's look at an example:

A sweater went on sale and now costs $25.20. If the original price was $42.00, what is the percent discount?

16.8%

20.0%

25.0%

40.0%

60.0%

Take a minute to work out the problem for yourself. If you get the wrong answer, it will be helpful to you to see where you went wrong – several of the answer choices are distinct traps that often appear on test questions like this.

SOLUTION:

With percentages, you can always set up a fraction.

First, you want to know what percent the sale price is of the original price. The reference point, or original price, will go on the bottom of the fraction. The numerator will be the sale price. The ratio of 25.2 / 42 is equal to 6 / 10.

The sale price, $25.20, is 0.6, or 60%, of the original price. A percentage is just the decimal times 100%. This is answer choice E. However, the question did NOT ask what percent the new price is of the original price. Read carefully: it asks for the percent *discount*. This language is commonly used for questions with prices. Here's what it means, in math terms:

Percentage discount = 100% - Percentage of the Sale Price

The percent discount is the amount less than 100% that the sale price is of the original price. We can use this equation to solve, which yields:

$$(42 - 25.2) / 42 = 0.40$$

Remember, a percent is a decimal times 100%. So, we can convert the decimal on the right side to a percentage by multiplying by 100%:

$$100\% * 0.40 = 40\%$$

The sale price is 40% *less than* the original price, which is answer choice D. Another mathematical reasoning approach would be to take the original fraction subtracted from 1:

$$1 - 25.2 / 42 = 0.4$$

From here, just recognize that if the sale price *is* 60% of the original price, then it is 40% *less than* the original price.

You can solve for the discounted amount and then find that as a percent of the original amount to solve for the percentage of the discount:

$$42 - 25.2 = 16.80$$
$$16.80 / 42 = 0.4$$

Those are three different ways to approach one problem, using the same concept of percentage and recognizing that a percent *discount* requires subtraction from the original. Here's another percentage problem, this time with a different trick:

168 is 120% of what number?

SOLUTION:
First, convert 120% to a decimal. Remember, converting a percentage to a decimal is done by dividing by 100%:

$$120 / 100 = 1.2$$

We are told that 168 is this percent *of* some other number. This means that 168 goes in the numerator of our percent fraction equation. Here is the resulting equation:

$$168 / x = 1.2$$

Here, x signifies the unknown number in the problem. Writing the percent equation is indispensable to solving this type of problem. Multiply both sides by x and then divide both sides by 1.2 to isolate the variable:

$$168(x) / x = 1.2(x)$$
$$168 = 1.2x$$
$$168 / 1.2 = 1.2x / 1.2$$
$$140 = x$$

Therefore, 168 is 120% of 140. We can verify this answer by plugging the numbers back into the original equation:

$$168 / 140 = 1.2$$

This problem is tricky because the percentage is greater than 100%, or greater than 1.0, so it violates our intuition that the bigger number should go on the bottom of the fraction. Usually, percentages are less than 100. However, when percentages are larger than 100, the numerator is bigger than the denominator. The inverse of this question could be the following:

168 is what percent of 140?

Many people, after reading this question, would automatically set up the following fraction equation:

$$140/168 = 0.83$$

83% would likely be an answer choice, but it's the wrong answer. The question is asking for 168 / 140. Read these questions carefully, and don't automatically place the larger number in the denominator.

Let's look at one more example, which combines these concepts, and then do a couple practice problems:
An ingredient in a recipe is decreased by 20%. By what percentage does the new amount need to be increased to obtain the original amount of the ingredient?

SOLUTION:

Here is a pro's tip for working with percentages:

When a problem is given only in percentages with no given numbers, you can substitute in any value to work with as your original amount. Since you are solving for a percent, you'll get the same answer no matter what numbers are used because percentages are ratios. The easiest number to work with in problems like this is 100, so use that as the original recipe amount. 100 what? Cups of flour? Chicken tenders? Chocolate chips? Doesn't matter. Here's how your equation should look:

$$x / 100 = 0.20$$

Solve for x, which gives the amount the ingredient has been decreased by:

$$x = 100 * 0.20$$

Remember that 20% is a decimal, so $0.20 * 100 = 20$. The ingredient has been decreased by 20 units. What is the new amount?

$$100 - 20 = 80$$

What was the question asking for? *By what percent does the new amount need to be increased to obtain the original amount of the ingredient?* Let's parse this mathematical language. We've found the new amount of the ingredient, 80. The original amount, we decided, was 100.

The next step in answering the question is to find the *amount* that we would need to add to get back to the original amount. This part is pretty easy:

$$80 + x = 100$$
$$x = 20$$

It's the same amount that we subtracted from the original amount, 20. But the question asks what percentage of 80 is required to add 20?

Set up the percentage equation. 80 times what percent (x / 100) will give that extra 20 units?

$$80 * x / 100 = 20$$

Solve as normal by dividing both sides by 80 and then multiplying both sides by 100:

$$x / 100 = 0.25$$
$$x = 25$$

The new amount must be increased by 25% to equal the original amount.

MATHEMATICS KNOWLEDGE

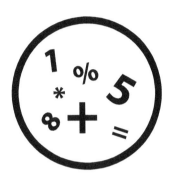

RATES AND SYSTEMS OF EQUATIONS

These are some of the most common questions on standardized math exams and also some of the most criticized. How many pop culture references are there to the nightmare of the "if train A is traveling west of Detroit at 70 miles an hour and train B is traveling north of Denver at 90 miles an hour, what is the weight of the moon" variety? Excluding the nonsensical nature of the joke (would we weigh the moon in terms of its own gravity, or Earth's? Do bodies in orbit actually weigh *anything*?? Wait, wrong subject), this is simply a rate problem! Train A has a speed and a direction, Train B has a speed and a direction, and given those facts, you can answer all kinds of questions easily.

A *rate* is anything that relates two types of measurement: distance and time, dollars and workers,

mass and volume, x per y. Exchange rates tell us how much of one currency you can get for a certain amount of another currency. Speedometers tell us how many miles we travel per unit of time. Growth rates tell us how much additional population we get over time. Rates are everywhere in the world, and they are everywhere on standardized math tests. To express a rate mathematically, think of the following:

All rates express one measurement *in terms of* another.

For example, *miles per hour* gives us a measurement of distance (miles) for one unit of time (an hour). "Per" is a term that means divide. It looks like this:

If a car is traveling 70 mph, it goes 70 miles for every one hour of time that passes.

All rates work this way. If you can get €0.81 (Euros) for one American dollar, the exchange rate is:

€0.81 (Euros) / 1 Dollar = 0.81 Euros per Dollar

A rate is written as a fraction. A rate *equation* gives you a value of one of the measurements if you know the rate and the value of the other measurement.

If a car travels 70 mph: Distance = 70 miles/hour * hours
This recipe for the equation always works for a rate problem:

Examine the mph example: when you multiply 70 miles/hour times a number of hours, the hours units cancel out, leaving you with a number of miles. This works for any type of rate. The thing being measured on the *top* (numerator) of the rate measurement is equal to the rate times the unit being measured on the *bottom* of the rate measurement.

To SOLVE A RATE PROBLEM, FOLLOW THESE STEPS:

1. Read the question carefully to determine what you will be solving for. Is it an amount of time? A distance? Something else? Make sure you understand this before anything else. It can be helpful to name the variables at this point.

2. Write equations to express all of the information given in the problem. This is just like we've demonstrated for percentage problems, averaging problems, etc. The ability to express information in an equation is one of the main mathematical reasoning abilities that you can demonstrate to succeed on tests like these. Remember the equation:
Distance = Rate * Time

3. Solve!
First, a simple example:

A train is traveling west at 75 mph. How long will it take to travel 60 miles?

Step 1: Identify what the question is asking for: in this instance, it's *how long*, or the time it takes to travel 60 miles.

Step 2: Write an equation: 60 = 75 * time

Step 3: Solve! We know that the rate is 75 miles per hour and that the miles traveled is 60. To solve for time, just plug those values into the equation:

Isolate the "x hours" by dividing both sides by 75 mph:

60 miles / 75 miles per hour = 0.8 hours
0.8 hours * 60 minutes per hour = 48 minutes

Rate problems can also require a system of equations. This just means that you need to write two equations to relate two unknown variables, instead of one equation to solve for one unknown variable, like the problem above. The algebra is not any more difficult for these types of problems. They just require the extra step of writing another equation.

For example: Jessica assembles one model airplane per hour. James assembles one model airplane per 45 minutes. If they work for the same amount of time and assemble twelve planes all together, how many planes did James assemble?

Step 1: Identify what the question is asking for: the number of planes that James assembled.

Step 2: Write equations:

x = 1 Airplanes per hour * T hours
y = 1/0.75 Airplanes per hour * T hours
x + y = 12

You convert "45 minutes" to 0.75 hours, since 45/60 = 0.75. If you'd rather not do that, you could leave the rate in minutes, but then change Jessica's rate to 60 minutes instead of one hour. The important thing is to use the same units for time across the whole equation.

Step 3: Solve! Notice that the "T hours" term is the same in both of the rate equations. The problem stated that the two of them worked for the same amount of time. To solve for the number of planes

James assembled, first we need to find T hours. The *number of planes Jessica assembles* and the *number of planes James assembles* can be added together since we know that the sum is 12. This is the new equation from adding those together:

$$12 = 1 \text{ Airplanes per hour} * T \text{ hours} + 1/0.75$$
$$\text{Airplanes per hour} * T \text{ hours}$$

The algebra here is a little bit hairy, but we can handle it! To solve for time, isolate T step by step. First, multiply every term in the equation by "1 hour":

Now, the unit "hour" cancels out of both terms on the right side of the equation. Remember, when you multiply *and* divide a term by something, that cancels out:

Now, we have:

$$12 \text{ plane hours} = 1 \text{ plane} * T \text{ hours} + 1/0.75 * T \text{ hours}$$

We need to isolate "T hours." Gather together the "T hours" terms on the right side of the equation. Right now, they are separated into an addition expression. If we add them together, they will be collected into one term. Since 1/0.75 is equal to 4/3, change that term first:

$$12 \text{ plane hours} = 1 \text{ plane} * T \text{ hours} + 4/3 \text{ plane} * T$$
$$\text{hours}$$

Now add:

$$12 \text{ plane hours} = (1 \text{ plane} + 4/3 \text{ plane}) * T \text{ hours}$$
$$12 \text{ plane hours} = (1 \text{ and } 4/3 \text{ plane}) * T \text{ hours}$$

You add together 1 and 4/3. This is the same as saying that $1x + 2x = 3x$. We just collected the like terms.

Now, divide both sides by 1 plane to isolate the T hours term. Since mixed fractions are difficult to work with, change this into an improper fraction:

$$12 \text{ plane hours} = (7/3 \text{ plane}) * T \text{ hours}$$

The planes unit cancels out on the right side. So we are left with:

$$12 \text{ hours} / (7/3) = T \text{ hours}$$

One arithmetic trick: dividing by a fraction is the same as multiplying by the inverse of the fraction. If you are comfortable dividing by fractions on your calculator, you can do the rest of the problem that way, or else you can flip the fraction over and simplify the arithmetic:

$$12 * 3/7 = T \text{ hours}$$
$$36/7 = T \text{ hours}$$
$$5 \, 1/7 = T \text{ hours}$$

The answer is $x = 5 \, ^1/_7$ hours, or approximately 5.14 hours.

That was a long problem! But it included rates, a system of equations, unit conversions (changing minutes into fractions of an hour) and algebra with complex fractions. That is about the most difficult type of rate problem you would ever see on a standardized math exam, so if you were able to follow along with the solution you're in good shape.

Remember, on exams like this, the vast majority of points come from the easier problems. The harder problems (which on most exams tend to be at the end of a section) are always worth giving a shot, but they are not necessary to get a good score. Problems like these are great for practice because they include a lot of different concepts. Don't be discouraged if you don't always get the tougher problems correct on the first try. They are preparing you to do well on a wide range of different problem types!

HESI A^2 - Spire Study System

MODULE 3

DAY, LOCATION, MUSIC

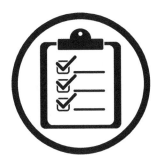

1 MONDAY, OCTOBER 12

COFFEE SHOP ON MAIN STREET

MY FAVORITE BAND

2

3

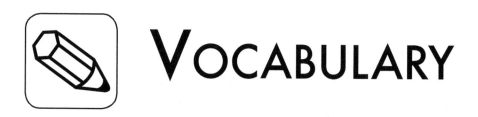

VOCABULARY

LET'S FACE IT. VOCABULARY JUST ISN'T THAT INTERESTING. SO, LET'S CHANGE IT UP! BELOW IS A CROSSWORD PUZZLE TO HELP YOU LEARN SOME NEW WORDS AND EXPAND YOUR VOCABULARY.

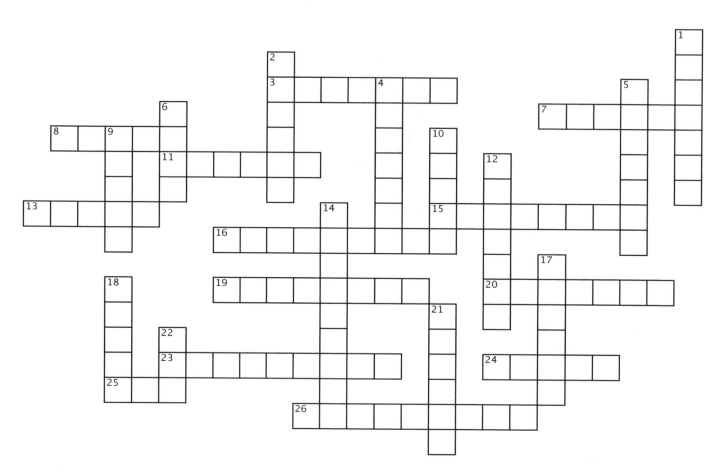

abhorrent bar chide debonair err frail glut haughty immerse jargon lofty malign abscond obscure parity ravage slander transpose unison vague amity ambiguous carcass hoist perpetual surmount

Across

3. to leave quickly
7. destroy or ruin
8. weak
11. together or at once
13. of considerable height
15. to overcome something
16. disgusting or hateful
19. stylish and charming
20. speaking falsely about someone
23. having more than one explanation
24. unclear or uncertain
25. to make a mistake
26. a state of being without change

Down

1. cover completely
2. specialized words
4. relatively unknown
5. arrogant
6. too much of something
9. friendly relations between two people
10. raise with a mechanical device
12. the remains of a dead animal
14. to change an arrangement
17. speak badly about
18. to scold
21. the equivalent of something
22. forbid or prevent

HESI A² - Spire Study System

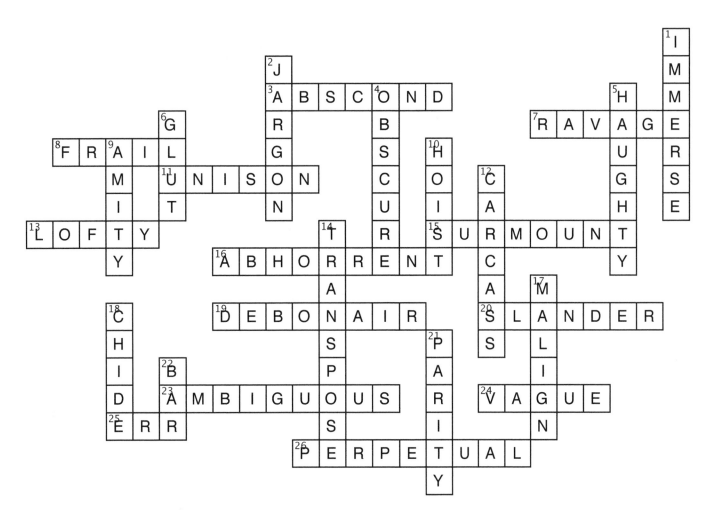

abhorrent bar chide debonair err frail glut haughty immerse jargon lofty malign abscond obscure parity ravage slander transpose unison vague amity ambiguous carcass hoist perpetual surmount

Across

3. to leave quickly [ABSCOND]
7. destroy or ruin [RAVAGE]
8. weak [FRAIL]
11. together or at once [UNISON]
13. of considerable height [LOFTY]
15. to overcome something [SURMOUNT]
16. disgusting or hateful [ABHORRENT]
19. stylish and charming [DEBONAIR]
20. speaking falsely about someone [SLANDER]
23. having more than one explanation [AMBIGUOUS]
24. unclear or uncertain [VAGUE]
25. to make a mistake [ERR]
26. a state of being without change [PERPETUAL]

Down

1. cover completely [IMMERSE]
2. specialized words [JARGON]
4. relatively unknown [OBSCURE]
5. arrogant [HAUGHTY]
6. too much of something [GLUT]
9. friendly relations between two people [AMITY]
10. raise with a mechanical device [HOIST]
12. the remains of a dead animal [CARCASS]
14. to change an arrangement [TRANSPOSE]
17. speak badly about [MALIGN]
18. to scold [CHIDE]
21. the equivalent of something [PARITY]
22. forbid or prevent [BAR]

CRITICAL READING

INFERENCES AND HOW TO MAKE THEM AND USE THEM

*Inference is a mental process by which you reach a conclusion based on specific evidence. Inferences are the stock and trade of detectives examining clues, of doctors diagnosing diseases, and of car mechanics repairing engines. We infer motives, purpose and intentions.

You use inference every day. You interpret actions to be examples of behavioral characteristics, intents or expressions of particular feelings. You infer it is raining when you see someone with an open umbrella. You infer that people are thirsty if they ask for a glass of water. You infer that evidence in a text is authoritative when it is attributed to a scholar in that particular field.

You want to find significance. You listen to remarks and want to make sense of them. What might the speaker mean? Why is he or she saying that? You must go beyond specific remarks to determine underlying significance or broader meaning. When you read that someone cheated on his or her income taxes, you might take that as an example of financial ingenuity,

daring or stupidity. You seek purposes and reasons.

Inferences are not random. While they may come about mysteriously with sudden recognition, you usually make inferences very orderly. Inferences may be guesses, but they are educated guesses based on supporting evidence. The evidence requires that you reach a specific conclusion.

Inferences are not achieved with mathematical rigor, and they do not have the certainty obtained with deductive reasoning. Inferences tend to reflect prior knowledge and experience as well as personal beliefs and assumptions. Thus, inferences tend to reflect your stake in a situation or your interests in the outcome. People may reason differently or bring different assumptions or premises to bear. This is why bias is addressed so carefully in our criminal justice system, so defendants are given a fair trial.

EXAMPLE

Given evidence that polychlorinated biphenyls (PCB) cause cancer in people and that PCB's are in a particular water system, all reasonable people would reach the conclusion that the water system is dangerous to people. But, given evidence that there is an increase in skin cancer among people who sun bathe, not all people would conclude that sunbathing causes skin cancer. Sun bathing, they might argue, may be coincidental with exposure to other cancer-causing factors.

*Daniel J. Kurland
(www.criticalreading.com/inference_process.htm)

INFERENCE QUESTIONS

Inference questions ask about ideas that are not directly stated, but rather are implied by the passage. They ask you to draw conclusions based on the information in the passage. Inference questions usually include words like "imply," "infer" or "conclude," or they may ask you what the author "would probably" think or do in a given situation based on what was stated in the passage.

With inference questions, it is important not to go *too far* beyond the scope of the passage. You are not expected to make any guesses. There is a single correct answer that is a logical, next-step conclusion from what is presented in the passage.

Let's take a look at some sample inference questions. Read through the following passages and use your inference skills to answer the questions. Remember that the inferences you make are not always obvious or directly stated in the passage.

SAMPLE 1

"Despite the fact that the practice is illegal in many states, some people set off their own fireworks at home each summer, especially on Independence Day. Most cities have public fireworks displays run by experienced professionals in a controlled environment, but many people still enjoy the thrill of setting off their own fireworks. However, this practice can be dangerous, and many people are injured each year from fireworks-related accidents. Having Independence Day fireworks in your own backyard is not worth the safety risk, especially when public fireworks displays are available in most areas."

THE AUTHOR OF THIS PASSAGE WOULD MOST LIKELY SUPPORT:

A. The complete legalization of fireworks nationwide
B. The reduction of public fireworks displays
C. More rigorous enforcement of restrictions on home fireworks
D. Promoting home fireworks use

ANSWER: C

In the passage, the author takes a negative tone toward home fireworks use, citing the fact that the practice is dangerous, illegal in some areas and unnecessary since many areas have safe public fireworks displays on holidays. Someone who is critical of home fireworks use would support strong enforcement of restrictions on their use.

SAMPLE 2

"A man took his car to the mechanic because the engine was overheating. The mechanic opened the hood to inspect the situation. He removed the radiator cap and could see that there was a sufficient amount of coolant in the radiator. He took the car for a drive and also noticed that the engine would overheat at a stoplight, but not on the highway."

ACCORDING TO THE PASSAGE, WHAT CAN YOU INFER ABOUT THE ENGINE?

A. The engine needs to be replaced
B. The radiator is leaking
C. The engine is operating normally
D. The radiator fan is broken

ANSWER: D

Although an overheating engine does indicate an abnormal condition, it does not necessarily indicate a catastrophic failure. Thus, the engine can be repaired instead of replaced. The radiator was full of coolant, so that eliminates the possibility of a leak. When a vehicle is moving, the airflow across the radiator cools the coolant. However, when a vehicle is stationary, the fan is responsible for cooling the coolant. If the fan is not working correctly, this would explain the overheating at a stoplight, but not on the highway.

ARITHMETIC REASONING

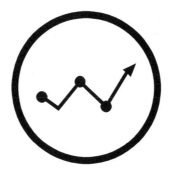

Working with Sets

All standardized math exams will touch on the basic statistical descriptions of sets of numbers: mean (the same as an average, for a set), median, mode and range. These are terms to know. Let's look at an example set and examine what each of these terms means:

Set of numbers: 42, 18, 21, 26, 22, 21

Mean/Average

The mean of a set of numbers is the average value of the set. The formula for finding the mean is:

$$\frac{\text{sum of the numbers in the set}}{\text{quantity of numbers in the set}} = \text{mean}$$

Use this formula to find the mean of the example set:

$$\frac{42+18+21+26+22+21}{6} = \frac{150}{6} = 25$$

You add together all the numbers that appear in the set, and then divide by the quantity of numbers in the set. The mean, or average, value in the set is 25. Notice that the mean is not necessarily a number that appears in the set, although it can be.

Median

The median of a set is the number that appears in the middle when the set is ordered from least to greatest. Therefore, the first step in finding the mean is to put the numbers in the correct order, if they are not already. You should always do this physically, on your scratch paper, to make sure that you don't leave any numbers out of the reordering. For the example set, that would be:

18, 21, 21, 22, 26, 42

Make sure you've included all the numbers in the order, even if there are duplicates. If a set with a lot of numbers, it's helpful to cross them off in the original set as you order them on your scratch paper. This helps ensure that you don't leave one out.

If there is an odd quantity of numbers in the set, the median will be the middle number. For example, if a set is comprised of nine numbers, the median will be the fifth number of the ordered set.

However, the example set has six numbers. Since no single number is in the exact middle, we average the two middle numbers to find the median:

$$\frac{21+22}{2} = 21.5$$

The median of this set is 21.5.

MODE

The mode of a set of numbers is the number that appears most often. Speakers of French will find this easy to remember: *mode* is the French word for style. The number that appears the most is "in style" for this particular set.

The example set has one number that appears more than once: 21. Therefore, 21 is the mode. Sometimes, it's easiest to see this after the set is ordered, when duplicate numbers appear next to one another.

If a set has two numbers that equally appear most often, such as two 21s and two 22s, then both 21 *and* 22 are the mode. We don't average them together, as we do to find the median. Therefore, the mode is the only descriptor of a set that must always be a number in the set. Since there are two modes, the set would be described as "bimodal."

RANGE

The range of a set of numbers is the distance between the highest and lowest values. Once you've reordered a set, these values are easy to identify. Simply subtract the two values to get the range:

highest value - lowest value = range

For the example set, this would be:

42 - 18 =2 4

The range of the set is 24.

Sets can include negative numbers, decimals, fractions, duplicates, etc. They may also appear in table form. Let's look at another example set to see what kinds of tricky questions you may encounter.

Month	Rainfall (inches)
August	0.8
September	1.3
October	2.1
November	1.3
December	3.7

What is the average rainfall for the months September, October, November and December?

SOLUTION:
Notice the first trick in this question – you are asked for the average of only four months, not all five listed in the table. This introduces two possible sources of error – you could add all five months' rainfall and/or divide by five when calculating the average. To find the average of only the four months stated in the question, the solution is:

$$\frac{1.3+2.1+1.3+3.7}{4} = 2.1 \text{ inches}$$

Here's another question for the same data table, but it uses a different approach to averaging:

The average monthly rainfall from July through December was 1.7 inches. What was the rainfall, in inches, in July?

SOLUTION:
This question gives you the average and asks you to find the missing rainfall value. This is a common way to make a mean/average problem a little tricky for the average (mean) test-taker. You can solve these types of questions by applying the basic equation for finding the mean:

$$\frac{\text{sum of the numbers in the set}}{\text{quantity of numbers in the set}} = \text{mean}$$

Next, fill in all the known values:

$$\frac{\text{July}+0.8+1.3+2.1+1.3+3.7}{6} = 1.7$$

Solve algebraically:

$$\text{July}+0.8+1.3+2.1+1.3+3.7 = 1.7 * 6$$

$$\text{July} = (1.7 * 6)-0.8-1.3-2.1-1.3-3.7$$

$$\text{July} = 1 \text{ inch}$$

Now, try to solve this question:

What is the difference between the mode and the median of the rainfalls for August through December?

SOLUTION:
Simply find the mode and median values. Remember, the first step is to order the set:

$$0.8, 1.3, 1.3, 2.1, 3.7$$

The mode is 1.3 because that is the only number that appears more than once.

The median is 1.3 because, of the five numbers in the set, 1.3 is the third (middle) number.

Therefore, the difference between the mode and the median is:

$$1.3-1.3 = 0$$

HESI A² - Spire Study System

MATHEMATICS KNOWLEDGE

PROBABILITY

Every probability is a ratio as described below.

Probability = $\dfrac{\text{Total number of desired events}}{\text{Total number of possible outcomes}}$

The simplest example of this type of ratio is found when tossing a coin. There are always two total outcomes, heads and tails, so the probability of either a head or a tail is always 1/2 for that coin.

Similarly, if you tossed that same coin 14 times, you would expect to see it land 7 times with the head showing and 7 times with the tail showing. Because these events are totally random, flipping the coin 14 times will not always provide an equal number of outcomes in a group of trials. So we say that the number of heads in a trial of 14 is the "expected value" of 7. Similarly, 7 would be the "expected value" for tails.

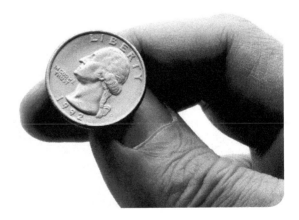

A common misconception is that there "has to be" a certain outcome based on the number of outcomes that have already occurred. In the repeated trial of an event, each outcome is it's own trial and is not influenced by the previous trial or trials.

The other common type of probability problem is with dice, where each of six faces of a cube has its own number from 1 to 6. Each of these numbers has the probability of 1/6 for a single roll of the die.

If we formulate a table of outcomes for two dice, thrown together, the details are slightly different. In this table, the individual numbers are shown across the top and vertically along the side. The entries in the table represent the total of the two dice.

	1	2	3	4	5	6	Cube "A"
1	2	3	4	5	6	7	
2	3	4	5	6	7	8	
3	4	5	6	7	8	9	
4	5	6	7	8	9	10	
5	6	7	8	9	10	11	
6	7	8	9	10	11	12	

Cube "B"

A look at the table shows that there are 36 possible outcomes when two dice are thrown together (6 * 6). The individual probabilities are shown below.

P (1) =	0		(never appears)
P (2) =	1/36	does not simplify	(appears once)
P (3) =	2/36	simplifies to 1/18	(appears twice)
P (4) =	3/36	simplifies to 1/12	(appears three times)
P (5) =	4/36	simplifies to 1/9	(appears four times)
P (6) =	5/36	does not simplify	(appears five times)
P (7) =	6/36	simplifies to 1/6	(appears six times)
P (8) =	5/36	does not simplify	(appears five times)
P (9) =	4/36	simplifies to 1/9	(appears four times)
P (10) =	3/36	simplifies to 1/12	(appears three times)
P (11) =	2/36	simplifies to 1/18	(appears twice)
P (12) =	1/36	does not simplify	(appears once)
P (13) =	0		(never occurs)

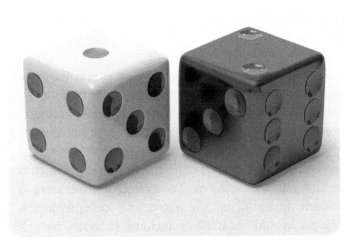

The symmetry of the table helps us visualize the probability ratios for the individual outcomes. By the definition of probability, any number larger than 13 will never appear in the table so the probability has to be zero. The probability of any impossible outcome always has to be zero. By the same reasoning, any event that must happen will have a probability of one. So, the probability of rolling a number from 2 to 12 is one.

If you are finding the probability of two events happening, the individual probabilities are added. For example, the probability of rolling a ten or eleven is the same as the probability of rolling an eight. The number eight appears in the table the same number of times as the combined total of appearances of ten or eleven.

The formulation of ratios for probabilities is simplest when using fractions. Often, the expression of a probability answer will be in a percent or a decimal. A coin from the first example would have the following probabilities P (heads) = 50% or .5 or 0.5.

Formulating probabilities from a word problem can always be structured around the ratio defined at the beginning of this section. However the words can mislead or misdirect problem-solving efforts.

For example, a problem that describes a class distribution may often be stated as the number of boys and the number of girls. The probability of selecting a boy in a random sample is defined as the number of boys divided by the TOTAL number of boys AND girls.

This is simple to see, but problems can be worded to mislead you into selecting the incorrect answer or to lead to the wrong conclusion when calculating an answer.

Another way that probability problems can be misleading is when multiple choices are used when simplified ratios are required. For example, if a class is made up of 6 girls and 10 boys, the probability of randomly selecting a girl from the classroom is $^6/_{16}$ or $^3/_8$. The misleading multiple choices that may be listed would often include 60%, (6/10) or 50% (since there are two outcomes — boys and girls). Reading a probability problem carefully is extremely important in both formulating the probability ratio and in making sure that the correct ratio is selected in the correct form. If the probability ratio for the example is formulated as $^6/_{16}$, the simplified form of $^3/_8$ is the only correct answer.

RATIOS AND PROPORTIONS

Ratios and fractions are synonymous when discussing numerical values. The ratios or fractions always imply division of the numerator by the denominator. In this section, the discussion is directed toward how words appear in ratio problems and how those words should be interpreted.

A commonly used ratio is contained in the term "miles per hour", usually abbreviated by mph. When the term "miles per hour" is interpreted numerically, it is the ratio of the total number of miles traveled divided by the number of hours traveled. The key word in this commonly used term is "per". It literally means for each hour of travel, a specific number of miles will be traveled. It has the same implication when the term is "gallons per hour" (how fast a tub is filled or a lawn is watered) or "tons per year" (how much ore is mined in one year).

Another way that ratios can appear is when a phrase defines a ratio as one value to another. A commonly used comparison is usually the ratio of "men to women" or "boys to girls". When this terminology is used, the first term is in the numerator, and the second term is in the denominator by convention.

There is an inherent problem when this terminology is used as illustrated by the example below:

In a classroom setting, the ratio of girls to boys is 3 to 4 (or 3:4 in strictly mathematical terms). How many boys are there in the classroom if the total number of students is 28?

There are two ways that this word problem may be easily solved. If the ratio of $(^{girls}/_{boys})$ is , the actual numbers may be or $^6/_8$ or $^9/_{12}$ or $^{12}/_{16}$ and so forth. These fractions are all equivalent fractions since they all simplify to the value of . The equivalent fractions are easily determined as the ratios of multiples of the numerator and denominator of the original fraction.

There is only one fraction where the numerator and denominator add to 28, and that is the ratio $^{12}/_{16}$. Therefore, the solution is the classroom has 16 boys and 12 girls.

Notice that the words specify which group (boys or girls) is the numerator and denominator in the original problem and in the solution. When choosing multiple-choice answers, make sure that the correct answer is chosen based upon the wording in the original problem. Most often, the correct ratio and its reciprocal are in the answer choices. For example, if the sample problem appeared on the exam, the multiple-choice answers would most likely include 16 boys and 12 girls AND 12 boys and 16 girls. But 16 boys and 12 girls is the correct answer choice.

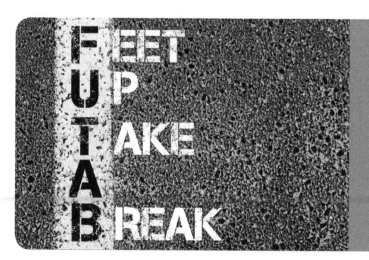

FEET UP TAKE BREAK

BREAK TIME (15 Mins)

PERFORM AN ENJOYABLE ACTIVITY TO DISTRACT YOU FROM STUDYING.
READ SOMETHING LIGHT, GO FOR A WALK —
WHATEVER YOU DO, TRY TO GET
YOUR MIND OFF THE MATERIAL
FOR A LITTLE WHILE.

BIOCHEMISTRY & CELL BIOLOGY

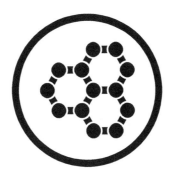

The majority of questions on the HESI are based on material from the HESI category identified as "Human Body Science". The Biochemistry & Cell Biology and General Human Anatomy sections cover the material equivalent to the HESI human body science topics. In Biochemistry & Cell Biology, we proceed logically from the general chemistry and begin to introduce the chemical reactions and molecular structures that can be classified as topics in biochemistry and cell biology. These topics are focused on the biochemical and cellular processes that include humans and are essential for a rational understanding of human body science that is continued in General Human Anatomy.

Biochemistry and Cell Biology

We concluded our discussion of Physics and General Chemistry with the topic of oxidation and reduction reactions and the prominent role that transition metals often play in these types of reactions. As we proceed to the chemical reactions that are associated with living organisms, we begin with a description of two critical

processes that serve as the foundation of all biological processes in mammalian cells (and therefore in humans).

These processes are the absorption of oxygen from the environment and the utilization of oxygen by cells to completely oxidize glucose to water and carbon dioxide. These oxidation processes generate the primary energy-rich molecules that are critical for for all bodily functions - ATP and the reducing compounds NADH and NADPH. Oxidation-reduction reactions involving transition metals (iron in particular) play key roles in both processes.

Hemoglobin-Oxygen Binding

Hemoglobin molecules are designed to bind O_2 molecules from air inspired in the lungs and to then release the O_2 molecules in regions of the body that require oxygen. To accomplish this the hemoglobin molecule contains iron (Fe) ions that are bound in the ferrous (Fe^{2+}) oxidation state. When O_2 binds to the Fe^{2+} it oxidizes the Fe^{2+} ion to the Fe^{3+} oxidation state.

Cytochromes and the Electron Transport Chain

Aerobic cellular respiration completely oxides glucose molecules to H_2O and CO_2. The final steps of this process occur in the mitochondria of human cells. End product molecules of the citric acid cycle - NADH and NADPH transfer electrons in the form of hydrogen atoms to the electron transport chain. The electron transport chain consists of a series of proteins called cytochromes which also contain iron ions bonded in a particular oxidation state.

As electrons are transferred from NADH or NADPH to the first cytochrome and then to subsequent cytochrome molecules in the chain, a series of oxidation and reduction reactions occur. In the process, the iron ions are alternatively oxidized and reduced. During this process energy is released and is used to pump hydrogen ions into a membrane compartment in the mitochondria. This builds up a **proton gradient** within the membrane-bound space that is used in subsequent diffusion processes across the membrane to generate large amounts of ATP molecules.

By this method aerobic cellular respiration reactions are able to capture almost 40% of the energy that is released by a combustion reaction of glucose and oxygen. Rather than the energy escaping in a single oxidation reduction reaction as thermal energy in a simple combustion reaction, the reaction is broken down into several smaller oxidation reduction steps through the electron transport chain and the energy produced from these redox reactions are captured and stored in the form of ATP molecules.

Oxidation Reductions and Chemical Functional Groups

In the human body, most of the molecules are **organic molecules** and most organic molecules are molecules that have a primary structural framework that consists of **chains of covalently bonded carbon atoms.** There are thousands of variations of these organic molecules in the human body. The difference is usually due to the other atoms or sub-unit molecular fragments that are also bonded to one or more of the carbon chain carbons. These molecular fragments are called functional groups. In the human body, most of the important functional groups are those shown below:

Hydrocarbons

We have already described the structures of the hydrocarbons which consist of chains of covalently bonded carbon molecules. In most cases, the carbon molecules are also single bonded to one or more hydrogen atoms. If all of the carbon-carbon bonds in a hydrocarbon are single bonds the hydrocarbon is classified as an **alkane**. If there is one or more carbon-carbon double bonds in the carbon chain the hydrocarbon is classified as a **alkene** and if there is one or more triple carbon-carbon bonds the hydrocarbon is classified as an **alkyne**.

Hydrocarbons generally are the skeletons or structural frameworks that form most organic molecules but they often can be functional groups of larger molecules as well When they are functional groups they are usually designated as such by the letter "R".

Alcohols R-OH

——OH

Alcohol functional groups are also carbon atoms bonded to hydroxyl groups (OH). The carbon atom is also covalently bonded to one or more carbons and or hydrogens.

Amines R-NH$_2$

——NH$_2$

Amines are important functional groups in biology because they are one of the functional groups of **amino acids**. The amine group of an amino acid can react with the carboxylic acid group of another amino acid (all amino acids have both an amine group and a carboxylic acid group) to form a peptide bond. This is the reaction that allows individual amino acids to form amino acid chain. These polypeptide chains are by definition **proteins**. Proteins are the most diverse and fundamental molecules that are used to create a living organism.

Aldehydes R-COH   Ketones R-CO-R

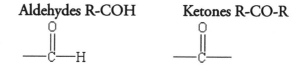

Aldehydes and ketones have an oxygen that is double bonded to a carbon. Together this carbon-oxygen unit is called a **carbonyl** unit. In ketones, the **carbonyl carbon** is also covalently bonded to two other carbons.

In Aldehydes, the carbonyl carbon is a terminal carbon - the last carbon of a carbon chain. It in addition to the oxygen double bond the carbonyl carbon is also bonded to one carbon and one hydrogen atom

Carboxylic Acids R-COOH

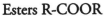

Carboxylic acids are aldehyde groups where the terminal carbonyl carbon is bonded to a hydroxyl group in place of a hydrogen. The carboxylic acid actually consists of two functional groups: an alcohol and a carbonyl group. It's always a terminal group since the carbonyl carbon has only one bond available to attach to a larger molecule. As discussed for the amines, amino acids have carboxylic acid functional groups which can react with the amine functional groups of other amino acids to form peptide bonds. This peptide bond formation process generates a polypeptide amino acid chain molecule called a protein.

Esters R-COOR

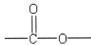

Esters can be thought of as carboxylic acid groups where the hydrogen of the alcohol or hydroxyl group has been replaced by an oxygen which in turn is bonded to another portion of the ester molecule, usually via a carbon-oxygen bond. Ester bonds are the bonds that occur between glycerol molecules and fatty acid molecules to form triglycerides.

General Types of Redox Reactions in Biology

In biological reactions oxidations and reduction in general often occur through a series of steps where a single molecule is progressively oxidized or reduced. Commonly these oxidation and reduction steps occur in the sequence that is illustrated below.

$R\text{-}CH_2\text{-}CH_3 \rightarrow R\text{-}CH{=}CH_2 \rightarrow R\text{-}COH\text{-}CH_3 \rightarrow R\text{-}CO\text{-}CH_3$

Alkane	Alkene	Alcohol	Ketone
CH_2 (-2)	CH (-1)	COH (+1)	CO (+2)

←-- Reduction

Oxidation---→

$R\text{-}CH_2\text{-}CH_3 \rightarrow R\text{-}CH{=}CH_2 \rightarrow R\text{-}CH_2\text{-}CH_2OH \rightarrow R\text{-}CH_2\text{-}CHO \rightarrow R\text{-}CH_2\text{-}COOH \rightarrow R\text{-}CH_3 +\text{-}CO_2$

Alkane	Alkene	Alcohol	Aldehyde	Carboxylic Acid	Carbon dioxide
CH_3 (-3)	CH_2 (-2)	CHOH (0)	CHO (+1)	COOH (+3)	CO2 (+4)

←-- Reduction

Oxidation---→

The first set of reactions shows - from left to right - a **progressive oxidation of an alkane to a ketone**. The oxidation (increase in oxidation state) is occurring at the red carbon and the oxidation state numbers of the carbon atom are shown in parenthesis. The second set of reactions shows - from left to right - a **progressive oxidation of an alkane to aa aldehyde**. The oxidation is also occurring at the red carbon. The red carbon then undergoes a final oxidation when it is converted into the carbon of a carbon dioxide molecule which separates from the original alkane molecule. This is called a **decarboxylation reaction.**

Of course, there are other participant molecules in the reaction sequences that are being reduced when the alkene is being oxidized (and vice versa if the reactions proceed from right to left as reductions toward an alkane) but these have been omitted to emphasize the main sequence of oxidation of alkanes and reduction to alkanes

In biology, redox reactions are very important but often they can be identified as those reactions that involve **oxygen molecules** that or consumed or produced by a reaction. Reductions usually occur by the addition of **hydrogen atoms or negative hydrogen ions (H^-).** The two most important sequences of redox reactions in biology are the reactions of photosynthesis and the aerobic (oxygen requiring) reactions of cellular respiration - the Krebs or citric acid cycle and the reactions of oxidative phosphorylation and the electron transport chain.

The two types of reactions photosynthesis and aerobic cellular respiration are actually the same reaction where the products of photosynthesis are the reactants of cellular respiration and vice versa. The detail of these multi-step reactions is very unlikely to appear on the HESI, but the overall reactions are an example of a combustion reaction (aerobic respiration) - which is a type of redox reaction and the reverse reaction of a combustion reaction (photosynthesis). A discussion of combustion reactions and the overall reactions for photosynthesis and aerobic respiration are provided below.

Combustion Reactions

Combustion reactions for the HESI are the oxidation-reduction reaction where oxygen molecules and molecules containing carbon hydrogen and sometimes oxygen are the reactants and carbon dioxide and water are the products. A typical combustion reaction is the reaction which occurs in an internal combustion engine with the reactants oxygen and the mixture of hydrocarbon molecules in gasoline.

An example of this type of combustion reaction - in which ethane and oxygen are the reactants - is shown below

$$2C_2H_6 + 7O_2 \rightarrow 4CO_2 + 6H_2O$$

This is a balanced reaction but it is more commonly written as

$$C_2H_6 + 3\frac{1}{2}O_2 \rightarrow 2CO_2 + 3H_2O$$

All combustion reactions are self-sustaining and highly exothermic, and therefore generate a large amount of heat energy.

Aerobic Cellular Respiration

The most important combustion reaction for the HESI is the overall reaction for aerobic cellular respiration where glucose is first processed by the reactions of **glycolysis** and next through the **Krebs or citric acid cycle** reactions and then **the electron transport chain** to produce carbon dioxide, water and energy. This overall reaction is

$$C_6H_{12}O_6 + 6O_2 + 38\ ADP + 38\ PO4^- \rightarrow 6CO_2 + 6H_2O + 38\ ATP$$

Glucose

The molecule $C_6H_{12}O_6$ is the **sugar** glucose. Sugars a class of molecules called **carbohydrates**. Carbohydrates are molecules that consist of carbon chains where carbons are also single bonded to hydrogens and double bonded to the oxygen (creating an aldehyde or a ketone functional group) or single bonded to oxygens of hydroxide groups (creating an alcohol functional group). Hydroxide groups consist of one oxygen atom single bonded to one hydrogen atom (O-H).   the carbon-hydroxide molecular subunit is called an alcohol. The chemical structure of glucose ($C_6H_{12}O_6$) is shown below.

Aerobic respiration occurs within the mitochondria of cells and the energy from the combustion reaction is stored as chemical potential energy in ATP molecules.

Overall Sequence of Reactions in Cellular Respiration
Glycolysis

The generation of chemical energy in human cells begins with a molecule of glucose. In the cytosol of a cell there are enzymes that catalyze a series of reactions in a process called glycolysis. The overall reaction for glycolysis is

Glucose ($C_6H_{12}O_6$) + 2 NAD^+ + 2 ADP + 2 P_i → 2 Pyruvate + 2 NADH + 2 H^+ + 2 ATP + 2 H_2O

The molecules that participate in this reaction, in addition to glucose are inorganic phosphate (P_i), the molecule pyruvate, the adenosine diphosphate (ADP) and adenosine triphosphate (ATP) molecules and the NAD^+ and NADH molecules. Inorganic phosphate is the phosphate ion PO_4^-. It is a solubilized ion that is present in solution in nearly all body fluids. Adenosine is a small organic molecule that can form a bond with a phosphate ion to form the molecule AMP (adenosine monophosphate). The phosphate group on AMP can bond with a second phosphate group to form ADP (adenosine diphosphate). The second phosphate group on ADP can bond with a third phosphate group to form ATP (adenosine triphosphate).

AMP + P_i ⇌ ADP; ADP + P_i ⇌ ATP

In biological solutions, particularly the solutions that occur within cells (the cytosol) The phosphate ion (PO_4^-) is a very stable ion. Energy is required to bond this ion in the form of ADP from AMP and ATP from ADP. Conversely when the phosphate-phosphate bonds are broken with a reaction with H_2O to form ADP from ATP or AMP from ADP (a hydrolysis reaction) energy is released. This is the mechanism that allows cellular respiration reactions to capture the energy stored in glucose molecules. The energy released from the metabolism of glucose molecules is used to create phosphate-phosphate bonds in ADP and ATP and that energy can be utilized by cells in reactions that require energy by coupling the energy requiring reactions with the energy producing reactions of ATP hydrolysis.

Anaerobic Metabolism of Pyruvate

Notice that glycolysis does not require oxygen. The products of the reaction in addition to 2 ATP, include molecules are 2 molecules of pyruvate and two molecules of NADH. Pyruvate molecules can be used as a source of energy when oxygen is not available to continue the next phases of cellular respiration. This commonly occurs in **skeletal muscle** cells during vigorous physical activities. The reaction that produces energy during this process converts pyruvate to lactic acid.

Pyruvate + NADH + H^+ ⇌ Lactate + NAD^+

This anaerobic process uses NADH to reduce pyruvate to lactic acid. Lactic acid buildup in muscles leads to fatigue and eventual muscle failure. The process of recovery requires the conversion of lactic acid back to pyruvate. Since this is an oxidation reaction, ultimately it requires oxygen to accomplish this task. The amount of oxygen required to convert this lactic acid to pyruvate is called the **oxygen debt** that is generated of the anaerobic metabolism of pyruvate.

The Krebs (Tricarboxylic Acid) Cycle

In the absence of oxygen, the metabolism of glucose to produce energy stored in the form of ATP molecules is extremely inefficient. One glucose molecule generates only two ATP molecules from the reaction of glycolysis. The reaction also produces two NADH molecules which are very important because NADH molecules can be used as reducing compounds in biological reactions.

NADH and NAD+

The transfer of a hydrogen atom to a molecule almost always results a reduction of the reactant molecule. A vast number of chemical reactions in the body include steps when reductions of molecules are required. This is usually accomplished by coupling a reaction with the conversion of NADH to NAD+. the coupling reaction reduces the target molecule and oxidizes the NADH molecule to NAD+. An extremely important additional role of NADH molecules is the role that they serve in the aerobic metabolism steps of cellular respiration

Acetyl-CoA

In the presence of oxygen, Glucose molecules can be completely oxidized to H_2O and CO_2. this process begins with the conversion of pyruvate (generated by glycolysis) to the molecule Acetyl coenzyme (Acetyl CoA). This process begins with the transport of pyruvate from the cytosol of the cell through the outer membrane of mitochondria and into the interior of the mitochondria. The overall reaction is

Pyruvate + NAD+ + CoA (coenzyme A) ⇌ acetyl-CoA + CO_2 + NADH + H+

Acetyl-CoA next enters the Krebs or tricarboxylic acid cycle. This is a series of reactions that begins with the bonding of acetyl CoA to the first molecule of the krebs cycle. A series of reactions within the cycle results in the regeneration of the first molecule of the krebs cycle (which can now bind another acetyl CoA molecule and repeat the cycle) and several other products as shown below

acetyl-CoA + (krebs cycle reactions) ⇌ 2CO_2 + 3 NADH + $FADH_2$ + ATP

Notice that one round of the krebs cycle converts two carbons a glucose molecule to CO_2. The cycle also generates one additional ATP molecule (actually a GTP molecule - but they are chemically equivalent) per acetyl-CoA molecule that enters the cycle. Most importantly the krebs cycle generates 3 additional

NADH molecules per acetyl-CoA molecule that enters the cycle and one NADH-like molecule, $FADH_2$.

Oxidative Phosphorylation

Notice that so far, the metabolism of one molecule of glucose by glycolysis has generated 2 ATP molecules 2 NADH molecules and 2 pyruvate molecules. Next each pyruvate molecule has generated one NADH molecule and been converted into one acetyl CoA molecule as it passes from the cytosol of the cell into the interior of a mitochondrial. Inside of the mitochondrion. One acetyl CoA molecule enters one round of the krebs cycle and generates one ATP molecule and three NADH molecules and one $FADH_2$ molecule.

Since glycolysis produces two pyruvate molecules, two rounds of the krebs cycle are required to metabolize one molecule of glucose. Overall the metabolism of glucose generates 2 ATP and 2 NADH molecules from glycolysis and 2 NADH molecules from the conversion of two pyruvate molecule to two acetyl CoA molecules and 2 ATP molecules, 6 NADH molecules and 2 $FADH_2$ molecules from two rounds of the krebs cycle. The total for metabolism of one molecule of glucose is therefore 4 ATP and 10 NADH molecules and two $FADH_2$ molecules.

Glucose ($C_6H_{12}O_6$) → glycolysis→ Krebs cycle → 6CO_2 + 4 ATP + 10 NADH + 2 $FADH_2$

Cytochromes and the Electron Transport Chain

The final steps in the aerobic oxidation of glucose to H_2O and CO_2 begins with the oxidation of NADH to NAD+ and $FADH_2$ to FAD. This occurs at the first cytochrome of the electron transport chain for NADH and at the second cytochrome for $FADH_2$. Cytochromes are iron-containing protein complexes that are designed to accept electrons (in the form of electrons of hydrogen atoms) - which reduces the cytochrome. The first cytochrome in the electron transport chain then transfers electrons to the next cytochrome in the chain. Notice this is an oxidation step for the first cytochrome and a reduction step for the second cytochrome.

The electrons continue to be passed to subsequent cytochromes in a series of oxidation-reduction steps.

The final cytochrome in the chain transfers electrons to molecular oxygen (O_2). This final reduction step results in the reduction of molecular oxygen atom's (oxidation state of zero) to oxygen atoms in the H_2O molecule (oxidation state -2). Oxygen is the final acceptor of the electrons that began as electrons of hydrogen atoms that participated in high energy covalent bonds within glucose molecules.

Processing of the End Products of Cellular Respiration

Overall the reactions of aerobic cellular respiration - glycolysis, the Krebs cycle and the oxidative transport chain completely oxidize glucose molecules to CO_2 and H_2O. These end products of cellular respiration - the carbons and oxygens of the glucose molecule in the form of CO_2 and the hydrogens of the glucose molecule - now bonded in H_2O molecules can now be eliminated from the body. CO_2 diffuses out of cells and into the circulatory system and then diffuses out of the circulatory system into air in the lung, which is finally expired into the external environment. Excess H_2O is eliminated by the kidneys ultimately leaving the body as solvent water molecules contained in urine solution. The NADH and $FADH_2$ molecules have be oxidized by the electron transport chain back to NAD^+ and FAD molecules that can now recycle through the cellular respiration cycle and continue to oxidize additional glucose molecules.

Of course, this process requires a continuous supply of O_2 molecules. These O_2 molecules are obtained from air inspired into the lungs. This oxygen in the lung air diffuses into the circulatory system where it binds with hemoglobin in red blood cells and is subsequently released by hemoglobin in low-oxygen regions of the body. The oxygen then diffuses out of the circulatory system and into cells and then into mitochondria where it can act as the final acceptor of electrons in the electron transport chain.

Proton Concentration Gradients and Phosphorylation of ADP

It is notable that the entire pathway of cellular respiration up to the final steps of oxidative phosphorylation have only generated 4 ATP molecules per molecule of glucose. This production of ATP is called **substrate-level phosphorylation**. The last steps of oxidative phosphorylation are where the majority of ATP molecules are produced from the phosphorylation of ADP molecules.

Nearly all of the energy from the metabolism of glucose in now stored in the form of NADH and $FADH_2$ molecules generated by glycolysis and the Krebs cycle. For the final steps, it is necessary to explain that **the molecular complexes of the electron transport chain are located on the inner surface of the inner mitochondrial membrane**. There is a space - **the intermembrane mitochondrial space** - located between the inner and outer mitochondrial membranes. As electrons are passed from NADH and $FADH_2$ molecules to the cytochromes of the electron transport chain and then through the chain to O_2 molecules. The oxidation reduction reactions that occur are very energetically favorable.

Each oxidation reduction reaction generates a large amount of energy. This energy is used by molecular pumps that are located alongside the cytochromes on the inner mitochondrial membrane. These membrane pumps use the energy from the oxidation reduction reactions to pump protons (H^+) through transmembrane pores of the inner mitochondrial membrane into the intramembrane space.

This **active transport** of protons creates a very large **concentration gradient of protons** within the intermembrane space compared to the interior of the mitochondria. Recall that chemical or internal energy can be stored in the form of concentration gradients. The energy required to create the gradient - from active transport of protons into the intramembrane - space is now stored as a concentration gradient of protons.

There is a second set of membrane pores on the inner mitochondrial membrane that allow protons to **passively diffuse** from the intramembrane space back into the interior of the mitochondria. This diffusion is driven by the proton concentration gradient and the energy of this diffusion process is utilized by molecular complexes at the membrane pores to phosphorylate ATP from inorganic phosphate (PO_4^-) and ADP. The phosphorylation process creates a high energy phosphate bond. This is the bond that stores most of the energy derived from the oxidation of glucose.

Net Production of ATP from Glucose by Aerobic Cellular Respiration

Overall, the oxidation each NADH molecule results in the production of three ATP molecules from ADP molecules and the oxidation each $FADH_2$ molecule results in the production of two ATP molecules from ADP molecules. Since the metabolism of each glucose molecule produces 14 NADH molecules and 2 $FADH_2$ molecules the total amount of ATP produced per glucose molecule through oxidative phosphorylation is $3 \times 10 = 30$ (for NADH) and $2 \times 2 = 4$ (for $FADH_2$) = 34 ATP molecules. Recall that 4 ATP molecules were already generated by the metabolism of glucose before the process of oxidative phosphorylation. **The net result of the aerobic metabolism of glucose is that each molecule of glucose generates 38 ATP molecules.**

Carbohydrate Chemistry in Biology

As we have seen in the previous discussion of the aerobic metabolism of glucose, carbohydrates play a crucial role in human biology. In addition to providing a source of chemical energy for cells, sugars and other carbohydrates have many other critical functions within living organisms. We briefly described the general chemical definition of carbohydrates as molecules that are individual sugars or are molecules that are composed of sugars. The sugars are in general classified as **saccharides** - a single sugar is a **monosaccharide**, two sugars covalently bonded form a **disaccharide** molecules and multiple sugars that are covalently bonded form **polysaccharide** molecules.

Monosaccharides (Single or Simple Sugars)

Nearly all monosaccharides are classified as "single" or "simple" sugars. They are the chemical subunits or building block of all more complex carbohydrates. The simplest monosaccharide is glyceraldehyde.

The **glyceraldehyde** molecule demonstrates the key molecular features of all monosaccharides. There is a central carbon chain that is the "backbone" of the

monosaccharide. The carbon chain is usually three to six carbons in length. The naming of monosaccharides that are sugars begins with the latin prefix of the number of carbons in carbon chain backbone the sugar - "tri" for three, "pent" for five and "hex" for six - and end in the suffix "-ose". The sugar "ribose" is a five-carbon sugar so it is a **pentose**. Glucose is a six-carbon sugar so it is a **hexose**.

When sugars are in a **linear configuration** (they are usually in a ring or cyclic formation). For most simple sugars (the major exception in biology is the sugar deoxyribose). all of the central carbons are bonded to to either a single hydroxyl group(-OH) or double bonded to an oxygen atom (forming a carbonyl group -C=O). The remaining carbon bonds are single bonds to hydrogen atoms. If the carbonyl group is at either terminal end of the carbon chain this is an aldehyde and if the carbonyl group is an internal carbonyl this is a ketone. Sugars with aldehyde groups are classified as **aldoses** and those with ketones are classified as **ketoses.** The central carbon chain of simple sugars or numbered beginning with the terminal carbon that is an aldehyde carbon or is nearest to a ketone carbon. This numbering system is shown below for glucose

We can see that glucose has an aldehyde group so it is an aldose and has a central six carbon chain so it is a hexose - overall glucose is therefore an **aldohexose**. In contrast, ribose - another important biological simple sugar has the molecular structure shown below

Ribose is a five-carbon sugar so it is a pentose and it has an aldehyde carbon so it is an aldose - overall ribose is an **aldopentose**.

Cyclic Configuration of Simple Sugars

In most cases, simple sugars in the body exist in their cyclic form. The terminal oxygen atom of the OH group on the terminal carbon or second from terminal carbon of pentose and hexose sugars forms a bond with the carbon of the ketone or aldehyde group of the same molecule, resulting in a five - or six-member ring structure.

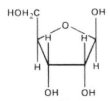 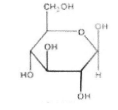

Ribose (ring configuration)   Glucose (ring configuration)

Glycogen

In the body, glucose, ribose, deoxyribose and many other monosaccharides in their ring configuration can be bonded to other molecules at any of the carbons of the sugar molecules. In one important example, in the liver glucose molecules are bonded to other glucose bonds by forming glycosidic bonds between glucose molecules at C-1, C-4 and C-6 glucose carbons. This synthesis of glycogen from glucose molecules is called **glycogenesis**. Glycogenesis results in a very large highly-branched glucose polymer molecule called glycogen. Glycogen is stored in liver cells (hepatocytes) and this glycogen can be readily broken down into individual glucose molecules that can then be released into the bloodstream. The breakdown of glycogen to glucose molecules is called **glycogenolysis**. Glycogen is therefore the most easily available reserve of glucose in the human body.

Gluconeogenesis

Glucose is absolutely essential for the maintenance of life in aerobic organisms including humans. Inadequate concentrations of glucose in the human body can lead to death within a matter of hours. When the ready reserve of glucose in the form of glycogen has been exhausted, the body begins to break down proteins into amino acids and triglycerides into fatty acids and glycerol. the liver begins to synthesize new glucose molecules from certain of these (glucogenic amino acids) amino acids and from glycerol molecules. These new glucose molecules are released into the circulation to maintain an adequate   supply of glucose for the continuation of cellular respiration. This process is called gluconeogenesis.

Starches and Cellulose

Dietary carbohydrates are usually consumed in the form of starches contained in grains and vegetables. Starches are another polymerized form of glucose. Cellulose is a glucose polymer that has glycosidic bonds that cannot be broken by human digestion. Cellulose forms the majority of non-digestible fiber in the human diet.

Nucleotides

Another critical role of cyclic sugars is the structural roles that the sugars ribose and deoxyribose provide into the genetic information storage molecule DNA and genetic information messenger and protein assembly molecule RNA. Both DNA and RNA molecules are very-large linear-chain polymers composed of nucleotide subunits. Nucleotides have the following structure

RNA nucleotide
PO_4-(C5)Ribose (C1)-(N)base

DNA nucleotide
PO_4-(C5)Deoxyribose(C1)-(N)base

The bases that are bonded to the C-1 carbon of ribose or deoxyribose are cyclic nitrogenous bases. We will discuss these bases in more detail shortly. The phosphate groups of nucleotides are bonded to ribose or deoxyribose at the C-5 carbons of either sugar. Phosphate groups are bonded to the C-5 carbon of either ribose or deoxyribose.

Sugar-Phosphate (Phosphodiester) Bonds in DNA and RNA

The structural backbone of DNA and RNA molecules are composed of a linear polymer of alternating sugars (ribose or deoxyribose) and phosphate groups. Phosphate groups form a phosphodiester bond between the C-3 and C-5 carbons of adjacent ribose or deoxyribose molecules. The formation of phosphodiester bond formed between two ribonucleotides is shown below.

Phosphodiester bond

$$(OH\text{-}C3)\text{-ribose-}(C5)\text{-}PO_4 + (OH\text{-}C3)\text{-ribose-}(C5)\text{-}PO_4 \rightarrow (3'\text{-ribose-}5')\text{-}PO_4\text{-}(3'\text{-ribose-}5')\text{-}PO_4 + H_2O$$

b	base	base	base	base

The phosphodiester bond Formed between two deoxyribonucleotides is identical except that the sugar is deoxyribose instead of ribose. Notice that this formation of phosphodiester bonds between nucleotides between the OH group at the sugar C-3 OH group and the phosphate group at the sugar C-5 carbon can continue with additional nucleotides bonded via phosphodiester bonds at either end of the enlarging sugar-phosphate chain molecule This polymerization process results in the production of the very-large biologically-functional DNA and RNA molecules. The RNA and DNA linear structures are diagrammed below (the ribose and deoxyribose molecules also each have one nitrogenous base bonded at the C1 sugar carbons - these are not shown in the diagram)

RNA ... -(3'-ribose-5')-PO$_4$-(3'-ribose-5')-PO$_4$-(3'-ribose-5')-PO$_4$-(3'-ribose-5')-PO$_4$-...

3'-to-5' direction→→→

←←← 5'-to-3' direction

DNA ... -(3'-deoxyribose-5')-(PO$_4$)-(3'-deoxyribose-5')-(PO$_4$)-(3'-deoxyribose-5')-(PO$_4$)-...

Notice that the phosphodiester linkages - indicated as the 3' (three prime) for the C3 carbon and the 5' five prime) for the C-5 between sugar molecules in DNA and RNA confer a directionality to both molecules. As diagramed above, the left end of the molecules is the 3'end and the right end of the molecules is the 5' end. The directionality of the molecules as shown is from - left to right- the 3'-to- 5' direction. From right to left it is the 5'-to-3' direction.

In summary, we see that sugars in the form of ribose and deoxyribose are the central molecular subunit of perhaps the two most important molecules in biology - DNA and RNA. These sugars form the covalent bonds between phosphate groups and between nitrogenous bases resulting in the complete RNA molecule and the complete single-stranded-form of the DNA molecule.

Glycoproteins

Glycoproteins are complex molecules composed of proteins bonded to sugars and/or modified sugar derivatives. Glycoproteins play a major role in countless numbers of molecular interaction in the body. Some of the most important are as cell membrane bound molecules that mediate cell-cell interactions. Most notable are the **major histocompatibility complex (MHC) glycoproteins** that are present on nearly all cell membranes in the human body. These molecules are critical to immune functioning they and are recognized by T-cell receptors and they identify cells as being "self" vs foreign or "non-self" cells. The A and B antigens of the **ABO blood types** on the surface of red blood cell membranes are glycoproteins. Many hormones are glycoproteins. This is only a tiny example of the thousands of types of glycoproteins that are involved in countless numbers of biological processes.

In addition to glycoproteins, there are a myriad of other classes of carbohydrate containing molecules in the body. These include glycolipids, proteoglycans and antibodies. It is more common than not that any biological molecule contains at least one carbohydrate functional group.

Lipid Chemistry in Biology

Lipids are a broad class of molecules that have a wide range of functions in the human body including energy storage in the form of triglycerides stored in adipose (fat) cells, major components of cell membranes in the form of phospholipid molecular subunits, cholesterol and cholesterol derivatives such as the steroid hormones, cell signaling and immune mediating molecules in the form of prostaglandins and other types of lipid based immunes system pathway molecules and as vital components of numerous cellular biochemical processes in the form of the fat-soluble vitamins A, D, E and K.

Fatty Acids

Nearly all of the types of lipids in biological processes are derivatives of either fatty acids or cholesterol. Fatty acids are single hydrocarbon chains - typically with chain lengths of between 16 and 26 carbon atoms and terminating in a carboxylic acid functional group

R-COOH

If the hydrocarbon segment of a fatty acid is an alkane the fatty acid is classified as a **saturated fatty acid**. If the hydrocarbon segment contains one or more carbon-carbon is classified as an **unsaturated fatty acid**.

Triglycerides

Most dietary fat and the storage form of fat in adipocytes is in the form of triglycerides. Triglycerides are formed by the reaction of a glycerol molecule and three fatty acid molecules. The glycerol molecule is a three-carbon molecule where each carbon is bonded to a hydroxyl group. These hydroxyl groups each react with a carboxylic acid group of a fatty acid forming an ester group that bonds the glycerol molecule and the fatty acid molecule. This reaction occurs at each of the three glycerol hydroxyl groups resulting in a triglyceride molecule.

Glycerol   Fatty acid

$$CH_2OH-CHOH-CH_2OH + 3\ R-COOH \rightarrow$$
$$H_2COOR-HCOOR-H_2COOR + 3H_2O$$

Triglyceride

Dietary triglycerides are hydrolyzed in the small intestine by the enzyme lipase to monoglyceride molecules and fatty acid molecules. After absorption, some fatty acids are recombined with monoglycerides to reform triglycerides. Most of these triglycerides are stored in fat cells but some remain in the circulation as free triglycerides. the remainder of fatty acids are packaged along with cholesterol molecules and proteins into circulating complexes called lipoproteins. Most notable of these are the **high-density lipoprotein (HDL)** and **low-density lipoprotein (LDL)** complexes. Fatty acids and cholesterol molecules are transferred from lipoprotein complexes in the bloodstream into cells where they serve raw materials for construction of cell membranes, as a source of energy production and many other functions.

The concentrations of triglycerides and lipoproteins in the bloodstream is a major factor in the risk for development of atherosclerosis and coronary artery disease. These two conditions are the primary causes of heart disease and cerebral stroke. Together these two conditions are by far the most common causes of death in the industrialized world. High levels of triglycerides and LDL increases the risk of these diseases and HDL lowers the risk of these diseases.

Cell Membrane Phospholipids

All human outer cell membranes and all intracellular membranes - nuclear membranes, mitochondrial membranes, endoplasmic reticular membranes, golgi membranes and vesicle and vacuole membranes - are composed primarily of phospholipid molecules. These molecules are derivatives of triglycerides where one of the fatty acids has been replaced with a phosphate group. This creates a phosphodiglyceride molecule - a molecule with a long linear " tail" consisting of the two hydrocarbon chains of the phospholipid molecule and a phosphate group "head". The hydrocarbon tails are nonpolar and the phosphate group is polar.

In the body, the phosphate group is hydrophilic (attracted to water molecules) in the surrounding extracellular solution and in the intracellular solution environment. The hydrocarbon tail of the phospholipid molecules is hydrophobic (insoluble in the water solution of the extracellular and intracellular solution environments) and as a result the phospholipid molecules form a bilayer envelope where the outer layer phospholipids phosphate groups face outward toward the extracellular environment and the inner bilayer phospholipid phosphate groups face inward toward the cytoplasm environment of the cell. The hydrocarbon tails of the inner and outer molecular layers form the internal or middle region of the membrane bilayer.

The formation of an outer cell membrane was almost certainly the critical and earliest event is the evolution of life. The cell membrane is the physical structure that allows cells to maintain a stable internal environment that is separate from the external environment. This is the essential requirement for life - the maintenance of cellular homeostasis

Cholesterol
Cholesterol is a four-ringed lipid-based molecule that is an important component of **cell membranes** and also a precursor molecule for the synthesis of the **steroid hormones** cortisol, aldosterone progesterone and the sex hormones testosterone and estrogen. It is also the precursor for the synthesis of **vitamin D**. Most of the cholesterol used in the body is synthesized rather that of dietary origin.

Arachidonic Acid
Arachidonic acid is a 20-carbon fatty acid that contains four carbon double bonds. It is the precursor molecule for the synthesis of a very important class of **cell-signaling and cell messenger molecules** that include **prostaglandins, leukotrienes and thromboxanes**. These molecules interact with cell membrane molecules and participate in various roles within the immune system, most notably in the inflammatory effects that occur as part of the intrinsic immune system response to cell injury and infection.

Amino Acids and Proteins
No class of biological molecules is more essential than the proteins. Amino acids are the small molecules that are used to assemble proteins. The general form of an amino acid is a central carbon atom single bonded to a hydrogen atom and to three functional groups - an amine ($-NH_2$) group, a carboxylic acid ($-COOH$) group and a side group designated as an "R" group.

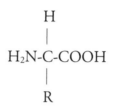

The R group is not the R group designated for hydrocarbons but is the amino acid side group that can be any of 20 unique functional groups. Each individual type of amino acid has a unique functional side group. The R or side group of the simplest amino acid - glycine - is a hydrogen atom. It is not likely that the HESI expects memorization of the R groups for all 20 amino acids, but it is useful to know that the R groups include hydroxyl groups $-OH$ as in the amino acid serine, hydrocarbon groups such as CH_3 in the amino acid alanine, amine groups $-NH_2$ as in the amino acid lysine, carboxylic acid groups $-COOH$ as in the amino acid glutamic acid (glutamate).

The amino acid cysteine R group has a sulfur atom that can form covalent bonds with the sulfur atom of the R group of other cysteine amino acids. In proteins, these disulfide bonds between cysteine amino acids often are critical to creating and maintaining a particular two or three-dimensional structure to protein molecules. Amino acids also have other critical functions in biology.

The amino acids glutamate and glycine can act as neurotransmitters, the amino acid tryptophan is the precursor for the neurotransmitter serotonin. Amino acids or amino acid derivatives are important components of many other biological molecules.

Proteins and Peptide Bonds

The simplest proteins are linear polymers of amino acids that are connected by peptide bonds. A peptide bond forms when the amine group of one amino acid reacts with the carboxylic acid group of an adjacent amino acid resulting in a carbon-nitrogen bond as shown below

$$H_2N-CH-COOH \ + \ H_2N-CH-COOH \ \rightarrow \ H_2N-CH-HC-NH-CH-COOH \ + H_2O$$

R1   R2   R1   R2

The continued formation of peptide bonds allows for the construction of a linear polypeptide chain (single chain protein) of any desired length. Typical lengths of single chain proteins in the human body range from a few hundred amino acids to over one thousand amino acids.

Protein Structure

With 20 different amino acids to choose from for every amino acid position in a single polypeptide chain corresponding to a complete biological protein the number of possible linear sequences of amino acids in the polypeptide chain is astronomical and therefore the range of different single-chain proteins is practically unlimited.

Primary Protein Structure

The primary structure of a protein refers only to single chain proteins. The primary structure is unique linear sequence of amino acids that comprise the single chain protein. Within an aqueous environment of the body the primary sequence of a protein directly determines the secondary structure and indirectly the tertiary structure and - in the case of multi-polypeptide chain proteins - the quaternary structure of functional proteins.

Secondary Protein Structure

The secondary structure of proteins again refers only to single chain proteins. This is often referred to as the two-dimensional structure of a polypeptide chain, but they are clearly a three-dimensional structure. There are two general types or motifs of secondary protein structures.

The β-Pleated Sheet

The first type of secondary protein structures is arguably a two-dimensional structure - the β-pleated sheet. This is a regular **saw-toothed structure where** each saw-tooth is about two amino acids in length. Typically, these β-pleated sheet segments are less than 10 amino acids in length, but often these segments are **hydrogen bonded with other β-pleated sheet segments** located in other regions of the polypeptide chain. This occurs when the polypeptide chain bends around and brings the β-pleated sheet segments close together. In this manner, β-pleated sheet segments of a polypeptide chain that are far apart in the linear sequence can be close together in space. This hydrogen-bond interaction between β-pleated sheet segments is one of the mechanisms where a tertiary structure of proteins can be formed.

The α-Helix

A helix is a tubular spiral configuration. The α-helix is a type of secondary protein structure that occurs when there is a particular short repeating sequence of amino acids in the primary structure. Within segments of a polypeptide chain where the α-helix secondary structure occurs every backbone N-H group of the sequence forms a hydrogen a hydrogen bond to the C=O group of the amino acid located three or four positions along the protein sequence. One complete turn of an α-helix is about 13 amino acids in length. As with the β-pleated sheet, the α-helix structure is stabilized by hydrogen bonds between amino acids that are close together in the helical configuration. **The α-helix segments of a polypeptide chain often precede or follow a** β-pleated sheet segment allowing the polypeptide chain to bend or change direction.

One very important mechanical feature of the **α-helix and of most helical molecular structures in the body is that the helix is able to stretch or compress along the long axis of the helix but resists stretching or compression in other directions**

Random Secondary Structure

A third type of secondary structure in a polypeptide chain is actual not a structure at all. It is a segment of amino acids that do not interact to form a stable structure such as a α-helix or a β-pleated sheet. These segments or often flexible in three dimensions acting like segments of rope. These sections allow the polypeptide chain to bend and flex wherever they occur. This gives the polypeptide chain the ability to form a vast array of complex configurations in three dimensions. Together the three forms of secondary structures determine the unique configuration that a polypeptide chain forms in three dimensions. This three-dimensional configuration is called the tertiary structure of a single chain protein.

Tertiary Protein Structure

The three-dimensional configuration of a single chain protein results from the interactions of the secondary structures of the protein. As the protein is being assembled within a cell, the secondary structures interact with the aqueous environment and with each other and the protein begins to fold in three dimensions. As the protein continues to be formed. Much more complex configurations begin to emerge as regions of the three-dimensional structure are brought close together. Hydrogen bonding among amino acids in these regions stabilize the larger structures and **covalent disulfide bonds** between cysteine amino acids form to provide permanent crosslinks of the polypeptide chain within the tertiary structure of the chain. This folding, hydrogen-bonding and disulfide-crosslinking of the polypeptide chain is incredibly complex and can produce a virtually unlimited number of complex protein structures that are capable of carrying out tens of thousands of unique structural and chemical functions within the human body.

Quaternary Protein Structures

While many functional proteins in the human body are single chain polypeptide proteins, many others are composed of two or more polypeptide chains. The geometric shape of the overall multi peptide-chain protein is the quaternary structure of the protein. It should be noted that the definition of a gene is a continuous region of DNA base sequences that code for a protein. This is true in the sense that all single polypeptide amino acid chains are by definition proteins. In the case of functional proteins composed of more than one type of single chain proteins it is not true that every functional protein in the body is coded for by one single gene. For instance, the protein hemoglobin is composed of four single chain proteins - two alpha chains and two beta chains. There are two different genes required to create a hemoglobin protein molecule. An alpha globin gene and a beta-globin gene.

Photosynthesis

Perhaps the most important biological reactions of all are the reactions of photosynthesis where chemical reactions within chloroplasts absorb energy in the form of photons of the visible light spectrum and use this energy to drive the reaction of carbon dioxide and water to produce glucose and oxygen. Notice that this is the reverse reaction of aerobic cellular respiration.

$$6CO_2 + 6H_2O + energy \rightarrow C_6H_{12}O_6 + 6O_2$$

With the introduction of photosynthesis and aerobic metabolism of glucose as examples of oxidation reduction reactions, we have transitioned to general types of chemical reaction to specific types of biochemical reactions. In the next section, we will discuss acid-base reactions and proceed to the important examples of acid base reactions that occur in the human body. This discussion begins with a review of the basics of acid-base reactions, beginning with a review of solution chemistry and the essential elements of acid and base dissociations in water.

Chemical Reactions in Solutions - Review
Nearly all biological chemical reactions occur in solutions. In a solution, the liquid that dissolves particles is called the solvent. For the HESI the solvent in a solution will almost certainly be water. The dissolved particles within the solvent are called solutes. Solutions where water is the solvent are called aqueous (aq) solutions.

Molar Concentration of Solutions - Review
The concentration of substances in solutions is usually given in unit of moles per liter. A mole is a numerical amount. The amount is 6.022×10^{23} particles. That is a huge number but atoms and molecules are incredibly small so it works out that this is a convenient number of particles to use experimentally for chemical reactions. A substance that has a concentration of 1 mole of substance/per liter of solution is defined to be a 1 molar solution of the substance or a 1M concentration of the substance

Aqueous (water) Solutions - Review
Liquid water is the ideal medium for acid-base reactions. Although water by definition is neutral, water exists in an equilibrium with hydrogen and hydroxide ions. This is because water undergoes the following reaction

H_2O (l) $\rightleftharpoons$ H+(aq) + OH-(aq)

At equilibrium, pure liquid water contains concentrations of 1×10^{-7} M of H+ and 1×10^{-7} M of OH- ions.

pH - Review
For solutions that contain hydrogen ions (H+), the negative log of the hydrogen ion concentration is defined as the pH of the solution. As we discussed, in pure liquid water, the hydrogen ion concentration is 1×10^{-7}. Therefore, the ph of pure liquid water is 7. This is by definition a neutral pH, Solutions with higher concentrations of H+ have pH values lower than 7. These solutions are defined as acidic solutions. Solutions with lower concentrations of H+ have pH values higher than 7. These solutions are defined as basic solutions. The pH of body fluids in humans is tightly regulated to an ideal pH of 7.4

Acids - Review
Acids are molecules that, in solution, partially or nearly completely dissociate into hydrogen ions and a conjugate base. One definition of an acid is that an acid is a proton (hydrogen ion) donor molecule.

A general formula an acid dissociation reaction is

HA(aq) $\rightleftharpoons$ H+(aq) + A- (aq)

HA is the acid and A- is the acid's conjugate base

Strong Acids
The strongest acids, in aqueous solutions at 1 molar concentrations, will completely or nearly completely dissociate into hydrogen ions and the acid's conjugate base. For the HESI, hydrochloric acid (HCl) is almost always the strong acid that is participating in chemical reactions. One should also know that sulfuric acid (H_2SO_4) is also a strong acid

For example, in an aqueous solution a 0.1 M solution of the strong acid HCL will completely dissociate as given by the following reaction

HCL $\rightarrow$ H+ + Cl-

Since one molecule of HCL dissociates into one proton and one Cl- ion, the concentration of H+ in the solution will be 0.1 M or 1×10^{-1} moles/liter, Therefore the pH of the solution will be 1

Weak Acids
In aqueous solutions, weak acids only partially dissociate into a hydrogen ions and conjugate bases. As a general example consider a 1 molar aqueous solution

of the weak acid HA with a measured pH of 5. The pH of the solution indicates that 1 mole of the weak acid HA partially dissociates into 1×10^{-4} moles of hydrogen ion and 1×10^{-5} moles of the conjugate base. This means only one acid molecule in 100,000 has dissociated into hydrogen ion and conjugate base. A 1M concentration of a strong acid such as HCL would nearly completely dissociate into 1 M of hydrogen ion and 1 M of conjugate base. This would result in a pH of 0 for the solution (since the H+ concentration written in exponential form is 1×10^{0} M). In this example, a 1M solution of HCl is 100,000 times stronger than the 1M solution of the weak acid HA.

Bases

Bases, by one definition, are molecules that accept hydrogen ions. Notice the general reaction for this definition of a base is the reverse of the general acid reaction

$$A- + H+ \rightleftharpoons HA$$

This is why A- is referred to as the conjugate base of an acid.

In aqueous solutions, the hydrogen ion acceptor is usually the hydroxide ion OH-. When this is the case, another way to represent a general dissociation of a base is

$$BOH \rightleftharpoons B+ + OH-$$

Strong bases will completely dissociate in 1 M solutions. For instance, a 1 molar solution of potassium hydroxide NaOH (a strong base) will completely dissociate as follows

$$NaOH(aq) \rightarrow Na+(aq) + OH-(aq)$$

For the HESI assume that strong bases have a 1 molar solution pH of 14. In contrast, weak bases do not completely dissociate and for the HESI assume that they have 1 molar solution pHs of greater than 7 and less than 14.

Acid-Base Reactions

The general formula for an acid (Ha) and base (BOH)

reaction is shown below

$$HA + BOH \rightleftharpoons BA + H_2O$$

The compound "BA" is referred to as the "**salt**" of an acid -base reaction.

An example of an acid base reaction between a strong acid (HCl) and a strong base (NaOH) is shown below

$$HCl + NaOH \rightarrow NaCl + H_2O$$

Notice that the salt produced by this reaction is an ionic compound; in this case the ionic compound NaCl. It is typical that salts formed by acid-base reactions are (in their solid form) ionic compounds. In water - which is a strong polar solvent - a substantial fraction of the salt that is produced by an acid -base reaction often is dissolved in the form of the ions that compose the crystal structure of the salt. In the case of the aqueous HCl/NaOH acid -base reaction, at equilibrium, there will be substantial amounts of Na+ and Cl- ions dissolved in the aqueous solution.

The actual amounts of dissolved ions in an aqueous solution for a given acid base reaction depend on the properties of the specific salt that is formed. Many salts are very insoluble in water and will precipitate out of the aqueous solution as solid salt crystals rather than remain dissolved as ions in the aqueous solution.

Acid-Base Reactions in Biology

In living organisms, there are very important acid-base reactions that must occur. Living organisms must maintain a carefully regulated narrow range of pH values for the fluids located inside of their bodies. This range for humans is between pH of 7.35 and 7.45. The metabolic processes of living organisms produce organic acids as waste products, and these acids must be neutralized or excreted from the body, otherwise the organism's internal fluids will become increasingly acidic and will rapidly reach fatally low pH levels. One of the most important series of reactions used by biological organisms to neutralize and/or excrete excess acid involve reactions involving the weak acid **carbonic acid.**

Recall that a fundamental reaction of aerobic metabolism is the production of carbon dioxide and water from the oxidation of glucose

$$C_6H_{12}O_6 + 6O_2 \rightarrow 6CO_2 + 6H_2O + energy$$

Within the fluids contained inside of an organism, carbon dioxide reacts with water to form carbonic acid.

$$CO_2 + H_2O \rightleftharpoons H_2CO_3$$

Carbonic acid is a weak acid and partially dissociates to hydrogen ion and the bicarbonate anion

$$H_2CO_3 \rightleftharpoons H+ + HCO_3-$$

As CO_2 is produced within an organism the concentration of CO_2 increases and this drives the forward reaction with water resulting in increasing amounts of hydrogen ion. If this process continues unchecked, ultimately the pH of the organism's internal fluids will reach toxic and eventually fatal acidic pH levels. To avoid this human remove CO_2 from the body via the respiratory system. This lowers the concentration of CO_2 to levels where the carbonic acid reactions produce acceptable levels of hydrogen ion at equilibrium.

In humans and many other organisms, the body can use the carbolic acid reactions to rid itself of excess hydrogen ions that are generated by organic acid waste products. The kidneys are able to excrete hydrogen ion and in the process, are able to generate bicarbonate anions in the body. These bicarbonate ions can react with hydrogen ions to produce carbonic acid which then can decompose into carbon dioxide and H_2O. The carbon dioxide produced in this fashion can also be exhaled. This further reduces the hydrogen ion concentration in the body and allows the body to maintain an optimum pH level. The pancreas also produces bicarbonate ion that is secreted into the intestine where it neutralizes the very acidic contents that pass into the intestines from the stomach.

Catalysts are substances that increase the rate of chemical reactions without themselves being transformed or consumed by the chemical reaction. In non-biological systems - usually involving industrial chemical processes. Catalysts are often finely ground metals that provide a huge surface area for reaction to occur. An example is the platinum pellets in an automobile's catalytic converter that increases the rates of combustion reactions so that the auto exhaust has reduced amounts of partially combusted gasoline products (the noxious fumes that comprise the majority of airborne "smog" pollution found in most large cities).

Reaction Yields and Reaction Rates

Catalysts do not increase the yield of a chemical reaction. The yield is the number of products produced by a chemical reaction and that is determined by the concentrations of reactants and products and by the energy that is produced by the reactions. If the products of a reaction are not removed the reaction eventually reaches equilibrium where no further increase in the number of products occurs. Catalysts increase the rate of these reactions. The rate of a reaction is the amount of product produced per unit time. When a catalyst participates in a chemical reaction, the reaction reaches equilibrium much faster than it would without the participation of the catalyst.

Activation Energy of Chemical Reactions

The rate of chemical reactions is determined by the activation energy of the reaction. This is determined by the physical **transition state** than occurs among atoms of the reactants as they are converted into products. This transition state is of higher energy than either the reactant or product molecules and represents an **energy barrier** that must be overcome for the reaction to proceed in either the forward or reverse direction.

Catalysts lower the activation energy of the transition state and consequently the forward and reverse chemical reactions are much more likely to occur. This results in an increase reaction rate. Inorganic catalysts such as the platinum in catalytic converters do this by providing huge surface area where reactant molecules can briefly bind to the catalyst and in the process, be brought very close to other reactants that are also briefly bonded to the catalytic surface. This makes the reaction much more probable and this effectively lowers the energy of the reaction's transition state.

Enzymes

Enzymes are **biological catalysts**. They are not simple metallic surfaces but extremely complex three-dimensional protein structures. They lower activation energies of biological reactions by attracting reactants to a specific site on the enzyme known as the **active site**. As reactants bind to the active site, the configuration of the site changes in a manner that orients the reactants in the optimum manner for the chemical reaction to occur. This process is called the **"induced fit" mechanism** for enzymatic activity. **The activity of an enzyme is defined as the rate at which the reaction catalyzed by the enzyme occurs.** The higher the enzyme activity, the greater the rate of enzyme catalyzed reaction

Enzyme Activity

The activity of an enzyme depends on the **concentration of the reactants and products** of the reaction and the **temperature** and **pH** under which the reactions occur. Enzymes will have an optimum temperature and pH range for maximal activity. In general, the reaction rate doubles for every increase of 10 degrees Celsius, but beyond an upper-temperature level the enzymes structure is thermally disrupted and the enzyme ceases to function. Similar structural disruptions occur at pH ranges outside of the enzymes activity range.

Enzyme Denaturation and Inhibition

The term for both **the thermal and pH disruptions that deactivate enzymes** is denaturalization. A denatured enzyme or other protein is usually permanently dysfunctional. The activity of enzymes can also be reduced by molecules that can interfere with the chemical reactions at the active site. This process is called enzymatic inhibition. Inhibitor molecules can reduce enzyme activity by various mechanisms, commonly by **physically blocking the active site**. This form of inhibition is called **competitive inhibition**. Other forms of inhibition are termed **noncompetitive or uncompetitive inhibition.** These other forms of inhibition are often utilized as a means for the body to regulate the activity of enzymes.

This concludes the discussion of the basic chemical level of organization that is found in living organisms.

The following section addresses the next level of organization the specific biochemical and chemical and physical processes that occur in living organisms

Proteins and Biology

We have now discussed most of the basic chemical reactions and the basic molecules involved in the processes that generate energy in cells and that form the physical building blocks of cells and extracellular substrates. We have also discussed the fundamental physics that underlie nearly all of the chemical and physical processes that are essential to the functioning of living organisms. In the next section, we will continue with discussions of proteins and their role in living organisms. These discussions will also be used to begin to introduce many of the most important aspects of human cellular and general anatomy and physiology.

Structural Proteins

One of the primary functions of proteins in the human body is to provide a physical structure for elements within the body. These may be microscopic structures inside of cells and in the extracellular spaces between cells or they may be macroscopic structures that extend over body surfaces These structural proteins are designed to provide the mechanical properties that are required by the structural role that they provide. These properties also are designed to respond in particular ways to the forces that the proteins experience in their structural roles. Some roles require that the proteins have the ability to stretch or flex in one or more directions, but to resist forces in other directions. In general, structural proteins have an overall **fibrillar** (fiber-like) shape - as opposed to globular proteins, which typically have enzymatic or transport functions.

Collagen

The most important extracellular structural protein is collagen. There are many different forms of collagen, each with its own unique mechanical properties. The collagen found in **bone** is rigid, in in tendons that connect muscles to bone, collagen is elastic and able to stretch and relax as muscles contract and relax. Collagen in **cartilage** has mechanical properties intermediate between rigidity and elasticity in its role of providing a protective layer over the ends of bones at movable **joints** and as structural elements in the nose, ears and within the skeletal system and elsewhere throughout the body. Collagen also is a major component of **ligaments** - which connect bones at joints - and in the **integumentary system** where it provides the ability of skin to stretch but to resist mechanical penetration by foreign objects and to contain the internal contents of the body. Collagen is also a major structural element of **blood vessels**.

Overall collagen comprises approximately 30% of the total protein mass of the human body. Collagen is synthesized by many types of cells but the most important producer is the **fibroblast cells**. These cells are found throughout the body and are constantly producing collagen particularly in **i**nflammation and **tissue regeneration and repair** processes.

Collagen is a **three peptide-chain protein** with a quaternary **triple-helix structure** composed of two alpha-1 single strand proteins and an alpha-2 strand protein. Therefore, two genes are required to produce collagen - an alpha-1 collagen gene and an alpha-2 collagen gene. As we mentioned helical molecular structures are often able to stretch and compress in response to mechanical forces but resist such forces in other directions. This is a primary structural property of collagen

After the collagen strands are constructed they undergo **post-translational modification** where some of the **amino acids of the collagen strand are hydroxylated** (a hydroxyl group is created on the amino acid). This type of modification of proteins is common in protein synthesis. In collagen, this hydroxylation process allows covalent bonds to form **cross-links** between the three collagen strands as they form a triple helix. **Vitamin C** is required to this cross-linking process. Vitamin C deficiency results in a failure of the collagen fiber crosslinking which severely weakens the strength of collagen leading to structural failure of the cartilage in skin, tendons, ligaments and blood vessels. This is the disease process known as **scurvy**. Scurvy is fatal if not corrected by adequate vitamin C intake.

Keratin

Keratin is the other major extracellular structural protein in humans. It provides protective and mechanical support to the outer layers of skin and also is the primary component of **hair and nails** in humans. In other animals, it also forms horns and claws. Keratin is composed of individual keratin filaments which are single polypeptide chains. These chains combine to form intermediate filaments which are multiple keratin filaments that are held together first by hydrogen bonds, then by disulfide bonds and finally by covalent fiber cross links similar to those found in collagen. The keratin intermediate filaments then form a three-dimensional **supercoiled helix** that is extremely tough but has very high elasticity in the long axis of the supercoiled helix. This can be seen macroscopically by plucking a hair from one's head and pulling the strand from either end. In young healthy persons, the hair strand when wet can be stretched to up to 50% of its original length.

Fibrillin and Elastin

Fibrillin is a protein and elastin is a glycoprotein that combine to form **elastic fiber** which is found throughout the extracellular regions of the body. Both fibrillin and elastin form fibers. In elastic fibers elastin fibers are randomly arranged and fibrillin fibers embedded linear arrangements. The result - elastic fibers are extremely resilient - they can flex, stretch and compress in all directions in response to external mechanical forces and then rapidly return to their original shape after the forces have dissipated. This ability allows elastic fiber to act as a **"shock absorbers'** in regions of the body subject to strong mechanical forces, such and the intervertebral discs of the spinal; column. Elastic fibers are found usually with collagen fibers in the skin and throughout the body. Elastic fiber is an important component of the **extracellular matrix** which forms **internal frameworks** for the cells that form tissues and organs and also form larger framework structures within the body. This structural matrix surrounds and supports internal organs and larger structures, allowing these structures to expand and contract, bend and shift positions within the body but to retain their overall relative positions within the body. Fibrillin also has many functions within cells as well.

Intracellular Structural Proteins

In humans, cells are not simple distensible balloon-like structures - they have an internal structure called the cytoskeleton. The cytoskeleton is a complex three-dimensional framework the provides structural support to the cell and also is involved in intracellular transport and other cellular functions. The cytoskeleton is not a static construct, it is constantly undergoing disassembly and reassembly in response to the needs of the cell. The cytoskeleton is composed of a cytoskeletal matrix. The matrix is primarily composed of **three types of protein filaments** (thread-like structures) - microfilaments, microtubules and intermediate filaments.

Microtubules

Microtubules are the largest diameter of the three general types of cytoskeletal filaments. Microtubules are hollow cylinders that are composed of two types of protein monomers (single-unit building blocks) -alpha-tubulin and beta-tubulin. The **tubulin proteins** are spherical and form alpha-beta pairs called dimers. These dimers often **self-assemble and disassemble rapidly** in response to various conditions within the cell. The microtubules participate in many functions of the cytoskeleton including vesicle transport but their most notable role occurs during **mitosis and meiosis** phases of a cell cycle.

During these **cell division** phases, microtubule organizing structures called **centrosomes** coordinate the formation of **microtubule "spindles"** that are composed of microtubules attached to chromosomes and two one of two centrosomes located at opposite poles of the cell during mitosis and meiosis. When the microtubules begin to disassemble near the centrosome, the tubules shorten and **chromosomes are pulled apart to opposite sides of the cell.**

Microtubules are also major elements of the **flagellum of sperm cells.** They form the core of the flagellum and interact with a centrosome-like microtubule organizing center at the base of the flagellum that coordinates sliding motions between microtubules within the flagellum. These sliding motions are powered by protein complexes called **dynein arms** located along the length of the microtubules. The sliding motions cause the flagellum to bend laterally - alternately in one direction and then the opposite direction. This results in a rapid whip-like motion of the flagellum that propels sperm cells in their journey through the uterus in an attempt to fuse with a female ovum.

Intermediate Filaments

Intermediate filaments are the most stable elements of the cytoskeleton. these filaments organize to form a complex three-dimensional framework throughout the cell that provides local support and spatial organization to all of the cell organelles - the nucleus, endoplasmic reticulum, golgi, mitochondria, cell vesicles and cell vacuoles. It also provides an underlying structural framework for the cell membrane which results in the specific **three-dimensional shape of the cell.** Intermediate filaments are formed from keratin like protein fibers. In addition to their structural role, the intermediate fiber framework also serves as a convey belt system for the transport of vesicles and their contents from the golgi or other regions inside to cell to the cell membrane, where the vesicles merge with the cell membrane and release the vesicle contents to the extracellular environment. This process is a specific example of the general process of exocytosis.

Microfilaments

Microfilaments are the smallest diameter of the three intracellular structural filaments. They are composed primarily of subunits of actin. **Actin** is a protein that has ATPase activity - it can hydrolyze ATP and use the energy of ATP hydrolysis to interact with other proteins and when organized into microfilaments - **actively move** along the length of the other proteins. This ability allows microfilaments to engage in a wide variety of functions within cells. It can serve as the "vehicle" that transports vesicles along the cytoskeleton of cell and can organize at the interior of cell membranes to dynamically reshape membranes - resulting in the ability of cells to phagocytize external substances (including other cells) by extending local regions of cell membrane around external substances and enveloping the external substance.

Actin Microfilament Related Cellular Processes

Cytokinesis

Actin microfilaments are also responsible for the physical separation of a single cell into two cells in a process that occurs at the end of a **mitotic or meiotic cell replication cycle**. The microfilaments create an encircling belt at the cell membrane that is drawn progressively tighter and eventually pinches the original cell into two new separate cells.

Cell Contraction
Many cell types are capable of actively contracting or shortening. All types of muscle cells - skeletal, cardiac and smooth muscle cells - are designed to contract and relax in response to various types of stimuli. In all cases actin microfilaments play a central role in the contraction and relaxation process.

Thin and Thick Filaments in Muscle Cells
In skeletal and cardiac muscle cells, **actin** and **tropomyosin** protein filaments and attached **troponin** protein molecules form a composite filament called a **thin filament**. During cell contraction, thin filaments slide between **myosin protein thick filaments**. This shortens or contracts the cell. The process is powered by ATPase (ATP hydrolysis) sites located on the myosin molecule. The free end of the myosin thick fibers has "heads" which are specialized regions of the protein that can swing back and forth and can also form crosslink bonds with troponin molecules, Troponin molecules are evenly spaced a short distance apart along the entire length of the thin fibers located on the thin fibers that are attached to actin microfilaments.

Electrical signal from nerves or adjacent muscle cell membranes trigger the **release of calcium ions** (Ca++) from a vesicular intracellular structure in the muscle cells called the **sarcoplasmic reticulum**. The calcium ions diffuse to and bind with troponin proteins which then **form crosslink bonds** with adjacent myosin fiber heads. The Myosin heads pivot or shift the crosslink bond site backwards and draws the thin filament further along myosin thick filament. The crosslink it subsequently broken during ATP hydrolysis occurring at myosin ATPase sites and the myosin head site swings forward and can then bind to another troponin molecule located further along the thin filament. In this manner actin fibers are grabbed like rungs of a ladder and pulled progressively further along the myosin fiber and the muscle cell progressively shortens.

Cell Motility
A wide variety of cell types in the human body are capable of independent locomotion. In particular, macrophages and other types of white blood cells, and fibroblasts are capable of actively traveling from virtually any region of the body to any other region of the body. This motion is accomplished by a coordinated extension and retraction of portions of the cell membrane. These local cellular extrusions are called pseudopods. **Pseudopods** are capable of attaching to various molecules in the extracellular matrix. This process is called cellular adhesion. Using pseudopod motions and cellular adhesion, motile cells are able to continuously creep along and squeeze through intercellular spaces. Pseudopod motion depends on a continuous reshaping of cell membranes that is produced by the activity of actin microfilaments.

Diapedesis
A closely related activity to pseudopod motion in motile cell is diapedesis. Motile cells generally begin their journeys to a particular target destination when they are circulating in blood vessels. When they detect signal molecules that have diffused from a target site that trigger the motile cells to leave the blood vessel and move into the intracellular space. This **movement out of the blood vessel** requires that the motile cell adheres to the interior wall of the vessel and then deform in a manner that allows it to ooze or **squeeze in between adjacent cells** that form the vessel wall. This process is called diapedesis and predictably it is also an active cell reshaping process that depends on the movements of actin fibers.

Chemotaxis
Chemotaxis is a process where motile cells are recruited to move to a region of the body where their particular functions are required. The process begins with the production of chemoattractant molecules at the target site that subsequently diffuse outward. This diffusion process creates a **concentration gradient** extending from the site where the chemoattractant was produced. When a motile cell detects a chemoattractant molecule that it is designed to respond to, the cell begins to move in the direction of the molecules. The cell continues moving towards the target site by selecting a direction of motion that corresponds to progressively higher

concentrations of the chemoattractant. In this fashion, the cell follows the chemoattractant molecules concentration gradient back to its source.

Endocytosis

Phagocytosis is an extreme example of the general process of endocytosis. While most cell types in the human body are not capable of phagocytosis, many cell types are capable of ingesting small molecules from the cell membranes and internalizing them in small membrane bound vesicles. This general process of endocytosis occurs in the same fashion as described for phagocytosis.

Phagocytosis

Usually, phagocytized substances are bacteria, injured or virally infected cells or remnants of cells and extracellular matrix substance fragments that require clearance during immune response and tissue repair and regeneration activities. Phagocytosis begins with the binding of a substance, virus or cell to the outer cell membrane. Actin microfilaments and other proteins begin to envelop the target substance, the enveloping cell membrane segment invaginates (draws into the cell) and pinches off, forming an intracellular membrane bound vesicle. These vesicles can be transported within the cell and other vesicles can be brought to the phagocytic vesicle and merged with the vesicle. Often this cellular vesicle is a **lysosome or a proteasome** - which contains powerful oxidizing chemicals or digestive enzymes. When the two vesicles merge the contents of the phagocytized vesicle are subjected to the effects of the lysosome or proteasome and the contents are chemically and enzymatically digested.

Exocytosis

The general process of transporting intracellular vesicles to an internal surface of a cell membrane and then fusing the vesicle membrane to the cell membrane so that the vesicle is turned inside out and empties its contents to the external environment is called exocytosis. Antigen presentation is a variation of exocytosis where the antigens within the vesicle remain bound to the vesicle membrane and thus become molecules attached to the external surface of the cell membrane. In all other cases the contents of intracellular vesicle are released into the extracellular environments. Nearly all of the products of cells are delivered to the rest of the body beginning with the process of exocytosis. The transport and vesicle-membrane fusion events of exocytosis are carried out by the movements of actin microfilaments.

Antigen Presentation

There are a wide variety of cell types in the human body that are capable of phagocytosis. The primary function of several of these cell types is phagocytosis. The most notable type of these in the human body are **macrophages**. Macrophages play central roles in tissue repair and regeneration activities and are critical to many immune system responses. This role is complex but it often begins with the phagocytosis of a foreign biological product - a virus infected cell, an infectious foreign cell such as bacteria or other foreign substances.

After these infectious elements are phagocytized and broken down into smaller digestive molecular remnants, actin filaments can transport these small molecular remnants to the cell membrane of the macrophage. These small molecular remnants are classified as **antigens**. Antigens have unique molecular structures that can be **recognized by other immune cells as foreign or non-self**. The detection of foreign antigens by the immune system triggers the body's immune response. These **antigens can be anchored to the external surface of the macrophage cell membrane.** This process is call antigen presentation and cell that have the ability to phagocytize foreign substances and then present the antigens derived from the ingested foreign substance are called antigen presenting cells. We will discuss additional features of antigen presentation shortly.

Cell-Membrane Associated Proteins

The adult human body is comprised of over 37 trillion cells Every one of these cells engages in complex function that are regulated and coordinated at the individual cell level, at the local cell region level at the level of tissue function, at the level of organ and organ system function and finally at a level of total body function. There are a staggering number of molecular interactions and chemical pathways that are involved in this orchestration of cooperative cell activity. An understanding of these processes can be appreciated by recognizing that most of this activity is mediated by cell-membrane associated proteins. These proteins can be classified as cell surface proteins, transmembrane proteins and inner-cell membrane proteins.

Cell Surface Membrane Proteins (Outer Cell Membrane Proteins)

Cell surface or outer cell membrane associated proteins are proteins that are embedded in the outer layer of the cell membrane phospholipid bilayer. They are exposed to the local external environment of the cell. They can be single proteins, modified protein molecules such as glycoproteins including membrane bound antibodies or members of multiprotein based molecular complexes. There are two general categories of protein and modified protein molecules that are localized to the outer cell membrane. These are the **cell surface markers** and **cell receptors.**

Cell Markers

Cell markers are displayed on the outer surface cell membrane. Most of these markers are considered to be **cell surface antigens**, that help identify and classify cells. The set of markers are unique to different cell types, for each cell type there are specific combinations of markers or antigens. These molecules serve not only as markers but they also have key functional roles as well. One of the distinctive features of most cell markers is that they usually are the targets of the other general type of protein-based cell surface molecule - cell receptors

Human Leucocyte Antigens (HLA)

One of the major categories of theses cell marker proteins are the **human leukocyte antigens (HLA)** protein cell markers. HLA cell markers are the proteins that are encoded in a set of genes called the **major histocompatibility complex (MHC)**. the MHC codes for 6 major HLA antigen-presenting proteins. Three of these are **MHC class I antigens** - HLA-A, HLA-B and HLA-C. The remaining three proteins are the **MHC class II antigens** - HLA-DR, HLA-DQ and HLA-DP.

There are a large number of different variations (alleles) of all six of the MHC genes. The particular set of MHC class I and II HLA proteins that are located on the cells of any particular individual are almost certainly different from any other non-blood related individual. (the offspring of the same two parents have a 25% chance of having the same set of HLA cell markers). This combination of the alleles of the 6 HLA type markers is therefore a fairly unique code or personal identification number that **identifies all the cells of an individual's body as "self"**. The immune system of an individual is programmed to recognize this code on the membranes of cells a proof that the cells are in fact member of the cells that belong to an individual's body. This HLA code is also referred to as an individual's **"tissue type"**. The tissue type of an individual can be precisely determined (phenotyping)For purposes of **organ or tissue transplant**s. Mismatches in HLA antigens from donor organs are the major trigger for **immune rejection** of the organ in transplant recipients.

Foreign Antigens

The primary role of the HLA antigens is in the immune system. Each of the six HLA class proteins are antigens. Antigens are usually small proteins or segments of proteins, glycoproteins or glycolipids. Most antigens are recognized by immune system cells - macrophages, natural killer cells and T-cells - as foreign or non-self molecular subunit structures. These foreign antigens are small molecular segments of a molecular toxin, virus or infectious organism. The immune system recognizes that these fragments do not normally exists as segments of the molecules that are produced by an individual's body. They indicate to the immune system that a specific foreign protein, virus or an infectious organism has invaded the body. Theses antigens trigger an immune response against these antigens and any other substance or organism that contains these antigens.

MHC Class I Antigens (HLA-A, -B and -C)

The HLA-A, B and C are involved primarily in immune responses where **a cell of the body has been infected with virus or other intracellular pathogen** (disease causing organism or other substance). Antigens resulting from intracellular digestion of the pathogen result in fragments of the pathogen that can be transported to the cell membrane surface where they can be recognized as foreign antigens. These **foreign antigens are presented in combination with a MHC class I HLA surface antigen**. This foreign antigen-HLA class I antigen complex attracts a specific cell type of the immune system - a **cytotoxic or killer -T Cell.** When a cytotoxic T-cell binds to this complex it is stimulated to kill the infected cell.

MHC Class II Antigens (HLA-DR, -DQ and -DP)

While the MHC I HLA antigens are involved in identifying cells of the body that have been infected and are therefore targets of destruction by cytotoxic T-Cells, the MHC class II HLA antigens - HLA-DR, DQ and DP - participate in immune responses to pathogens that have invaded the body but are located outside of cells.

Antigen-Presenting Cells

Antigen-presenting cells (APCs) are a class of immune cells that mediate the cellular immune response by processing and presenting foreign antigens that they have acquired - usually by phagocytosis or endocytosis - from the extracellular environment for recognition by certain lymphocytes such as T cells. We have already discussed the topic. of antigen presentation for macrophages but other cells also can present antigens as well - these cell types include dendritic cells, Langerhans cells and B cells.

T-Helper Cells

Ingested pathogens, products of pathogen and fragments of pathogens are digested within the antigen presenting cells and the antigen fragments resulting from this intracellular digestion are then transported to the cell membrane and presented on the cell surface along with a MHC class II HLA antigen. This **foreign antigen- MCH class II HLA antigen complex** is recognized by another type of T-cell - the **T-helper cell.** The T-helper cell that recognizes this complex has been pre-formed or primed to recognize only the specific foreign antigen presented on the cell.

The T-helper cell T-receptor has a precise region that is a molecular structure that almost perfectly conform to the molecular structure of the foreign antigen. This allows the T-cell receptor to fit to the antigen like a glove over a hand. This may seem to be an impossible coincidence since there are millions of possible molecular structures for foreign antigens, but T-helper cell receptors come in tens to hundreds of thousands of different variations. Antigen presenting cells always can encounter at least a few T-cells that have receptors that will be sufficiently complementary any particular foreign antigen molecular structures that is presented by the antigen presenting cell.

Once the antigen presenting cell finds a complementary T-cell for its foreign antigens, the T-helper cell binds and this activates the T-cell to initiate the processes that lead to the production of large amounts of antibodies that then circulate throughout the body in search of any cell or other substance that contains the foreign antigen. These antibodies are perfectly designed to bind to the specific foreign antigens whenever and wherever they encounter the antigens anywhere in the body. This is called the **antigen-specific immune response.**

Classification Determinant (CD) Cell Surface Markers

CD (cluster of designation or classification determinant) cell surface marker classification is a protocol used for the identification and investigation of cell surface molecules providing targets for immunophenotyping of cells. In terms of physiology, CD molecules can act in numerous ways, often acting as receptors or ligands (the molecule that activates a receptor) important to the cell. A signal cascade is usually initiated, altering the behavior of the cell. Some CD proteins do not play a role in cell signaling, but have other functions, such as cell adhesion.

Cell Biology

The cell is the fundamental living unit of all organisms. In the case of single-cell organisms, the cell is obviously the entire living organism. When many cells are organized to create a multicellular organism, the individual cells are usually specialized to serve specific functions within the organism. The broadest category of these functions is summarized below.

Primary Functions of Living Organisms

On a continuous basis, complex multicellular organisms must continuously adapt to external conditions in order to identify and acquire needed resources and to identify and avoid risks to survival that are present in the external environment. For animals, this includes the abilities of the nervous system to sense the external environmental conditions and to adapt as needed to these conditions.

Adaptation and Voluntary Movements

An important method that animals use to adapt - as the nervous system deems necessary - to their environment is locomotion – are voluntary movements generated by the musculoskeletal system. Pursuit of prey, avoidance of predators and gathering all manner of physical resources requires locomotion. At a higher level, the propagation of a species requires that male and female members sexually reproduce and subsequently rear offspring. All of these activities require continuous adaptation and physical activities of the voluntary muscle to generate these long-term and complex behaviors.

General Body Functions

At a more fundamental level, the physical acts of ingesting water and nutrients and of obtaining oxygen and expelling carbon dioxide via breathing are also functions that require muscular motion. The absorption of water and processing of nutrients into a form that can be distributed throughout the body require digestion and the transport of oxygen, water, nutrients and waste products requires a circulatory system. The elimination of wastes requires an excretory system. Production of offspring requires sexual reproductive systems and the regulation of overall body functions requires both a nervous and an endocrine system.

The Cell

The cell is the smallest unit of life. There are other biological entities that show many characteristics of living organism. Most notable of these are viruses and infectious protein particles called prions. Viruses and prions are incapable of survival without parasitizing living cells.

Universal Features of Cells

Cell Membranes - Review

We have discussed the details of the structure of human cells membranes. In Summary: All cells have a number of universal features. First all cells have a cell membrane that separates the internal contents of the cell from the cell's external environment. This membrane is a bilayer of long, linear phospholipid molecules -hydrocarbon chains that are attached as chain pairs to a phosphate group at one end of the molecule. The phosphate "heads" of molecules face outward in the outer layer of the membrane bilayer and inward in the inner layer; thus, forming the exterior and interior surfaces of the cell membrane. The hydrocarbon chains or "tails "of the molecule aligned and face inward toward the center of the bilayer.

Cytoplasm: All cells contain cytoplasm. Cytoplasm consists of the material enclosed within a cell membrane with the exception of the material enclosed within the membrane of the cell nucleus (the nuclear membrane). The contents of the nucleus are called the **nucleoplasm.** Cytoplasm includes all of the cell organelles and the **cytosol** which is the gel-like aqueous (watery) solution the fills the interior of the cell. The cytosol consists primarily of water but also contains countless other dissolved chemicals and proteins.

Nucleic Acids, Enzymes and Other Proteins: All cells contain nucleic acids - DNA and RNA molecules These are the genetic information molecules of the cell. All cells have proteins that can replicate DNA within the cell. All cells have enzymes that can convert an energy source - sunlight or chemicals obtained from the outside environments - into high energy molecules that can drive other chemical reactions within a cell.

Ribosomes: All cells contain ribosomes. Ribosomes are small spherical complexes of proteins and RNA that can read messenger RNA transcripts and assemble the proteins coded for in the mRNA. The ribosomes assemble these proteins from individual amino acids that are dissolved in the cell cytosol. The ribosomes of bacterial cells are considerably different in structure compared to the ribosomes of human cells. For this reason, **many antibacterial drugs are designed to attack the bacterial ribosome**. The differences between the bacterial ribosome and human ribosomes are sufficient that the antibacterial drugs will not affect the human ribosomes

Cytoskeleton -Review

All human cells contain a cytoskeleton. We have

discussed the elements of the cytoskeleton in detail, to summarize this structural system provides mechanical support and numerous other intracellular functions. The three primary components of the cytoskeleton are actin-protein microfilaments, intermediate filaments and microtubules.

Common Features of Cells

Cell Walls

Depending on the type of cell, there are common structures and organelles that cells often possess. Cell walls are physical barriers or envelopes that exist exterior to the cell membrane. They are constructed of various types of molecules and are several times thicker than a cell membrane. **Bacterial cells** have cell walls are composed of complex structural arrangements of several types of molecules. **Plants** have cell walls composed of **cellulose** - a relatively simple sugar polymer and fungal cells have cell walls composed of **chitin** - another relatively simple sugar polymer. Animal cells do not possess cell walls. **Human cells do not possess cell walls.**

Bacterial cell walls are significant for medical science because they are not a feature shared with human cells and are therefore **a prime target for antibiotics** and other antibacterial treatments. A primary classification system for pathogenic (disease causing) bacteria is based on the **Gram-stain**. The Gram stain identifies two types of cell walls in bacteria - the **gram-positive** and the **gram-negative** bacteria have different molecular cell wall structures. This feature is very useful in the early stage of diagnosis and treatment of bacterial infections. In addition, a molecular component of gram-negative bacterial cell walls is **lipopolysaccharide (LPS)** is an extremely potent **toxin** that is a primary cause of **gram-negative sepsis** and **toxic shock**. Gram-negative sepsis a major cause of medical complications and death in hospitalized patients.

Flagella, Cilia and Pilli

Flagellum cilia and pili are extensions of cell membranes or attachments of cell membranes. Flagella are long whip-like energetically driven structures that can generate locomotion of a cell. The structure varies greatly. The flagella of bacteria are completely different than the flagella of protist or animal cells. Cilia are found on many unicellular organisms and on many specialized cells of multicellular organisms. They often have powered independent movement ability. Pili are tubular structures found in most bacterial cells that can transfer DNA from one bacterial cell to another.

Internal Organelles

The Nucleus

The nucleus is a major intracellular organelle. Cells that contain a nucleus are defined as **eukaryotic cells**. Those without a nucleus are defined as **prokaryotic cells**. Nearly all human cells contain a nucleus (mature red blood cells are a notable exception). Bacterial cells do not have a nucleus and are therefore prokaryotic cells. All other cells - plant, animal, protist and fungal cells - contain a nucleus and are therefore eukaryotic cells.

The nucleus is a **membrane-bound** structure that contains the **DNA** of a cell and the **nucleolus**. The nucleolus is a structure where ribosomes are constructed. There are **membrane pores** in the nuclear membrane that allow various small molecules to enter - primarily building blocks of DNA and RNA molecules. Nuclear pores also allow messenger RNA (mRNA) molecules and ribosomes to exit from the nucleus into the cell cytoplasm.

A much simpler, non-membrane-bound structure called the **nucleosome** contains the majority of DNA in **prokaryotic cells**.

Mitochondria and Chloroplasts

Mitochondria and chloroplasts are complex organelles that possess with both an inner and outer encapsulating membrane. Mitochondria are found in most of the cells of every eukaryotic organism. Chloroplasts are found in cells of all plants and a few types of protist cells. Chloroplasts contain the enzymes that are involved in photosynthesis -the conversion of sunlight water and carbon dioxide into carbohydrates and oxygen.

Mitochondria are present in nearly all eukaryotic cells including most human cells (again - as is the case with the cell nucleus - mature red blood cells are a notable exception.) We have discussed in detail the metabolic pathways of aerobic cellular respiration that occur in mitochondria - the Krebs or citric acid cycle, the electron transport chain and oxidative phosphorylation in detail to review: Mitochondria contain enzymes that extract chemical energy from nutrients - usually glucose molecules - and convert the energy into potential energy stored in high energy molecules - usually ATP or NADH. These high energy molecules are coupled to chemical reactions that require energy to proceed. Without this coupling, most of the synthesis of complex chemicals in the cell could not occur. Mitochondria and chloroplast are never found in prokaryotic cells.

Rough and Smooth Endoplasmic Reticulum (ER)

The endoplasmic reticulum (ER) is found in eukaryotic cells and is a convoluted network of membrane passageways that is connected to the cell nucleus and then continues extensively into the cell cytoplasm. **Smooth ER is involved in synthesis of lipid compounds** and the transport and packaging of various compounds produced by the cell. Smooth ER functions in close coordination with the Golgi apparatus. Rough ER (RER) is so called because **ribosomes are distributed in the RER membranes**, giving a granular or rough appearance to the RER membranes. Cells that produce large amounts of proteins for transport outside of the cell contain prominent amounts of RER.

The Golgi Apparatus (the Golgi)

The Golgi apparatus is found in almost all eukaryotic cells and in a much simpler form in prokaryotic cells. The Golgi is a highly folded series of membrane compartments that resembles a stack of pancakes. The Golgi functions with the smooth ER to **process, package and transport** a wide variety of products synthesized with the cell. Most often these products are packaged into **secretory vesicles** that are subsequently carried to the cell membrane and then secreted out of the cell into the external environment. In some types of cells, these vesicles remain inside the cell and are involved in intracellular digestion of phagocytized substances.

Centrosomes

Centrosomes are structures in eukaryotic cells that assemble and **organize microtubule structures**. These are required for a wide variety of purposes within the cell. They are for example central elements in the construction of **flagella in human sperm** cells and in the construction of the **spindle apparatus** during **mitosis and meiosis** stages of cell division.

Cellular Functions

At the most basic levels all of these higher adaptive and general functions require cellular functions - growth (cell division) cellular differentiation (production of specific cell types) and cellular repair mechanisms. All of these cellular functions require cellular metabolism and the ability of cells to process the genetic instructions encoded on DNA into proteins and to replicate DNA.

Homeostasis

Homeostasis for living organisms is the maintenance of a stable and specific internal environment that is distinctly different from the external environment. All living organisms must achieve homeostasis as a necessary condition for continued life.

Homeostasis for all living organisms must be achieved first at the cellular level. For unicellular organisms - such as bacteria, this is sufficient. For multicellular organisms, there are several additional levels of homeostasis that must be achieved. For humans, these mechanisms for the maintenance of higher levels of homeostasis are described in the human physiology sections.

Cellular Homeostasis

Cell Membranes

For biological cells, homeostasis requires a physical barrier in the form of a cell membrane to separate the cell's internal environment from the surrounding external environment. The external cell membrane is a selective, semi-permeable membrane. The cell membrane is permeable to water, oxygen and carbon dioxide molecules. These molecules are free to cross the membrane but most other atomic ions and molecules are not.

Osmolality

We have discussed the general topic of osmolality in detail. In the context of human cellular biology, all intracellular processes occur in solutions where the solvent is water. The particles dissolved in intracellular water include oxygen, carbon dioxide, electrolytes, small molecules such as glucose and a vast number of other chemicals and proteins. The total concentrations of all of these dissolved particles is defined as the osmolality of the intracellular fluid or simply the osmolality of the cell

Hypertonic and Hypotonic Solutions

Outside of the cell there is usually a liquid environment as well - and this environment also has an osmolality. The tendency of water is to diffuse between regions so that the osmolality of regions equalizes. For cellular homeostasis, the internal and external osmolality levels are slightly different. The internal cellular osmolality is artificially maintained at a slightly higher concentration level. This tends to draw water into cells via **osmosis** and the result is that the cells have a higher internal fluid pressure. The desired homeostatic state for cells is that they are surrounded by a hypotonic solution. - meaning the surrounding external solution of the cell has lower osmolality than the cell's internal osmolality.

If the external environment has higher osmolality this is called a hypertonic external solution environment. In this case water moves out of the cell via osmosis and the cell shrivels - if the situation continues the cell will die. Conversely, if the outside osmolality is too low -a hypotonic external solution environment - so much water will enter the cell that the cell membrane will burst. This phenomenon can be observed microscopically by adding red blood cells to a Petri dish filled with pure water - which has no (zero) osmolality.

Simple Diffusion

We have discussed the details of diffusion in general. To review: All dissolved particles in a solution will, if possible, move by diffusion spontaneously from regions of higher particle concentrations to regions of lower particle concentration. This is referred to a movement with or down a concentration gradient. This diffusion process does not require energy. In fact, **diffusion processes can be a source of chemical energy that drives chemical reactions**. Within the human body oxygen will typically diffuse into and carbon dioxide will typically diffuse out of the cells via simple diffusion.

Facilitated Diffusion

Other solubilized particles -those which are impermeable to the cell membrane- can move across the cell membrane down their concentration gradients, but this diffusion requires the participation of **transmembrane cell structures** that provide a pathway through the membrane. This type of diffusion is called facilitated diffusion. It is a process that does not require energy use by the cell.

Active Transport

The cell and organelles inside the cell have membrane pores and associated proteins that can pump various dissolved particles into out of or into the cell against the particles' concentration gradients. This process is called active transport. It requires energy in the form of ATP to actively transport particles across a cell membrane.

Transmembrane Pores and Transmembrane Pumps

Transmembrane pores and transmembrane pumps are protein complexes that extend through the cell membrane and have a central canal or passageway that is designed to allow for the movement of specific ions or molecules across the cell membrane. This movement can be from the inside to the outside of the cell or vice versa. Any substance that cannot freely diffuse through the cell membrane requires access to a specific transmembrane channel to move into or out of a cell.

These transmembrane channels are usually associated with a surface membrane protein -based complexes that often includes a surface receptor complex and a regulatory complex that can open or close the transmembrane channel. Transmembrane channels that can be selectively opened and closed are referred to as **"gated"** channels. On the interior cell membrane surface, there is often another protein based complex associated with the internal opening of the transmembrane channel. This complex frequently includes a **second messenger system** of molecules that generate internal molecules called second messengers that diffuse through the cell cytosol and initiate a variety of often very complex cellular responses to the second messenger molecules.

When the functions of the transmembrane channels and their associated molecular complexes include energy requiring activities, the transmembrane complex also frequently includes **ATPase complexes** that can hydrolyze ATP molecules to ADP molecules and couple these hydrolysis reactions to power the overall functions of the transmembrane complexes. This is often required when the transmembrane channels are transporting substances against the substances transmembrane concentration gradient. The Transmembrane transport complexes that have functions that include transport of substances against their transmembrane concentration gradients are generally referred to as transmembrane pumps.

Notice that although the internal and external osmolality of a cell may be nearly equal the difference in the internal concentrations of specific particle may be large and therefore there will be a large force tending to drive these particles across the cell membrane. A large fraction of the energy usage of cells is devoted to continuously maintaining several of these large individual concentration gradients across the cell membrane

Cotransport

In human cells, there are several transmembrane transport systems that couple the transport of one molecule down its transmembrane concentration gradient with the simultaneous transport of another molecule against its transmembrane concentration gradient. The diffusion of the one molecule type down its concentration gradient provides some or all of the energy required to transport the other type of molecule against its concentration gradient.

When both types of molecules are transported in the same direction across the cell membrane, the process is called **symport**. When both types of molecules are transported in the opposite directions across the cell membrane, the process is called **antiport.**

Transmembrane Ion Channels

A fundamental feature of cellular homeostasis and an important feature required for a wide variety of cellular functions is the maintenance of a transmembrane concentration gradient of several atomic ions, most notably the sodium ion (Na+), the potassium ion (K+) the calcium ion (Ca2+) and the chloride ion (Cl-).

These ions along with several others are generally referred to as electrolytes. There are active and passive transmembrane transport systems for all of these electrolytes.

The Sodium-Potassium Pump

One of the most important transmembrane ion channel complexes is the sodium-potassium ATPase pump. This transporter complex includes an **ATPase subunit** that powers the transport of sodium ions out of the cell and potassium ions into the cell. Both ions are transported against their transmembrane concentration gradient. **The transporter pumps three sodium ions out of the cell for every two potassium ions pumped into the cell.** The result is that the concentration of sodium ions is higher outside of the cell compared to inside of the cell and the reverse is true for potassium ions.

Symport of Glucose and Amino Acids

The establishment of a transmembrane sodium gradient has several important consequences. The first is that the passive movement of sodium down its concentration gradient back into the cell is used as the energy favorable cotransport sequence of the transport of glucose and amino acids into the cell (a symport mechanism). Cotransport mechanisms that use passive sodium transport are found in many other symport and antiport processes in specialized cells throughout the body.

Transmembrane Electrical Potentials

The second important consequence of the creation of transmembrane concentration gradients of electrolytes in general and of sodium ions in particular is the generation of a transmembrane cellular electrical potential - also called a potential difference. When there is a difference in the concentration of positive and negative electrical charges in a region There exists a electrical potential - the electrical forces between charges acts to restore the system to a neutral state - one without regions of differing charge. This is the process that drives electrical currents in batteries. The greater the magnitude of the charge difference and stronger the potential difference and the more energy that is stored in the electrical potential.

This electrical potential can perform work when the

system is allowed to return to a neutral state by the movement of charged particles down their concentration gradients. The overall separation of charge that occurs across cell membranes due to the creation of electrolyte transmembrane concentration gradients results in a transmembrane potential of approximately -70 millivolts (mV). where the interior of the cell has a negative charge compared to the exterior of the cell. Most of this potential is due to the transmembrane concentration gradient of sodium ions that is created by the sodium-potassium ATPase pump. All cells generate this transmembrane potential, but it is particularly important for the function of a class of cells called electrically excitable cells.

Electrically Excitable Cells

Electrically excitable cells have a complement of membrane receptors, membrane channels and second messenger systems that allow them to generate electrical currents that travel along the cell membrane and also allow the electrical currents to trigger secondary processes - such as the release of chemicals into the external environment in the case of neurons and the contraction of the cells by interactions of thick and thin filaments in the case of muscle cells.

The phenomena of the generation and transmission of electrical signals on electrically excitable cell membranes and the coupling of these electrical signals with fundamental cell functions illustrates the integration of cell receptors transmembrane channels, second messenger complexes and specialized intracellular processes that underlie nearly all of the biochemistry and cell physiology that occurs in the human body.

Neuron Anatomy

The classic electrically excitable cell is the neuron - the cell type that carries out the electrical functions of the human nervous system. Although there are many variations of the overall structure of neurons the generic anatomy of a neuron consists of a central cell body - the soma which contains the majority of the cell organelles and cell cytoplasm and two extensions of the soma - one being a tree like branching region composer of terminal branchings called dendrites and extending from the opposite pole of the soma - the axon. The axon is a cable -like extension that terminates in several

branches with bulb like endings. Typically, both dendrites and the terminals of axons are in close proximity with axons and dendrites of other neurons or with effector cells - muscle cells or glandular cells.

Synapses and Neurotransmitters

The synapse is the region where the ends of dendrites from one neuron closely approach the terminal of an axon of another neuron. The narrow region of space between the axon and dendrite is called the synaptic cleft. The neuromuscular junction refers to the local region where axon terminals approach the cell membrane of a muscle cell. There is also a narrow space between axon terminal and the muscle cell membrane that is analogous the the synaptic cleft.

Ligand-Gated Ion Channels

At a chemical synapse (there are also electrical synapses) small molecules called neurotransmitters are released from the terminal of the axon of one neuron and diffuses across the synaptic cleft where they bind with cell membrane receptors on the dendrites of another neuron. There are many different types of neurotransmitters and there are many types of receptor designed to bind to each specific type of neurotransmitter - often there are many different types of receptors that can bind to a single specific neurotransmitter. In neurons, these receptors are part a membrane complex that includes a transmembrane ion gate.

When the neurotransmitter binds to the receptor the ion gate is triggered to respond - usually by opening but occasionally by closing. This type of receptor ion gate complex is called a **ligand-gated ion channel** (a ligand is any molecule that can bind to a cell receptor). Most often the ion channel is a sodium ion channel, but frequently it is a potassium or a calcium ion channel. If the channel is a sodium channel, and the neurotransmitter binding results in an opening of the channel then sodium ions diffuse into the cell.

This diffusion is driven both by the concentration gradient of the sodium ion and by the electrical potential difference between the positively charged sodium ions and the relatively negative charge of the interior of the cell. As sodium ions rush into the cell the cell interior becomes near to the channel becomes less negative. This lowering of the transmembrane potential is called depolarization. The opposite effect can also occur of the binding of neurotransmitters opens other channels - such as potassium ion channels or closes sodium channels that were previously open. In this case the interior of the cell becomes more negative. This process is called hyperpolarization.

End-Plate Potentials
Ligand gated depolarization or hyperpolarization typically occurs on the dendritic region located at a synaptic cleft. This region of the dendrite is called the end-plate regions and the small changes in the polarity of the membrane are called **miniature end-plate potentials (MEPPS)**. If the MEPPs are depolarizing potentials they are **excitatory** and if they are hyperpolarizing they are inhibitory. Excitatory MEPPs can lead to the generation of a large electrical spike called an action potential. Inhibitory MEPPs can reduce the likelihood that an action potential will be generated by a neuron. This explains how a neurotransmitter can be excitatory or inhibitory depending on what type of ligand gated channel the is activated by the binding of the neurotransmitter molecule to the dendritic membrane neurotransmitter receptor.

Membrane Thresholds and Action Potentials
Excitatory MEPPs can travel as localized regions of membrane depolarization outward along a neuron cell membrane. When they arrive at the region of the cell where the neuron soma and the neuron axon meet (the axon hillock), the excitatory MEPPS can add together and create a much larger local region of membrane depolarization. If this depolarization reaches a critical level called the **threshold depolarization level** another type of ion channel located in the axon hillock called **voltage gated sodium channels** will be activated

Action Potential Depolarization and the Voltage Gated Sodium Channel
The voltage gated sodium channel opens in response to the voltage changes associated with threshold depolarization of the local membrane. This results in an inflow of sodium ion that further depolarize the local membrane region. This further depolarization triggers

nearby voltage gated sodium channels to open. The axon hillock has a high density of these voltage gated channels and as the opening of one channel triggers the opening of nearby channels there is a chain reaction that creates a very large inflow of sodium ion resulting in a reversal of membrane polarity.

Action Potential Hyperpolarization and the Voltage Gated Potassium Channel
The local region membrane depolarization suddenly surges and the interior of the cell becomes positive relative to the outside of the cell. This positive spike of membrane potential is called an action potential. An action potential typically has a value transmembrane potential of +35-to +45 millivolts (mV). At the peak of the action potential spike, the sodium channels close and another voltage gated ion channel - the **potassium gated ion channel** opens in the same membrane region as the spike. Potassium ions - which have a positive charge - have a higher concentration inside of the cell. When the potassium channels open, potassium ions rush out of the cell - driven by their concentration gradient.

Refractory Periods and Propagation of Action Potentials
This movement of positive potassium ion charges from inside of the cell to the outside causes a sudden fall in the membrane potential. This sharp drop again reverses the membrane polarity and actually drops the value to around -80 mV. This hyperpolarization of the cell makes the local membrane region that generated the action potential causes the local membrane region to be resistant to the generation of another action potential for a short period of time. This is referred to as the refractory period for the generation of an action potential.

Meanwhile the adjacent region of the axon membrane has voltage gated sodium and potassium channels as well. The initial action potential triggers a new action potential in the adjacent axonal membrane region and the process called action potential propagation - continues down the entire length of the axon fiber.

Neurotransmitter Release and Voltage-Gated Calcium Channels

When an action potential reaches the end of an axon voltage-gated calcium channel are activated. Calcium channels open and calcium ions - which have a higher external concentration - rush down their concentration gradients and enter the cell.

Once inside the cell, these calcium ions trigger a complex series of actions that cause vesicles containing neurotransmitter molecules to move to the axonal membrane at the synaptic cleft. The vesicles then fuse with the cell membrane and the neurotransmitter molecules diffuse across the synaptic cleft where they bind to their receptors located on dendrites of the postsynaptic neuron.

This binding in turn can generate a new action potential in the postsynaptic neuron in the same manner as we have just described for the presynaptic neuron. This is the process of electrical signal transmission that occurs among all neurons throughout the nervous system of the body

The Neuromuscular Junction

For neurons that are involved in generating contractions of skeletal and cardiac muscle cells, the first step in generating muscle cell contraction occurs at the neuromuscular junction. As an action potential reaches the end of an axon terminal at a neuromuscular junction, the release of the neurotransmitter **acetylcholine (ACh)** occurs.

ACh diffuses across the neuromuscular junction space and binds to receptors on the membrane of the muscle cell. This results in the generation of action potentials that propagate outward along the muscle cell membrane (the sarcolemma) and into **T-tubules.** T-tubules are membrane extension into the cell that carry the action potential to regions that are close to intracellular calcium containing vesicle structures called the **sarcoplasmic reticulum.** The action potential triggers internal cellular processes that lead to the **release of calcium ions into the cell cytoplasm.** The subsequent process that results in the contraction of the muscle cells has been described in detail in the contractile protein section of our review.

Molecular Genetics and Protein Synthesis
Nucleic Acids

We have already discussed several aspects of nucleic acids in the carbohydrate biology section of or review. Namely the role of the sugars ribose and deoxyribose in the sugar-phosphate backbones of DNA and RNA molecules and of the structural roles of theses sugars in nucleotides - the subunits of DNA and RNA molecules that a polymerized to form complete RNA and DNA molecules. The integrated roles of DNA and RNA in human biology are discussed below.

Nitrogenous Bases

All cells contain the nucleic acids DNA and RNA. The DNA molecules within a cell contain all the genetic information required to synthesize all of the proteins that the cell requires to carry out its metabolic, physiological and structural functions. This information is stored as a linear sequence of nitrogenous bases. The nitrogenous bases occur in two forms, purines and pyrimidines. Both forms are small nitrogen-containing molecules that have either one structural ring - the purines, or a double ring - the pyrimidines.

The nitrogenous bases in DNA are the purines adenine (A) and guanine (G) and the pyrimidines thymine (T) and cytosine (C). The nitrogenous bases found in RNA molecules are the same as those found in DNA molecules with the exception that in RNA, another pyrimidine, uracil, is substituted for thymine.

The DNA Double-Helix

The structure of a DNA molecule in a cell is usually the double-stranded form of DNA. This double-stranded structure is a spiraling (helical) ladder consisting of linear backbones of alternating deoxyribose sugars and phosphate groups. One deoxyribose phosphate polymer backbone forms the left side rail of the DNA ladder and another one forms the right-side rail of the DNA ladder.

Complementary Base Pairing in Double-Stranded DNA

Each deoxyribose sugar is also bonded to a single nitrogenous base. Additionally, in double-stranded DNA, each of these bases is hydrogen bonded to its complementary base, which is similarly bonded to a deoxyribose sugar on the opposing sugar-phosphate backbone of the DNA molecule. These hydrogen-bonded nitrogenous base pairs form the rungs of the double stranded DNA ladder.

The term "complementary" in complementary base pair bonding refers to the fact that each nitrogenous base will pair bond with one and only one specific complementary base, Adenine (A) will only pair bond with thymine (T) and guanine (G) will only pair bond with cytosine (C). There are two hydrogen bonds formed between base-pairing adenine and thymine and three hydrogen bonds formed between base-pairing guanine and cytosine in double stranded DNA.

Nucleotides - Review
A "nucleotide" is the term for a nucleic acid molecular subunit consisting of either a ribose or a deoxyribose sugar bonded to a phosphate group and to a nitrogenous base is referred to as a nucleotide. Any DNA molecule can be assembled entirely from deoxyribose containing nucleotides. Any RNA molecule can be assembled entirely from ribose containing nucleotides.

Chromosomes
In eukaryotic cells, DNA is usually in an extended linear form that allows the cells to access the nitrogenous base sequences for DNA replication and for transcription of DNA base sequences into messenger RNA molecules. During cell division, these DNA strands are highly condensed into structures called chromosomes. The formation of chromosomes during cell division cycle involve a series of coiling and supercoiling actions of the DNA molecule This process involves the physical wrapping of the DNA molecule around specialized spherical proteins called histone proteins or "**histones**".

Chromatids
Each chromosome can exist in two forms. One is as a single condensed strand of DNA. The other form consists of two condensed identical strands of DNA. These two condensed DNA strands are called chromatids individually, and together they are called "sister chromatids". The sister chromatid form occurs

only after replication of an entire DNA strand is completed.

Homologous Chromosomes
Human somatic cells have 46 chromosomes. These 46 chromosomes occur as 23 pairs of chromosomes - 22 pairs of autosomes and 1 pair of sex chromosomes. The pairs of chromosomes are called homologous chromosomes. The sex chromosome pair in males is not an actual pair - it consists of one "X" chromosome and one "Y" chromosome. In females, the sex chromosomes are a chromosome pair - consisting of two X chromosomes.

Alleles
Each single chromosome in an autosomal homologous chromosome pair contains the same genes - but the two chromosomes of a homologous chromosome pair are not necessarily exact copies of one another. There are often two or more variations of a gene. These gene variants are called alleles.

Frequently the individual chromosomes of a homologous chromosome pair will contain different alleles of a given gene. At a molecular level alleles have variations in the base sequences that code for a particular single-chain protein that is designed to severe a specific function within an organism. Alleles of a particular gene will ultimately generate single chain proteins that have variations in their amino acid sequences. This will often result in an alteration in the protein's function.

Often the variant proteins will not be optimally functional but sometimes they have enhanced functional abilities. This is how the succeeding generations of organisms are able to continuously evolve more effective biological adaptations to their environment.

Diploid and Haploid Cells
Cells that contain a full set of chromosome pairs are called diploid cells. All human somatic cells are diploid cells. Most organisms including humans can create haploid cells - cells that contain only single chromosomes rather than homologous chromosome pairs - These haploid cells have exactly half of the total

number of chromosomes as a corresponding diploid cell.

Germ-Line Cells

In humans, haploid cells are produced by germ-line cells, the cells that undergo meiosis to produce gametes. Gametes are the sex cells of the male and female that can fuse to form a new hybrid diploid cell called a zygote. The zygote is capable of developing into a new individual organism. In humans the gametes are, in the male - sperm cells and in the female - ova or egg cells. These haploid cells contain 23 chromosomes; one of each of the 23 chromosome pairs of a human somatic cell. During successful fertilization, the human gametes fuse - one sperm and one ovum - to form a zygote with 23 pairs of chromosomes.

Notice this is now a new human diploid cell with a total 46 chromosomes in the form of 23 homologous pairs of chromosomes. Each homologous pair of chromosomes includes one chromosome from the male sex cell and one from the female sex cell

In Humans, when male and female gametes fuse during fertilization, the resulting cell - the zygote- contains a full complement of 46 chromosomes, 22 pairs of homologous autosomes and 1 pair of sex chromosomes. In female zygotes, exactly half of the DNA is contributed by the mother and half by the father (in male zygotes, slightly more DNA is contributed by the mother. Her X chromosome contains somewhat more DNA than the father's Y chromosome. Y chromosomes can only be contributed by the father. In male zygotes, the X chromosome is always contributed by the mother. This method of generating offspring is called sexual reproduction.

The purpose of sexual reproduction is to vastly increase the range of genetic variability among offspring. This allows a species to enhance the chances of continued survival through the process of natural selection. Increased genetic variability in a species increases the likelihood that some offspring will have an optimum set of genetic traits to more successfully adapt to the external environment and to outcompete other species for the limited essential resources available in the environment.

During the replication of new complementary DNA strands or during the transcription of DNA gene sequences into mRNA molecules, the DNA is not organized into a chromosome since chromosome are a highly condensed configuration of the DNA molecule - one whose base sequences cannot be accessed by DNA or RNA polymerases.

Protein Synthesis

When a cell begins the process of constructing a protein, it first must expose the DNA base sequences of the gene that codes for the desired protein. During protein synthesis, the region of the DNA that contains the gene that will be transcribed is exposed by disrupting the hydrogen bonds between the nitrogenous base pairs. This separates the left and right halves of the DNA ladder as if it were being unzipped down the middle of the nitrogenous base pair rungs.

Transcription of DNA into mRNA - The 3' to 5' Direction

A protein complex called RNA polymerase then inserts itself into the cleft created by the disruption of the hydrogen bonds between complementary base pairs. The RNA polymerase then begins to assemble a single-strand RNA molecule that is complementary to the DNA strand that contains the base sequence code for the protein that will be constructed. The DNA strand that is transcribed is transcribed beginning at the 3' end of the DNA molecule and continues in the 5' direction.

The Sense and Antisense Strands of DNA

The DNA strand that is transcribed by RNA polymerase is called the "antisense strand" The other DNA strand - the complementary strand of the sense strand - is called the sense strand. Since the base sequence of the sense strand is the complementary sequence of the antisense strand, the sense strand does not code for functional proteins and it is not read by RNA polymerase. The mRNA base sequence is identical to the sense strand DNA sequence with the exception that the nitrogenous base uracil in the mRNA base sequence replaces the nitrogenous base thymine in the sense strand of the DNA molecule

Genes

The base sequence in the sense strand that codes for a

single-chain protein is called a gene. One gene always codes for one and only one polypeptide chain - a polypeptide chain is a linear molecule composed of amino acids. All polypeptide chains are single-chain proteins. Some complex proteins are composed of more than one type of polypeptide chain.

Codons

The individual amino acids that will form the protein's chain are coded for by three-base sequences. These three-base sequences are called codons. Since there are four different bases that can occur at any point in the DNA base sequence, there are statistically 64 possible combinations of three-base sequences. Therefore, there are 64 possible codons. There are only 20 amino acids that are used to assemble proteins, so there may be more than one codon that specifies for a given amino acid. The reverse is NOT true - None of the individual codons ever codes for more than one specific amino acid.

Transcription of DNA

As RNA polymerase assembles an RNA molecule, a new nitrogenous base, uracil (U), is used in place of the base thymine, Uracil is the RNA base that is complementary to adenine. The process of constructing an RNA molecule that contains a complementary base sequence to a DNA gene sequence is defined as "transcription".

Anticodons and Ribosomes

Once a complete RNA transcript of a gene has been completed, the transcript, known as a messenger RNA (mRNA) molecule leaves the nucleus and enters the cell cytoplasm. Eventually the mRNA molecule encounters a ribosome that attaches to the mRNA transcript. The ribosome then reads the RNA as three-base compliments of the DNA codons. These three- base RNA sequences are called anticodons.

Translation of mRNA

When the ribosome reads an anticodon, it inserts the amino acid that corresponds to the anticodon onto a growing polypeptide chain. When the entire mRNA molecule has been processed by the ribosome the result is a newly synthesized single chain protein. This polypeptide chain is the protein coded for by the gene that was transcribed at the beginning of this process. The reading of mRNA by ribosomes and the construction of the corresponding protein is called "translation".

Transfer RNA

During the assembly of a protein chain at a ribosome, the individual amino acids are transported to the ribosome by transfer RNA (tRNA) molecules. These molecules are short segments of RNA that have a three-leaf-clover configuration. One end of the "stem" of the clover binds to a particular amino acid. There are 20 different types of tRNA molecules and each binds to one and only one type of amino acid. There is a complementary tRNA molecule type for each of the 20 amino acids.

DNA Replication

During DNA replication, the unzipping of double-stranded DNA is accompanied by the construction of a new complementary DNA for each of the original strand of the double stranded DNA. The synthesis of these two new complementary strands continues for the entire length of the DNA molecule. The result is that exact two copies of the original DNA molecule are created. Each of the new DNA molecules contains either the right or the left strand of the original DNA molecule and a complete newly synthesized complementary strand. This type of replication of DNA is called semi-conservative replication.

DNA Polymerase

During the replication of DNA, DNA polymerases are the enzyme complexes that insert themselves into gaps created by disruption of complementary base pair hydrogen bonds. These DNA replication molecules synthesize complementary DNA strands to both the original DNA sense and antisense strands simultaneously.

Mutations of the Genetic Code

During the replication process, the polymerase molecules occasionally make errors. For example, as the polymerase molecule is synthesizing complementary DNA strands, it may erroneously emplace or mismatch a complementary base. For instance, an adenine on an original DNA strand may be mismatched on the complementary DNA strand. This mismatch would be a substitution of guanine or a cytosine in place of the correct complementary base -thymine.

This is a mutation at the genetic level. The mismatched base will probably (but not necessarily) code for a different amino acid in the gene of which it is a part. If the error is in the antisense strand, then upon the next round of DNA replication, the new sense strand will base pair correctly with the mutated base. This will likely result in an alteration in the amino acid that is coded for in the mRNA molecule.

Even more seriously, some codons are "stop" codons that signal that signal RNA polymerase to terminate the transcription of a gene sequence. This stop codon is placed at the end of a normal gene sequence. If the stop codon is created within the gene sequence by a mismatch or other type of mutation, RNA polymerase will terminate transcription of the gene at the moment that it reads this stop codon. This almost always results is a completely nonfunctional and possibly toxic gene fragment protein.

DNA Repair Mechanisms
Mismatch errors are substitution errors -one base (the correct base) is substituted for by another base (an incorrect base). DNA polymerases have a highly accurate method of repair for this type of mutation. Essentially the DNA polymerase double-checks the base pairing and nearly always detects this type of error before the replication process goes much further. The error is then corrected by DNA polymerase. This type of error correction is called "proofreading repair". When the proofreading repair mechanism for a substitution error fails, there is a second type of error correction that DNA polymerase also utilizes before completion of replication. This mechanism is called mismatch repair.

Somatic Cell Mutations
The overall substitution error rate in human DNA is very low due to proofreading and mismatch repair mechanisms. Some errors - mutations - are not corrected by proofreading or excision repair functions. These mutations can become permanent alterations in the genetic code of all subsequently replicated DNA. If

this occurs in a somatic cell the mutation may be amplified over many mitotic cycles resulting in a clonal population of mutated cells. These may be dysfunctional cells or even cancerous cells.

Germ-Line Cell Mutations
When mutations evade detection and correction by proofreading and excision repair in a germ-line cell, the mutation becomes a hereditary mutation that can be passed to future generations. These mutations will commonly be present in nearly every cell of organisms that developed from a mutated germ-line cell. While it is most likely these mutations will be harmful or at least harmless - some actually result in better versions of genes.

Mutagens and Carcinogens
After the replication of a DNA molecule is complete, there are numerous ways that the DNA can be damaged or altered. During mitosis or meiosis, sections of chromosomes can be lost or fail to separate resulting in chromosomal abnormalities. Radiation and chemicals can cause direct damage to DNA. Agents that have been shown capable of inducing mutations to DNA are called mutagens. Those that have been shown capable of inducing cancerous mutations are termed carcinogens.

Excision Repair of DNA
There are several types of DNA repair genes and DNA repair processes that can correct various types of post-replication damage to DNA. One of these is the excision repair mechanism. This mechanism can identify short segments of damaged DNA and can then snip the damaged DNA section out. The repair enzymes then use the complementary segment as a template to create a correct DNA base sequence replacement for the excised damaged DNA segment.

Genetic Adaptation and Natural Selection
These mutated versions of gene are alleles of genes found on chromosomes. This mutation process is how different alleles of a gene are first created. And the creation of new alleles is the means through which natural selection and evolution of species occurs. Therefore, some level of germ-line DNA mutation must occur so that the offspring of organisms may

continue to successfully adapt to a changing environment and to survive the competitive challenges of other species that are themselves continuing to adapt through genetic mutations. This is essentially the definition of the process of natural selection through genetic adaptation.

Cell Division

The Cell Cycle

Cells that are capable of replication have a cell cycle that corresponds to specific activities related to cell replication. The cycle consists of interphase and mitosis/meiosis. The interphase phase of the cell cycle consists of two growth phases (G1 and G2) that are separated by an intervening synthesis (S) phase. The G1 and G2 phases correspond to the periods where there is active transcription of DNA into mRNA and the translation of mRNA into proteins. Replication of the entire cell genome occurs during the S phase. Mitosis (and meiosis 1) begins upon the completion of the G2 phase of the cell cycle.

Mitosis

Prophase

In prophase of mitosis, the nuclear membrane begins too disintegrates, and a centrosome - a microtubule assembly structure - forms and divides into two centrioles. The centrioles begin to move to opposite poles of the cell. Microtubule spindle fibers begin to form and DNA begins to condense into chromosomes.

Since the DNA of every chromosome has been replicated, the mitotic chromosomes at this stage have twice the amount of DNA that they possess during the interphase stage of the cell cycle. This is apparent in the structure of the chromosomes which consist of two sister chromatids connected at their central region. Each sister chromatid of a given chromosome has an identical sequence of base sequences (unless one or more mutations had occurred during the replication process).

Chromosomes with duplicated sister chromatids have an X shape (but they are not X chromosomes - the X chromosome is one of two forms of the sex chromosome. The other form is the Y chromosome)

Metaphase

During metaphase of mitosis, all 46 individual chromosomes form a single file line arrangement at the center of the metaphase plate. Centrioles- have settled at opposite poles of the cell to the left and right of the aligned chromosomes. Microtubule spindle fibers then begin to form between the centrioles and between the centrioles and the chromosomes. Spindle fibers to attach to the central connecting regions of the sister chromatids of every chromosome with a single spindle fiber attached to theses central regions from the right centriole and a single fiber from the left centriole.

Anaphase

In anaphase of mitosis, the left and right microtubule spindle fibers attached to each central region of every chromosome begins to shorten. This action pulls the sister chromatids of each chromosome apart. The left chromatids are pulled toward the left centriole and the right chromatids are pulled toward the right centriole. At this time, the entire cell begins to divide into two separate daughter cells. This process is called cytokinesis,

Telophase

During telophase of mitosis, cytokinesis progresses to completion. The chromatids drawn to the left are separated into the left daughter cell and the chromatids drawn to the right are separated into the right daughter cell. Nuclear membranes then form to contain each daughter cell's compliment of 46 individual chromosomes. Once cytokinesis is complete, the original cell has now divided into two daughter cells that have a full set of chromosomes that are identical to the full set of chromosomes contained in the original cell. With subsequent generation of mitosis, a single progenitor cell can generate a huge number of identical daughter cells.

Meiosis

The cells that participate in meiosis are called germ-line cells. All other cells in the body are somatic cells. Meiosis consists of 2 separate stages, and two rounds of cell division. The first stage of meiosis, meiosis 1, occurs during the first round of cell division. Meiosis 2 occurs during the second round of cell division.

In contrast to mitosis, meiosis does not produce identical daughter cells; rather it produces gametes, sex cells that have exactly one half of the number of individual chromosomes as the progenitor cell. Rather than 23 pairs of chromosomes (homologous chromosome pairs), these cells, beginning with the first two daughter cells resulting from the first cell division of meiosis (meiosis I), contain only one of the two chromosomes from each of the 23 homologous chromosome pairs contained in the progenitor cell.

Meiosis 1

Meiosis I begins with a diploid, germ-line progenitor cell. The progenitor cell replicates its entire chromosomal DNA just as occurs in somatic cells prior to mitosis. During metaphase of meiosis 1, in contrast to mitosis, the chromosomes align at the metaphase plate not as a single file line of individual chromosome but instead as homologous chromosome pairs. The chromosome pairs then separate in the same fashion as occurs in mitosis. Notice this does not result in the separation of the sister chromatids of individual chromosome. Instead, one chromosome from each homologous chromosome pair, with each chromosome still consisting of both sister chromatids, is separated into separate daughter cells. These daughter cells now contain one chromosome from each of the 23 pairs of chromosomes contained in the progenitor cell.

Genetic Variability

Recall that homologous chromosome pairs do not in general have identical genes, but often have variants of each gene, different versions of a gene called alleles. Therefore, the two daughter cells resulting from the first cell division of meiosis have one half of the total number of chromosome - 23 instead of 46 and these cellular sets of genes, but these are not identical sequences of DNA. The individual chromosomes from homologous chromosome pairs which are now in different cells, almost certainly have a wide variety of differing alleles for a wide variety of individual genes. Also, during the pair separation process in anaphase of meiosis 1, small segments from chromatids on different chromosomes of the homologous pairs can be exchanged. This creates hybrid chromatids. This process is called "crossing over" and it increases the genetic variability of the chromosomes.

Meiosis 2

The next round of cell division follows immediately without any replication of DNA. This is the Meiosis 2 phase of meiotic cell division. The events of Meiosis 2 cell division are identical to the events of mitosis cell division. In each of the two daughter cells created by the meiosis 1 cell division, the 23 individual chromosomes align at the metaphase plate of each daughter cell and individual sister chromatids of each chromosome are pulled apart and separated into the second generation of daughter cells.

This process - beginning with the original diploid progenitor cell - results in the production of four haploid cells. Each haploid cell contains one chromosome on the form of a sister chromatid, from each of the 23 pairs of chromosomes contained in the progenitor cell. In the human male, meiosis results in the production of sperm cells. In the human female, meiosis results in the production of ova,

Molecular Genetics

In individual members of a species, the total amount of genetic information contained in the genes of a diploid cell of the individual represents the individual's genome. The specific types of genes within the genome are the individual's genotype. The manner in which an individual's genotype is expressed in physical form is the individual's phenotype.

Calculating Gene Frequencies

For species where there are multiple alleles for a given gene, individual members of the species may have different combinations of these alleles in their individual genomes. When there are two alleles for a given gene - for instance if we indicate these to be the alleles "A" and "a" for a specific gene, individuals may possess one of three possible combinations of the two alleles within their genotype. These are "AA", "aa" and "Aa". The combinations AA and aa are the two possible homozygous genotypes and the combination Aa is the heterozygous genotype. This type of mating is often described as an "Aa x Aa" cross. When a mating

Aa male and Aa female pair of a species create a zygote (an Aa x Aa cross), the probability or predicted frequencies of the alleles in the zygote can be calculated using a Punnett square.

	A	a
A	AA	Aa
a	Aa	aa

A Punnett square representation of a cross between two heterozygous (Aa) parents (an Aa x Aa cross).

The Punnett square above shows the possible combinations of zygotes resulting from a mother and father where both are heterozygous for the gene with alleles A and a. Since each parent can contribute only one allele to any particular zygote, the alleles for one parent are separated into an "A" column and an "a" column. The other parent's alleles are represented by an "A" row and a little "a" row. The four squares show the combination of alleles that results from combining a parental row with a corresponding parental column.

Notice that for two heterozygous individuals there is one AA square, one aa square and two Aa squares. This indicates that there is a 1 in 4 probability (25% chance) that the parents with produce a zygote with AA alleles, a 1 in 4 probability (25% chance) that the parents with produce a zygote with aa alleles and a 2 in 4 probability (50% chance) that the parents with produce a zygote with Aa alleles. Since zygotes can develop into children, for humans these are the probabilities of heterozygous parents having children with the AA, Aa and aa genotypes.

The expected gene frequencies resulting from matings between parents with other genotypes can be calculated in the same fashion using the Punnett square technique. The gene frequencies for the gene with two alleles A and a in the offspring of one heterozygous (Aa) parent and one homozygous (AA) parent (an AA x Aa cross) is shown in the Punnett square below.

	A	A
A	AA	AA
a	Aa	Aa

A Punnett square representation of a cross between one heterozygous parent(Aa) and one homozygous parent (AA) - an AA x Aa cross.

There is only 1 possible gamete for the homozygous parent (AA) for the gene. this is the allele A. The homozygous parent gametes are represented in the horizontal orientation as A and A at the top margin of the 2x2 Punnett square. The heterozygous parent (Aa) can produce two different gametes for the gene - either the allele A or the allele a. The heterozygous parent gametes are represented in the vertical left margin orientation as A and a.

We see that there are two possible zygotes from this heterozygous/homozygous cross - AA and Aa. Of the four possible crosses (represented by the allele pair in each of the four individual squares), two are AA and two are Aa. The gene frequencies for both AA and Aa are 2/4 or 50%. Notice that there is a zero percent chance of a homozygous aa offspring.

There is another possible cross for the homozygous/heterozygous state. This would be a cross between a parent homozygous for the a allele of the gene (aa) and a parent heterozygous for the gene (Aa). This would be an Aa x aa cross.

	A	a
a	Aa	aa
a	Aa	aa

Notice the gene frequencies are the same as for an AA x Aa cross except that it is the aa homozygous state that is 50% (instead of the AA homozygous state) and that there is a zero percent chance of an AA homozygous state (instead of an aa homozygous state) state. The heterozygous state (Aa) has the same 50% probability as it does for the AA x Aa cross.

There are three other possible crosses for a single gene with two alleles (A and a). Two are homozygous crosses of aa x aa and AA x aa. It should be obvious that each has only one possible zygote outcome. For the aa x aa cross, there is only an a allele, and so all offspring must be homozygous for the a allele (aa). By similar reasoning only one combination of alleles AA is possible for offspring of an AA x AA cross. The final possible combination for a cross of a single gene with two alleles (a and a) is the cross between a homozygous AA parent and a homozygous aa parent

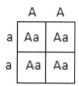

A Punnett square representation of a cross between two homozygous parents one parent is homozygous for the allele A (AA) and the other parent is homozygous for the allele a (aa).

There is only one possible combination of zygotes from this cross - the heterozygous combination (Aa).

Dominant and Recessive Alleles

Often the phenotypic appearance or the physical trait that results from a gene depends on whether the alleles for the gene are dominant or recessive. The classic example is eye color - where the brown allele is "B" and blue allele is "b".

Brown (B) is the dominant allele and blue (b) is the recessive allele. Homozygous brown eyed individuals - those who are BB, and heterozygous individuals - who are Bb, always have brown eyes. Only homozygous blue (bb) individuals have blue eyes. Notice that the offspring of parents who are heterozygous for eye color (Bb), will have the same expected genotype frequencies as shown in the Punnett square example above; but the blue-eyed phenotype is only the bb genotype. Therefore, heterozygous brown-eyed parents will have a 1 in 4 or 25% chance of having a blue-eyed child.

Notice that two blue-eyed parents will never have brown-eyed children, since both parents possess only the blue eye color allele. Finally notice that in any

couple where at least one parent is homozygous brown (BB), there is no possibility of offspring who will be homozygous blue (Bb) and therefore these parents have no chance of having a blue-eyed child.

Dihybrid Crosses

A classic topic in mendelian genetics is the calculation of the types of different gene combinations that can occur in offspring of parents for two genes - each with two alleles that assort independently. This type of cross is classified as a dihybrid cross.

If we represent the two alleles for these two genes as A and a for the alleles of the first gene and B and b as the alleles for the second gene, then we can construct a Punnett square to calculate the possible gene combinations and frequencies for the offspring of any two parents with any possible combination of the alleles for the two genes (A, a, B and b).

We have partially completed the construction of a Punnett square to calculate these gene combinations and frequencies for a dihybrid cross where both parents are heterozygous for both genes. This would be a diploid state of AaBb for each parent. As the Punnett square illustrates, each parent can generate gametes with four possible combinations of the alleles for the two genes.

These possible combinations are AB, Ab, aB and ab. Each of the four combinations is listed at the top margin for one parent and at the left margin for the other parent. Notice that the possible zygote for any square is the combination of the horizontal and vertical gametes that correspond to the row and column of the square.

	AB	Ab	aB	ab
AB	AABB			
Ab		AAbb		
aB			aaBB	
ab				aabb

There are sixteen squares for a dihybrid cross, but the

actual number of different combinations of alleles that are possible for the parental offspring depends on the particular alleles of the genes possessed by each parent. For instance, in our example of a dihybrid cross where both parents are heterozygous for both genes, several of the 16 possible combinations are equivalent. For example, an AaBb combination is identical to an aAbB combination. Both combinations have exactly one of each allele (A, a, B and b) - it makes no difference which parent contributed a particular allele.

	AB	Ab	aB	ab
AB				AaBb
Ab			AaBb	
aB		AaBb		
ab	AaBb			

The Punnett square above shows that there are four squares that have the equivalent allele combination of AaBb. The frequency for this combination is therefore 4/16 (or ¼) or 25%. At this point we have partially completed the Punnett square as shown below.

	AB	Ab	aB	ab
AB	AABB			AaBb
Ab		AAbb	AaBb	
aB		AaBb	aaBB	
ab	AaBb			aabb

If we continue the process of assigning allele combinations to the remaining empty squares the result is the square shown below.

	AB	Ab	aB	ab
AB	AABB	AABb	AaBB	AaBb
Ab	AABb	AAbb	AaBb	Aabb
aB	AaBB	AaBb	aaBB	aaBb
ab	AaBb	Aabb	aaBb	aabb

We have listed capital alleles (A, B) before lowercase alleles (a and b) in the squares to make it easier to identify equivalent combinations. It is still difficult to recognize all of the possible combinations by looking at the squares. The HESI will unlikely ask a question of the degree of difficulty required to determine exactly the frequencies of all the allele combination from this type of dihybrid cross, but one should be able to construct the Punnett square itself for any dihybrid cross and to identify frequencies for simpler examples of a dihybrid cross.

Cell Differentiation
Once a human sperm cell and a human ovum have fused to form a zygote, the process of the development of a new human being begins. During this process, the zygote will undergo countless rounds of cell division. As the zygote proliferates into a large collection of cells, the process of cell differentiation begins. This process involves a vast, complex and still poorly understood interaction of cell markers, cell receptors, extracellular matrix molecules and cell signaling molecules That cause undifferentiated cells to begin to change into specific mature cell types and to begin to organize into tissues and organs. The first stage of this process is called embryogenesis

Embryogenesis
Almost immediately after a zygote is formed the first stage of embryogenesis - the development of an **embryo** begins. First, the single-cell zygote undergoes an initial mitotic cell division. The two daughter cells then undergo a second round of mitotic cell division. Each new generation of daughter cells continues this cycle of mitotic divisions. During these early rounds of cell division, the daughter cells undergo divide simultaneously. This results in a doubling of the number of cells derived from the original zygote with each round of cell division.

The Morula Stage
During these divisions, there is little if any individual cell growth so the increasing mass of cells retains a total volume that is approximately equal to the original zygote. These types of divisions are called cleavages. After the first four rounds of cleavage the original zygote has become a solid spherical cell mass consisting

of 16 cells. This cell mass is called a morula - The morula stage is the first stage of embryological development. These 16 (or so) cells are completely undifferentiated, each cell has the capacity to differentiate further into any mature cell type in the human body. Cells that have this capacity are called totipotent stem cells.

As subsequent rounds of cell division occur the progeny cells of the cells of the morula begin the process of cell differentiation. Through cell-cell interactions, these progeny cells begin to rearrange themselves into a more complex structure. As this structure develops the cells also begin to express new cell markers and cell membrane receptors. Further increasingly diverse cell-cell interactions and other intracellular processes lead to selective activation and deactivation of genes within individual cells. This allows cells to become further differentiated with subtypes of cells emerging that are capable of new functions. This increasingly diverse cell mass transforms from the morula stage to the next phase of embryogenesis - the blastula stage.

The Blastula Stage
At the beginning of the blastula stage of embryological development, the cells of the morula begin to increase in mass with subsequent cell divisions and the cell divisions are no longer simultaneous. Cells in differing local regions of cell mass begin dividing faster than others. Cells also begin to develop the ability to move or migrate from one location to another. This process leads to the formation of two separate cell layers - an inner cell layer and an outer cell layer. The outer layer is called the **trophoblast** and the inner layer is called the **inner-cell mass**. The two layers separate except at one specific site called the **embryonic pole.**

The Embryonic Disc
The cells of the trophoblast and most of the cells of the inner cell mas will proliferate and differentiate into extraembryonic structures - those that do not continue as part of the developing embryo. Instead these go no to form the yolk sac, amniotic sac and portions of the placenta and fetal umbilical cord. The cells that do proliferate and differentiate into the developing embryo are the cells of the inner cell mass located at the embryonic pole. The space created between the two cell

layers begins to expand and fill with fluid. After the seventh round of cell division the resultant 128 cell mass has differentiated into a structure called the blastula. In humans, the blastula consists of a spherical outer cell layer called the **blastoderm** and an inner fluid-filled cavity called the **blastocoel.** In humans, a local region of the blastoderm begins to differentiate into an inner-cell mass called the blastocyst. The blastocyst further proliferates and differentiates into a fluid-filled substructure that includes cells that will form the amniotic sac and a small region of cells the **embryonic disc.** The cells of the embryonic disc are the cells that will proliferated and differentiate into the human embryo. This differentiation process begins with the formation of the cells of the **primary germ layers.**

The Gastrula Stage and the Primary Germ Layers
The blastoderm cells of the embryonic disc continue to proliferate, differentiate and migrate to form three layers of cells. The upper layer of cells are ectoderm cells. **Ectoderm** is one of the three primary germ layers. The middle cell layer is composed of mesodermal cells. **Mesoderm** is the second of the three primary germ layers. The bottom layer of cells is composed of endodermal cells. **Endoderm** is the third of the three primary germ layers. All subsequent cells, tissues and organs of the human body are composed of cells derived from these three primary germ layers. This three-layer cell structure consisting of the three primary germ layers is called the **gastrula.**

Differentiation of the Primary Germ Layer Cells
With the creation of the three primary germ layers of the gastrula, the development of the human embryo proceeds with further cell proliferation and differentiation of the three primary germ layer cells. There are two methods to describe the differentiation process of the germ layer cells. One is to describe the germ cell derivation of the four primary tissues. The other is to describe germ cell derivation of the organs of the human body.

The Four Primary Tissue Types
Tissues are organized collections of one or a few types of cell that share the same functions and by many definitions have the same primary germ-cell origins.

The four primary tissue types are epithelial, connective, muscle and nervous tissues. It is important to recognize that functional tissues are composed of a not only a particular type of cells but also of an extracellular component that includes structural matrices of proteins and other substances. Together these form an organized assembly of cells and extracellular material that are integrated to provide a common set of functions within the body. There are many subsets of the four basic tissue types and theses tissues can perform many different functions throughout the body. In many cases a particular tissue is composed primarily of extracellular materials with actual tissue cells only sparsely distributed throughout the tissue.

Epithelial Tissue

The definition that a tissue is - in part -comprised of cells that are derived from the same germ layer is somewhat confused since epithelial tissues by most definitions include epithelium derived from **ectoderm** - which forms the epidermis of the skin, subcutaneous glands, mammary glands; from **endoderm** - which forms the linings of the digestive tract. The respiratory tract, the urinary bladder and urethra; and from **mesoderm** - which forms **endothelium**, the cells that line the interior surfaces of blood vessels the chambers of the heart and lymphatic vessels and **mesothelium**, the cells that line the surfaces of internal body cavities such as the peritoneum, the pleura and the pericardium.

The alternative view is that epithelia tissue of mesodermal origin - endothelium and mesothelium - are not true epithelial tissue. Regardless of either definition there is agreement that true epithelial tissue includes types of epithelium derived from ectoderm and epithelia tissue derived from endoderm.

Structural and Functional Characteristics of Epithelial Tissue

Epithelial tissue is typically organized in one of two general structural forms; one is as **sheets of tissue**, Where the tissue may provide structural /protective functions, absorptive functions, filtering functions and secretory functions. the other form is as globular arrangements of epithelial tissue called **glandular epithelium** where the tissue functions as glandular tissue. The primary role of glandular epithelium is the secretion of substances, such as sweat, sebaceous material, mucous, digestive fluids and enzymes, and hormone molecules.

Epithelial tissue cells are notable for their **high regenerative capacity** - they can and do frequently undergo mitosis to replace cells that have been damaged or lost due to mechanical or other types of injury. Another notable feature of epithelial cells is that they **do not have a direct blood supply** but **they are innervated** (have connections to the nervous system)

Characteristics of Epithelial Cells

A primary feature of all epithelial cells is the **three-dimensional shape** of the cells; **squamous** epithelial cells are flattened and have an irregular polyhedral shape. **Cuboidal** epithelial cells are -as the name implies - shaped like a cube and **columnar** epithelial cells are elongated in the form of a rectangular solid - with the height of the sides of the cell being significantly greater than the length and width of the top or apical surface of the cell and of the length and width of the bottom or basilar surface of the cell.

Within a particular type of epithelial tissue, the sheet or membrane form of epithelial tissues can have one of several arrangements of the epithelial cells. **Simple epithelial** tissue consists of a **single layer** of cells. Simple epithelium is usually found in regions where the function of the epithelium is to absorb or to filter substances such as in the alveoli of the lungs, in the glomerulus of the renal tubules of the kidney in the digestive tract and in the capillaries of the circulatory system. Simple epithelium can have secretory functions particularly as the epithelial linings of the peritoneal cavity of the abdomen and the pleural cavity of the chest where they secrete pleural and peritoneal fluid which acts as a lubricant and shock absorbing substance. **Stratified epithelium** consists of **two or more layers** of epithelial cells. Stratified epithelium is typically located where the tissue serves a protective or structural role and therefore is subject to mechanical, chemical or environmental or other types of stress. **Stratified cuboidal** epithelium is located in the ducts of **sweat glands and mammary glands** and typically has two layers of cuboidal cells.

Together epithelial tissue can be described as a combination of these two features- These include simple squamous, cuboidal and columnar tissue and stratified squamous and stratified cuboidal. In some cases, the epithelial tissue is a stratified arrangement where the lowermost layer is columnar or cuboidal and progressively higher layers become more squamous shaped. This is most notably seen in the dermis and epidermis of the skin. Columnar epithelial cells are almost always arranged is a single layer as simple columnar tissue. In some cases, columnar tissue is irregularly shaped and arranged in a fashion that creates the appearance that there are two layers of cells. This arrangement is known as **pseudostratified columnar** tissue.

In addition to the shape of epithelial cells and to the number of layers of epithelial cells there are several other features of non-glandular epithelial tissue that most or all specific epithelial tissues have in common. A near universal feature of non-glandular epithelium is that the epithelium has a barrier function - this requires that the tissue prevent substances from crossing between epithelial cells and passing into underlying regions of the body.

Tight Junctions and Desmosomes
The bottom or basal layer of such epithelial tissue (and the only layer in the case of simple epithelium) are densely packed and connected to adjacent cells by specialized intercellular structures called tight junctions and desmosomes. Tight junctions are located at the upper or apical regions of the epithelia cells. Tight junctions form a leak proof seal between epithelial cells and also help to keep specialized elements of certain cells localized to the apical region of the cell. Desmosomes are "spot-welds between epithelial cells, were intermediate filaments inside adjacent cells are linked together by intercellular connections. Desmosomes provide a remarkable degree of tensile strength to the epithelial tissue while allowing the tissue to remain flexible.

Basement Membranes
At the base of the epithelial cells the cells are attached to an extracellular membrane consisting primarily of collagen fibers. The basement membrane serves as an additional barrier to the leakage of substances past the epithelial cells and also provides additional structural support and mechanical resilience to the epithelial tissue. The basement membrane is semipermeable - this is important because epithelial cells do not have a blood supply Oxygen, nutrients and other essential molecule are able to diffuse through the basement membrane and then gain access to the epithelial cells. Similarly, substances that are absorbed by epithelial cells and waste products from epithelial cells are able to diffuse across the basement membrane into the interior of the body.

Polarity of Epithelial Cells
Another key feature of non-glandular epithelium is cell polarity. The apical surfaces of epithelial cells that facing outward toward the interior of lumen (passageways) of anatomical structures - such as the bronchial airways of the lungs and the lumen of the gastrointestinal tract - frequently have specialized structural and molecular features that enable the cells to perform absorptive or transport functions. Since these features are localized to the apical surface the cells are described as polar - one end of the cell is different than the other end of the cell. Polarity is most commonly seen in simple columnar and pseudostratified columnar epithelium.

Cilia and Microvilli
Two of the most common polar specializations of the apical end of endothelial cells are cilia and microvilli. Cilia are densely packet thread-like extensions of the apical membrane that are capable of active movement. As a group on a cell and as a continuous layer on epithelial tissue surfaces, cilia generate a coordinated wavelike motion that move across epithelial surfaces. This is particularly important in the **airways of the lungs**, where this cilia-generated motion moves substances within the airways progressively out of the lungs and into the trachea and then the oropharynx. This phenomenon is called the **mucociliary conveyor belt**. The ciliated epithelium in the bronchial airways are **pseudostratified** epithelium.

Microvilli are the other common specialized feature of the apical region of epithelial cells. These are also densely packed tubular extrusions of the cell membrane. In the small intestine microvilli greatly **increase the surface area of the epithelial cells** increasing their ability to absorb water and nutrients. Microvilli form an outermost region of the epithelial tissue called a **brush border**. In addition to increasing the absorptive capacity of the epithelial cells, there are several types of digestive enzymes - called the **brush border enzymes** - that are attached to the microvilli of epithelial cells in the small intestine. The majority of these are **disaccharidases** - enzymes that break disaccharides down into simple sugars. The epithelium of the digestive tract is a simple columnar epithelium.

Connective Tissue

Connective tissue is **derived from mesoderm**. The adjective "connective" if frequently misunderstood as a description of the functions of connective tissue. Some connective tissues - literally connect - in the mechanical sense - separate structures to one another within the body. This is a function of some types of connective tissues in some cases, for instance ligaments and tendons are composed of connective tissue and they do physically bind bones to bones and muscles to bones. Connective tissues have many other functions however. They can connect in a broader sense - by providing protective and structural support to organs and other body structures as well as providing an interactive biological ground substance that extends throughout the body - filling the spaces between body structures and providing the underlying framework the results in the shape of the body.

Connective tissues networks are the source of the many of the overall mechanical and physical properties of the body. The distribution of substances throughout the body and many of the functions of organs and organ systems depend on processes that occur within this continuous and complex network of connective tissue.

Connective tissue is also an important component of organs, blood vessels and lymph nodes where among other functions, they provide a structural framework of **reticulin fibers** that organize the cells within organs, blood vessels and lymph nodes.

Ground Substance

General features of most types of connective tissues is the ground substance of connective tissue. Ground substance is an extracellular often gel-like mixture of fluids and various embedded proteins such as **elastic and collagen fibers** as well as and other molecules and molecular complexes including **proteoglycan** and **glycosaminoglycan** molecules. Proteoglycans and glycosaminoglycans are macromolecules that serve as osmotic particles to retain water within the ground substance and also provide various structural and cell-signaling functions. The connective tissue cells are also embedded within this ground substance. There is a wide range of variation in the specific types of materials, concentration of materials, organization of structural components and types of connective tissue cells that comprise the ground substance of any particular type of connective tissue. The actual overall content of the ground substance depends on the structural and functional roles that the connective tissue is designed to provide at any given location within the body.

Dense Connective Tissue

Dense connective tissue has a high content of fibrous proteins within the connective tissue ground substance. These fibers are composed primarily of collagen and also of variable amounts of elastic fibers. Fibroblasts are distributed among the extracellular fibers. Dense connective tissue forms **ligaments, tendons and cartilage** and the lower structural layers of the dermis of the skin.

Loose Connective Tissue

The composition of loose connective tissue varies widely but in general loose connective tissue includes a high content of ground substance fluid, with lesser amounts of fibrous proteins, adipose cells, fibroblasts, monocytes, macrophages and neutrophils. **Adipose tissue** is connective tissue with a high content of adipose (fat) cells. Fibroblast synthesize and secret most of the proteins including collagen and elastin that is found in the ground substance of loose connective tissue. Macrophages and neutrophils are white blood cell leukocytes that clear the connective tissue matrix of cellular debris through phagocytosis and also engage in immune system surveillance and response functions. Several other types of immune system cells are frequently distributed within loose connective tissue including mast cells, eosinophils and plasma cells.

Adipose Tissue

Adipose tissue is a specific type of loose connective tissue. Large collections of adipose tissue function as a fat storage depot for the body by more loosely arranged adipose tissue is distributed throughout the body where it provides cushioning, shock absorbing functions and a flexibility and freedom of movement to the organs and other body structures which the adipose tissue surrounds. Other types of connective tissue provide similar functions throughout the body.

Bone and Blood

Although bone can be considered to be a dense connective tissue and blood can be considered to be a loose connective tissue, this is not a very helpful definition for either. Bones have a high content of dense connective tissue but they also or composed of several other types of tissues and most authorities consider bones to be organs. Bones also play key roles in the immune system and in the endocrine system and in the overall metabolic homeostasis mechanisms of the body. Blood has many of the characteristics of a loose connective tissue - where the fluid component of the blood - plasma - can be considered the ground substance and the circulating cells - red blood cells white blood cells and platelets are the cellular components. Blood is a dynamic substance and a key element of the circulatory system. The extracellular proteins and cells of the blood are critical participants in the immune system as well as nearly all of the organs and organ systems of the body. We will therefore discuss bones and blood in the context of their function within these systems.

Nervous Tissue

Nervous tissue is derived exclusively from ectoderm. Neural tissue of the primary tissue of the central nervous system - the brain and the spinal cord - and of the peripheral nervous system. Nervous tissue is almost entirely composed of nervous tissue cells - **neurons and glial cells**. We have described the anatomy and physiology of neurons in the context of the creation and transmission electrical impulses. Glial cells are nervous tissue cells that play critical roles in the development maintenance and repair of nervous and

enhance the functional roles of neurons. The a severa different types of glial cells. These are oligodendrocytes, astrocytes, ependymal cells and microglia, and in the peripheral nervous system cells, Schwann cells and satellite cells.

Microglia are not technically nervous tissue cell because they are derived from mesoderm. They are **phagocytic cells** that are mobile and constantly patrol nervous tissue for cellular debris and infectious agents and participate in immune and cell repair activities within the central nervous system. **Astroglia (astrocytes)** are notable for their shape which includes numerous branching arm-like structures. Astroglia or astrocytes are arranged around blood vessels within the CNS and form an important element of the **blood-brain barrier;** they also regulate the levels of electrolytes in the extracellular regions of the CNS. **Schwann cells and oligodendroglia** provide extensions of their cell membrane, which encase the axons of neurons, providing an insulating layer to the axons that is called **myelin.**

Muscle Tissue

Muscle tissue is exclusively derived from mesoderm. There are three distinct types of muscle tissue - skeletal/voluntary muscle, cardiac muscle and. **Skeletal or voluntary muscle** is a syncytium - individual cells have intercellular connections called **gap junctions** that allow the cytoplasm of cells to move freely among the other cells of the syncytium. **Cardiac muscle** is the muscle tissue that forms the heart. Cardiac muscle is also a syncytium. We have discussed the structural and biochemical process that occur during the contraction of skeletal and cardiac muscle. **Smooth muscle** is the muscle type that is located throughout the body particularly in the muscular layers of the **respiratory airways**, the walls of the **digestive tract** and in the walls of **circulatory vessels**. Cardiac and smooth muscle are not under voluntary control but are regulated by the **autonomic nervous system.**

HESI A^2 - Spire Study System

MODULE 4

DAY, LOCATION, MUSIC

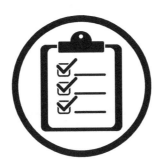

① 1

MONDAY, OCTOBER 12

COFFEE SHOP ON MAIN STREET

MY FAVORITE BAND

② 2

③ 3

GENERAL HUMAN ANATOMY

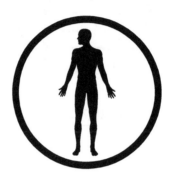

Anatomical Positions

The anatomy of the human body and the discrete structures within the human body are described in part by their spatial orientations and relationships. The terms used to describe the relative positions of anatomical structures to one another are also used to describe specific regions of individual anatomical structures. There is some overlap in the definitions of these terms and occasionally they may be used interchangeably. Most of the terms are best understood as pairs of opposing directions or relative locations.

<u>Dorsal vs. Ventral:</u> Dorsal means towards the back of the body and ventral means towards the front of the body. At the outer body surface, the back of the head, neck, torso, upper and lower legs and arms, the back of the hands and the upper surface and the top (vs. the soles) of the feet are the dorsal exterior surfaces. The most significant dorsal region landmarks are the midline of the spine and the shoulder blades or left and right scapulae.

The exterior ventral surfaces are the front of the neck, chest, abdomen, pelvis, upper and lower arms and upper and lower legs and the soles of the feet. Prominent ventral surfaces landmarks include the trachea (or windpipe) in the midline ventral neck, the sternum (or breastbone), the clavicles (or collarbones), the breasts in the ventral thorax (chest), the umbilicus (belly button) in the midline of the ventral abdomen, and the external genitalia in the ventral pelvis. The ventral surfaces of the arms are the surfaces that face upward when the arms are extended straight out with palms facing upward.

Important dorsal/ventral regions are the dorsal and ventral regions of the spine and spinal cord, and the dorsum of the hands and feet (vs. the palms of the hands and the soles of the feet).

<u>Anterior vs. Posterior</u> These terms are to a large extent analogous to the terms dorsal and ventral, but they are usually the terms preferentially used to describe relative positions. It is common to describe one structure as being "anterior to" or "posterior to" another structure rather than to say "dorsal to" or "ventral to". For instance the esophagus is correctly described as being located "dorsal to" the heart, but usually the esophagus is described as located "posterior to" the heart and conversely the heart is described as being located "anterior to" the esophagus.

Notable anatomical regions identified with these terms include the anterior and posterior pituitary (sub regions of the pituitary gland) and the coronary arteries (arteries that supply oxygenated blood to the muscle tissue of the heart), the left anterior descending coronary artery for example.

Lateral vs. Medial: Lateral means "to the side" or "the side(s) of". Medial means "toward the center" or "closer to the midline". Lateral and medial are often used in combination other positional terms to produce a more precisely defined location such as dorsolateral, ventromedial, anterolateral etc. The ventromedial hypothalamus is a notable region described in this manner.

It is common to say that one anatomical structure is located "lateral to" or "medial to" another anatomical structure. Externally, the major lateral regions are the lateral chest regions, the lateral abdominal regions and the lateral thigh and knee regions. The prominent medial regions of the external surfaces of the body are the medial thigh and medial knee regions.

Inferior vs. Superior: Superior means "above", "over" or "towards the top of the head". Inferior means "below", "underneath" or "towards the feet". These terms can be combined with other positional terms to identify more precise and discrete anatomical regions, such as the anterior-superior ischial spine region of the pelvis.

Rostral vs. Caudal: This pair of descriptive terms is somewhat analogous to the terms superior and inferior. Rostral means "towards the head or cranium" and caudal means "towards the pelvis or the base of the spine". These terms are comparatively rarely used. They are most often used in reference to the regions between the head and pelvis and are not used to describe the appendages (arms and legs).

Superficial vs. Deep: Superficial means "shallow" or "towards the surface of" or "closer to the skin". Deep means "closer to the center of" or "farther from the surface of". Superficial body structures include skin, hair, facial structures such as the eyes, nose and mouth; nipples of the breast, the umbilicus and external genitalia.

The deepest structures in the appendages of the body (arms and legs) include the medullary cavities of the long bones. The deepest regions of the skull are the ventricles at the center of the brain. The heart, the digestive organs, the kidneys, urinary bladder and female reproductive organs are deep structures with respect to the external body surfaces.

When describing relative positions of two or more anatomical structures or locations, the superficial structure or location is closer to the external surface of the body compared to the deep structure or location. The esophagus is posterior to the trachea, but it is equally correct to describe the esophagus as being deep to the trachea.

Proximal vs. Distal: Proximal means "close" or "nearer to" and distal means "distant", "further away from" or "towards the end of". The reference point that is used to define what is proximal or distal varies depending on what is being described. In the broadest sense, proximal is closer to the center of mass of the body within the deep chest or abdomen. Distal is nearer to the tips of the toes or fingers or the top of the head.

Usually the reference point is more specific; the main artery of the body, the aorta begins at the heart and passes from the chest into the abdomen with a first major branch at the femoral arteries. The reference point in this case is the heart; the abdominal aorta is proximal to the femoral arteries and distal to the thoracic aorta with respect to their proximity to the heart. In the kidneys, small filtering units have structures called renal tubules. The tubule is divided into proximal and distal renal tubule segments. In this case the reference point is Bowman's capsule, a central region of these filtering units of the kidney.

Prone vs. Supine: This term pair defines two general positions of the entire human body. The supine position is when one is lying flat on one's back, the arms and legs are extended (straight, not bent at a joint such as the knee or elbow) The palms of the hands are facing upward, and the heels of the feet are in contact with the ground.

The prone position is the reverse of the supine position, occurring when one is lying flat and face down, with the palms of the hands and the tops of the feet in contact with the ground. In the supine position, all of the ventral anatomical surfaces of the body are facing upward. The reverse is true for the prone position where all of the dorsal surfaces of the body are facing upward (except for the upper arms, where the lateral surfaces face upward).

Cross Sections

The anatomy of the body can be visually displayed as cross sections, either of the entire body or of body structures, (the heart or the brain for example). These sections are defined in relation to a human body that is in an upright standing position. There are three primary types of cross-sectional views; the transverse, the sagittal and the coronal cross-sectional views.

Transverse sections are the views represented as if the body has been sliced cleanly in two on the horizontal plane - a mid sagittal view will divide the upper body - head, arms, chest and upper abdomen and the lower body - lower abdomen, pelvis, and legs at about the waistline of a typical individual. Cross-sections of the body may occur at any higher or lower horizontal height either moving toward the top of the head or toward the soles of the feet.

Sagittal sections divide the body into a left and a right side. The mid-sagittal section will divide the body into equal right and left sides, as if a knife had cut cleanly through the body beginning at the top of the head and then proceeded downward through the midline axis of the body. The left section will include the left side of the face, neck, chest, abdomen, pelvis and the left leg. The reverse is true for the right section of the body.

Coronal sections are identical to sagittal sections except that the dissection plane is rotated by 90 degrees. This results in a transection of the body that results in a front, ventral or anterior section and a back, dorsal or posterior section. A mid-coronal section divides the body into front and back sections at the midline of the body.

Any sagittal section of the body may be obtained by moving the dissection plane parallel and lateral to the midsagittal section. Any coronal section of the body may be obtained by moving the dissection plane parallel and lateral to the mid-coronal section.

Direction of Motions of the Parts of the Human Body

Nearly all voluntary movements of the human body occur through muscle contractions that result in motions of bones at joints that are designed for body movement (notable exceptions are facial expression movements and the motion of the diaphragm during breathing).

Generally, these motions refer to movement of the arms and legs (the appendages), but considerable numbers and types of movements occur along the skull -spine and spine-pelvis axis. The appendages in particular are capable of quite complex motions, particularly at the shoulder, wrist and ankle regions.

For the HESI the primary types of motions one should know are abduction vs. adduction and flexion vs. extension.

Flexion vs. Extension: At a joint, the adjacent ends of bones may be able to move such the joint angle between the bones increases (opens) or decreases (closes), in a simple hinge-like fashion, usually within a maximum range of 180 degrees. This simple, hinge-like joint motion notably occurs at the elbow and knee joints, but most joints can produce this motion.

Extension is the increase in the angle of the joint (opening or extending out). Flexion is the opposite or reverse of extension. Flexion at a joint causes the bones at the joint to move in a manner that causes the joint angle to decrease (close or bend inward).

Abduction vs. Adduction: This type of motion is almost always in reference to motion of the upper arms at the shoulder joints and the upper legs at the hip joints. Abduction results in movement of the arms or legs outward or away from the midlines of the body. Adduction is the reverse of the motion of abduction, the movement of arms or legs towards the midlines of the body.

The Axial Skeleton
The axial skeleton consists of the bones of the skull and the spinal column, the ribs and the sternum.

The Spine
The spine is in many respects the fundamental structural element of the human body. It consists of individual bones known as vertebrae arranged linearly to form a continuous, flexible, bony column.

There are 5 regional spinal segments, the cervical, thoracic and lumbar spinal segments, the sacrum and the coccyx. The cervical segment begins with the vertebra that articulates with the base of the skull (this vertebra has a specific name - the "atlas") There are seven cervical vertebrae. These are the vertebra found in the neck.

The thoracic spinal segment begins with the 8th vertebra. There are 12 thoracic vertebrae. They are notable in that they articulate laterally with the 12 pairs of ribs that are important structural components of the chest or thoracic walls. The lumbar vertebrae begin with the 19th vertebrae, there are 5 lumbar vertebrae.

The final lumbar vertebra connects to the sacrum (which is actually 5 or 6 fused vertebrae). The sacrum is fused medially to the other bones of the hip and together they form the bony pelvis. At the most distal end of the sacrum are four small partially fused vertebrae that together are referred to as the coccyx. In many other species, the coccyx is the base of the tail. The terminal vertebra of the coccyx represents the caudal end of the spine.

The Vertebral Canal
The surfaces and underlying sub-regions of the spine and the individual vertebrae are identified as the dorsal, ventral, lateral and central regions. The central vertebral-spinal region is hollow and forms the vertebral canal. The vertebral canal contains the spinal cord of the central nervous system. The spinal cord begins as the distal extension of the brainstem and enters the vertebral canal through the foramen magnum - a large opening in the posterior base of the skull.

The spinal cord does not extend for the entire length of the vertebral canal. It terminates distally (or caudally) at the junction level of the 1st and 2nd lumbar vertebrae. The dorsal and ventral spinal nerve roots that combine to form the 31 sets of spinal nerves of the somatic or voluntary nervous system emerge from the spinal cord at the dorsolateral and ventrolateral intervertebral junctions in the cervical, thoracic and lumbar spinal regions.

The Skull
The skull consists of the tightly fused bones that form the cranial vault, which contains the brain and pituitary gland, and the facial bones; including the upper jaw bones - the maxillae and the lower jaw - the mandible. The mandible is the only moveable bone of the skull. The inner surfaces of the bones that form the cranial cavity (cranial vault) correspond to the adjacent underlying regions of the cerebral cortex of the brain. The frontal bone overlies the left and right frontal cortices. The midline parietal bones overlie the parietal cortices. The laterally positioned temporal bones overly the temporal cortices and the posteriorly positioned occipital bones form the back of the skull and overly the occipital cortices.

The cerebellum and brainstem of the brain also occupy the occipital region of the cranial cavity at the base of the brain. A small depression called the sella turcica is located in the medio anterior inner surface of the base of the skull. The pituitary gland is partially contained within the sella turcica. The 12 pairs of cranial nerves emerge from the brain through various openings in the skull. Together with the 31 pairs of spinal nerves, these form the peripheral portion of the somatic nervous system.

The Thoracic Skeleton
The thoracic (the chest and upper back) skeleton is comprised of the thoracic vertebrae, 12 sets of ribs, the sternum (breastbone) and the medial sections of the clavicles (collarbones). The ribs connect to the lateral surfaces of the thoracic vertebrae then extend laterally to form the dorsal thorax. Next, the ribs curve anteriorly to form the lateral walls of the thorax and then curve medially, continuing to their medial articulations with the sternum. The sternum is located in the midline of the anterior (ventral) wall of the

thorax. The medial ends of the clavicles articulate to the superolateral angles of the sternum.

The thoracic skeleton creates a cage-like structural framework. When the associated muscles and connective tissues are added to this framework, an interior thoracic cavity is created. This cavity will contain the heart, lungs and several other important anatomical structures. The floor of the thoracic cavity will be formed by a single dome-shaped sheet of muscle - the diaphragm.

The Appendicular Skeleton

The upper appendicular (attached) skeleton consists of the bones of the shoulder girdles, arms, wrists, hands and fingers. The shoulder girdles are formed by the clavicles and the scapulae. The medial ends of the clavicles articulate with the superolateral angles of the sternum. This is the only direct bony connection of the upper appendicular skeleton to the axial skeleton. The distal end of the scapula and a lateral extension of the clavicle - the acromion, articulate distally and, along with the proximal end of the humerus, together form the bony elements of the rotator cuff - the complex shoulder joint.

The distal end of the long bone of the upper arm - the humerus, forms the elbow joint with the proximal ends of the two lower arm bones - the radius and the ulna. The distal ends of the radius and the ulna articulate with several of the wrist bones -the carpals, to form the complex wrist joint. The carpals articulate with the metacarpal bones of the hand. The distal ends of the metacarpals articulate with the bones of the fingers - the phalanges.

The Lower appendicular skeleton consists of the bones of the pelvis (except for the sacrum -which is part of the axial skeleton), and the bones of the legs, ankles, feet and toes. The left and right portions of the bony pelvis are fused to the axial skeleton medially at the lateral edges of the sacrum. The proximal end or "head" of the femur fits into a semicircular depression of the inferolateral borders in the bones of the pelvis. Along with associated muscles and connective tissues, these form the ball and socket joint of the hip. The distal end of the femur articulates with the proximal ends of the

tibia and fibula at the knee joint. The distal ends of the tibia and fibula articulate with several tarsal bones to form the complex ankle joint. Tarsal bones in the ankle region articulate with proximal ends of metatarsal bones in the foot. Distal ends of metatarsal bones articulate with the bones of the toes, the phalanges.

Skeletal Muscles

Most of the skeletal structure of the body is covered by layers of muscles. The anterior surface of the tibiae or shins and the wrists, ankles, cranium and dorsal surface of the spine the ribs and the sternum and the clavicles have comparatively thin or extremely thin overlying layers of muscles. Major skeletal muscle groups include the upper arm muscles, the biceps and triceps; the deltoid muscles of the shoulders, the large muscles of the anterior chest - the pectoralis major muscles; the large lateral muscles of the back - the latissimus dorsi; the large muscles of the pelvis (hips) - the gluteal muscles; the anterior muscles of the upper leg - the quadriceps; The large muscles of the posterior upper leg - the hamstrings, and the largest muscle of the lower leg - the gastrocnemius (calf) muscles.

Body Cavities

There are two major cavities of the human body - the dorsal and the ventral body cavities. These cavities are almost completely sealed off from the external environment by surrounding bone and or muscle and other connective tissue. The dorsal body cavity consists of the cranial cavity and the spinal canal. The dorsal cavity is enclosed by the inner surfaces of the bones of the cranium and the vertebra walls of the central vertebral canals. The dorsal cavity contains the brain and the spinal cord. The ventral cavity is enclosed by the inner walls of the thorax - thoracic muscles, ribs sternum and thoracic vertebrae - the inner surfaces of the ventral, lateral and dorsal abdominal wall muscles, and the inner surface bones and associated muscles of the pelvis. The ventral cavity is divided into an upper cavity - the thoracic cavity - and a lower cavity - the abdominal/pelvic cavity - by a transverse dome-shaped muscle - the diaphragm. Major contents of the thoracic cavity are the heart and lungs. Major contents of the abdominal/pelvic cavity are the intestines, associated digestive organs - liver, gallbladder and pancreas - the urinary bladder and, in females, the uterus and ovaries.

The Integumentary System

The integumentary system of the human body - or simply "the integument" - is a multilayered sheath of tissues and associated cells and extracellular structural and functional components that completely encloses the interior of the body. The most superficial layer of the integumentary system is exposed to the external environment and forms the external surface of the body. Two of the most general primary functions of the integumentary system are to provide a physical containment of the internal body contents and to provide a physical and biochemical barrier to elements of the external environment. There are several secondary functions of the integumentary system as well. Most of these functions as a group can be categorized as homeostatic functions in the sense that they all provide mechanisms to maintain a controlled and stable yet adaptable internal environment that is distinctly separate from the external environment.

Defensive Barrier Functions

The external surface of the integumentary layer in humans is relatively impermeable to water and atmospheric gases. This feature prevents the loss of water (dehydration) and soluble substances from the body. The surface layer of the integument is resistant to radiation damage by ultraviolet wavelength light which is a component of sunlight. The surface layer of the integument is also resistant to penetration by potentially harmful toxic chemicals and infectious biological agents such as viruses, bacteria, fungi, and other eukaryotic unicellular and multi-cellular parasites. Therefore, the integument provides a critical role as the first line of defense in the body's immune system.

Thermoregulation

Another important homeostatic function of the integument is thermoregulation - which allows the body to maintain a constant optimum internal temperature range. The integument regulates internal body temperature by several mechanisms. The lowest layer of the integument - the hypodermis contains adipose tissue that has poor thermal conduction and therefore acts as an **insulator** to protect against excessive heat transfer between the internal regions of the body and the external environment.

Sweat and Evaporative Heat Loss

The insulation capacity of the integument is a passive form of thermoregulation but there are several active thermoregulatory mechanisms possessed by the integument. The integument possesses sweat glands which transport an aqueous solution (sweat) to the surface of the skin. The secretion of sweat can be regulated by neural and hormonal signals. The evaporation of sweat from the skin surface absorbs heat energy from the body as it undergoes a phase change from the liquid phase to the gas phase, thereby lowering the internal body temperature when it exceeds the optimum internal temperature range.

Vasoconstriction and Dilation

The integument is also highly vascularized and the dense capillaries near the skin surface can constrict or dilate in response to local conditions and also in response to neural and hormonal signals. When the internal body temperature is too high, superficial blood vessels dilate and blood flow increases near the surface of the skin. Heat energy can flow from the blood via conduction to the skin surface where it can radiate to the environment or be removed via sweat evaporation. Conversely when internal body temperature is too low, superficial blood vessels constrict and decrease the loss of heat from the body via the bloodstream.

Somatosensory Functions

The integument plays a major role in the sensory functions of the nervous system. The middle layers of the skin are richly innervated and contain several types of sensory cells that are distributed throughout the entire volume of these integumentary layers. The sensory receptors are designed to provide nearly all of the specific types of sensory information that comprise the **somatosensory sense** including sensations of pain, heat, cold, light touch, pressure and vibration. Specific examples of these integumentary sensory receptors include Meissner's corpuscles which detect changes in texture and slow vibrations, Pacinian corpuscles which detect deep pressure, fast vibrations, and Merkel's discs which detect sustained touch and pressure and free nerve endings which are pain receptors.

Excretory Functions

The integument does arguably play a minor role is as an excretory organ. Alcohol and several metabolic waste products including **urea** and several types of **organic acids** are excreted from the bloodstream onto skin surfaces and **excess body water and electrolytes** contained in sweat may be excreted in the form of sweat. It should be noted however that the primary method of clearing **alcohol** by the body is by metabolic functions provided by the liver and excretion of urea and organic acids is a primary function of the kidney which is completely capable of providing excretion of these substances without any contribution of excretion through the skin. The excretion of these substances through the skin is simply a result of the forces of diffusion. They are not regulated excretory process of the body.

The secretion of some types of organic acids are a design feature of the integument, but not as an excretory process but as an element of the **innate immune system** - where the organic acids generate a **low surface skin pH level** that is unfavorable to the growth of fungi and bacteria. The loss of water and electrolytes through sweat is more likely to result in excessive loss of water and electrolytes leading to dehydration and electrolyte abnormalities within the body which can be dangerous and even fatal. In this sense, this form of excretion is undesirable and is disruptive to the maintenance of homeostasis of the body.

Non-Barrier Immune Functions

The extracellular matrix and highly keratinized cells of the outer surface of the integument provide physical barriers in the form of tight cytoskeleton-keratin protein and extracellular phospholipid interconnections. Hydrolytic enzymes, short polypeptide segments with antimicrobial activity and organic acids provide biochemical resistance to infectious organisms. Active immune functions of the integument are provided by other cells and molecular substances located within the integument including antigen presenting cells called dendritic cells, T-cells and other cells of the immune system.

Vitamin D Synthesis

The integument has metabolic functions, most notably in the synthesis of vitamin D where ultraviolet radiation travels into the skin where it participates in chemical reaction stage required for the conversion of vitamin D precursors - which are also located in the skin to -to vitamin D. The hypodermis of the integument stores energy in the form of fat contained in adipose cells.

Layers of the Integument

The integument consists of a dermal or cutaneous layer and a subcutaneous or hypodermal layer. The dermal layer consists of two sub layers- the dermis and the epidermis.

The Hypodermis (Subcutaneous Layer)

The lowermost or deepest layer of the integument the hypodermis or the subcutaneous layer of the integument consist primarily of loose adipose connective tissue, blood vessels, lymphatic vessels and nerves. The hypodermis provides a transitional connective zone between the overlying dermal layer and the adjacent underlying body contents, usually outer skeletal muscle layers, but in some areas bony structures - particularly over the knee and elbow joints and the anterior surfaces of the lower leg (the shins).

The adipocytes of the hypodermis are organized into small collections called lobules that are enmeshed in collagen fibers. Fibroblasts are sparsely distributed throughout the hypodermis. The hypodermis- dermis boundary is a continuous series of interdigitating invaginations of both layers into the other with direct structural connections provided by collagen and elastic fibers. One of the four major types of mechanoreceptors - Lamellar or Pacinian corpuscles, are located at the boundary region between the hypodermis and the dermis. These sensory receptor cells provide tactile information those results in the perception of pressure or vibration.

The Dermis

The dermis is the middle layer of the three major integument layers. It is composed of three primary cell types, fibroblasts, macrophages and adipocytes, but there are numerous other types of cells interspersed within the dermis, including chromophores or melanocytes and various cells associated with the immune system including dendritic cells and T-cells.

The extracellular matrix of the dermal layers contain collagen, elastin and reticulin fibers and several types of macromolecules that help to retain water within the matrix and also serve other functions. The most common types of these extracellular macromolecules are glycosaminoglycans, proteoglycans and glycoproteins.

The Dermal Reticular Layer

The dermis consists of two sub layers - the deep layer - adjacent to the hypodermis - is the reticular layer. The reticular layer is composed of dense connective tissue. This tissue contains dense amounts of collagen fibers and elastic fibers and reticular fibers. These fibers provide the mechanical properties of tensile strength and elasticity to the integument. The roots of hair follicles, sweat glands, sebaceous glands and sensory receptor cells are also implanted within the reticular layer of the dermis.

The Dermal Papillary Layer

The second sub layer of the dermis - the papillary layer - is immediately superficial to the reticular layer. The primary type of tissue contained in the papillary layer is **areolar connective tissue**. Areolar connective tissue is a very loose arrangement of adipocytes and collagen and elastin fiber with an abundance of gel-like extracellular matrix. These features of areolar connective tissue allow substances to readily diffuse through the tissue.

The Dermal-Epidermal Interface

At the interface between the papillary layer of the dermis and the overlying superficial layer of the integument - the epidermis - the papillary layer projects numerous knob like extension of tissue called **papillae** between interdigitating ridges of the epidermis -called **rete ridges**. The result is a tight enjoining of the two integumentary layers. The papillae of the papillary layer contain tufts of capillaries or Meissner's corpuscles. Meissner's corpuscles are sensory receptor cells that are adapted to provide information that is interpreted in the CNS as the sensation of light touch. Mid portions of hair follicles, sweat and sebaceous glands nerves and

lymphatic vessels also travel through the papillary dermis toward the epidermis.

The Epidermis

The most superficial layer of the integument is the epidermis. The epidermis has **no direct blood supply** and depends on diffusion for the supplies of oxygen and nutrients and for transport of CO_2 and other waste products. The epidermis begins immediately adjacent at the superficial surface of the papillary layer of the dermis. The two layers are separated by a basement membrane. The **basement membrane** is a common feature of almost all epithelial tissues and serves as an attachment surface for the lowermost layers of epithelial cells and also creates anchoring connections with loose connective tissue located beneath the basement membrane.

The basement membrane of the epidermis provides the biomolecular features that allow the epidermis to adhere to the dermis. The basement membrane has several additional functions including immune system functions and cellular repair functions. The basement membrane has a complex structure consisting of multiple layers of fibrous proteins including anchoring collagen fibers, substrate **adhesion molecules (SAMS)** integrins and several other types of macromolecules. The basement membrane is also the last line of defense of the spread of cancerous cells that originate within the epithelium.

Regions of the Epidermis

The epidermis is composed of either four or five stratified regions depending on the local anatomical areas where the epidermis is located. Most areas consist of four regions - the stratum basale stratum spinosum, stratum granulare and the stratum corneum. The epidermis of the palms of the hands and the soles of the feet soles is known as "thick skin" because it has 5 epidermal regions and is referred to as thick skin. The additional region of thick skin is the stratum lucidum which is interposed between the stratum spinosum and the stratum granulare.

The Malpighian Layer

The deepest layer of the epidermis is the **Malpighian layer** which is subdivided into the stratum basale or inner basal layer and the overlying stratum spinosum layer.

The Basal Layer (Stratum Basale)

The basal layer is composed of columnar epithelial cells that are attached to the superficial surface of the underlying basement membrane by connective structures called hemidesmosomes. These cells are germinal epithelium that undergoes mitotic division to produce a continuous supply of cells which migrate toward the outer surface of the epithelium. As these cells migrate, they undergo progressive stages of differentiation with varying characteristics that define the overlying regions of the epidermis.

Melanocytes, Merkel cells and associated cutaneous nerves and cells that participate if the inflammation reactions of the immune system are also present in the basal layer. Melanocytes connect to keratinocytes and provide the pigment melanin to keratinocytes. Melanin provides a barrier to ultraviolet radiation and is also the pigment that determines the degree of darkness of skin tone that is a component of human racial characterizations. Merkel's cells and associated cutaneous nerves provide sensory information associated with the perception of light-touch.

The Stratum Spinosum (Spinous or Prickle Cell Region)

The stratum spinosum is the second of the two sub layers of the Malpighian layer of the epidermis. The stratum spinosum region is located directly superficial to the inner basal layer. This region consists of polyhedral-shaped cells that are daughter cells of the basal epithelial progenitor cells. The stratum spinosum cells also undergo mitotic division contributing to the approximately five layers of epidermal cells within the region. The cells have a spiny or prickly appearance due to microfilament shortening within desmosomes that interconnect among the cells.

The stratum spinosum cells synthesize large amounts of fibrillar proteins called **cytokeratin**. Cytokeratin aggregates within the cells to form **tonofilaments**. Tonofilaments are assembled into desmosomes which form tight junctions between the epidermal cells as they continue to differentiate and migrate toward the epidermal surface.

As keratinocytes within the stratum spinosum continue to migrate upward and differentiate, the Golgi within the keratinocytes begin to produce **lamellar bodies** that contain a complex assortment of phospho and glycosphingolipids, free fatty acids and enzymes that have antibiotic activity. These products will eventually participate in the formation of the complex extracellular matrix of the outer epidermal layers.

The Stratum Granulosum

The region of the epidermis adjacent and superficial to the stratum spinosum is the stratum granulosum. The region is three to four cells in thickness. The cells of the granular region have a high content of keratin granules that produce a granular microscopic appearance - hence the name "granulosum" that is given to this layer. The cells of the stratum granulosum are classified as keratinocytes. Keratinocytes do not divide - in contrast to the cells of the stratum basale and the stratum spinosum. As keratinocytes continue to be displaced toward the outer surface of the epidermis, they become progressively flatter and more tightly compacted. In the palms and soles of humans the **stratum lucidum** is a two-to-three cell-thickness region of the epidermis is adjacent and superficial to the stratum granulosum.

The Stratum Corneum

The most superficial region of the epidermis is the 10 to 30 cell-layer-thick stratum corneum. Keratinocytes proceed through the final stages of cell differentiation to become corneocytes as they move from the stratum spinosum or stratum lucidum region to the stratum corneum. **Corneocytes** have ejected their cell nucleus (mature red blood cells also eject their cell nuclei) and are enveloped in a keratin protein matrix that in turn is surrounded by stacked layers of lipid molecules. The keratin proteins are connected to the cytoskeleton of corneocytes by structures called **corneodesmosomes**. This interconnection of corneocytes through keratin-corneodesmosomes-cytoskeleton networks provides the exceptional mechanical durability of the epidermis.

Extracellular Matrix of the Stratum Corneum

The contents of the lamellar bodies within corneocytes are transported out of the cells and serve as the raw materials for the construction of the extracellular matrix of the stratum corneum. The lipid molecules within this matrix are arranged parallel to the skin surface and form a barrier that is impermeable to water. Organic acids, hydrolytic enzymes and short chain peptides with antimicrobial activity are interspersed throughout the extracellular matrix and provide an environment that is hostile to disease causing organisms including bacteria and fungi.

The stratum corneum has very low water content and supports a community of non-harmful microorganisms that provide additional hostile conditions to potentially harmful microorganisms. Finally, the continuous shedding and replacement of superficial skin cells enhances the protective functions of the epidermis. The entire epidermal region above the basal layer is completely regenerated approximately every 48 days.

Glands of the Integument

The integument contains a variety of glands, most notably apocrine and eccrine sweat glands and sebaceous or oil glands. All of these glands are **exocrine glands**. Exocrine glands secrete substances through a glandular duct (tube) onto the **surface of epithelial tissue**, either on the surface of the skin on the luminal surface of an epithelial-lined hollow organ such as the small intestine. In contrast, **endocrine glands** secrete substances directly into the **bloodstream or lymphatic system.**

Holocrine, Apocrine and Merocrine Glands

Glands are also categorized based on the manner in which they secrete substances. There are three general types of secretory process, holocrine, merocrine and apocrine. **Holocrine** secretion occurs through the **disintegration of the secretory cells** - the disintegration of holocrine glandular cells releases the secretory substances present in the cytoplasm of the cells. **Sebaceous glands** of the integument are holocrine glands. The fragments of disintegrated glandular cells are also constituents of the secretions of holocrine glands.

Apocrine secretion occurs through a **budding of cell membrane** segment which form vesicles that contain the secretory substances of the gland. **Apocrine sweat glands** are one of the two types of sweat glands located in the integument. The cell membrane segments that bud off of apocrine glandular cells are constituents of apocrine secretions. Human **mammary glands** are also apocrine glands.

The cellular fragment components of both holocrine and apocrine glands can obstruct the ducts of the glands. Obstructed glandular ducts can result in the formation of abscesses of the gland. The contents of these abscesses may become infected by bacteria resulting in **acne** and other types of localized infections within the integument.

Merocrine glands utilize **exocytosis** to secrete their glandular products. No disintegration or budding of cell membranes occurs in the secretory cells of merocrine glands. The exocrine glands of the pancreas and virtually all endocrine glands are merocrine glands. The second type of sweat glands found in the integument - the **eccrine sweat glands** - are merocrine glands.

Sebaceous (Oil) glands

Sebaceous or oil glands are widely distributed within the integument with the exception of the soles of the feet and the palms of the hands. Sebaceous glands have ducts that most commonly communicate with the spaces adjacent to hair shafts within hair follicles but a small percentage open directly onto the external epidermal surface. The glandular cells are located in the dermis usually adjacent to a hair follicle. Sebaceous glands are holocrine glands that synthesize and secrete a substance called **sebum.** Sebum is an oily or waxy substance consisting of triglycerides, lipid esters and free fatty acids.

Sebum provides an oily medium that contributes to the composition of the sweat layer on the surface of the skin. The oily component of sweat extends the cooling effects of evaporative sweating and prevents dehydration by increasing the adherence of the sweat layer to the surface of the skin. The free fatty acids contained in sebum lower the pH of the skin surface to a range of 4.5 to 5.0 - a level that strongly inhibits the growth of potentially harmful microorganisms.

In addition to the indirect antimicrobial effect provide by the lowering of skin pH, free fatty acids in sebum also provide strong, direct antimicrobial activity. The production of sebum can be influenced by various hormone levels, in particular, testosterone stimulates sebum production and estrogen inhibits sebum production.

Eccrine Sweat Glands

Eccrine glands are merocrine glands. They are by far the most numerous and widely distributed type of sweat glands. Eccrine sweat glands secrete a watery solution containing sodium and chloride ions. In addition, eccrine sweat contains bicarbonate ions, cytokines, immunoglobulins and short-sequence polypeptides that have antimicrobial activity. The secretory cells of the glands are coiled deep in the dermis. Myoepithelial cells surround the secretory cells and contraction of these cells propels sweat solution through the eccrine duct and onto the skin surface. Eccrine sweat glands are innervated by autonomic nerve fibers that modulate sweat secretion in response to core body temperature levels and to emotional stress such as excitement or fear.

Apocrine Sweat Glands

The secretory cells and surrounding myoepithelial cells of apocrine sweat glands are located in the dermis near the dermis-hypodermis interface. The duct of apocrine sweat glands - like those of most sebaceous glands- communicate with the spaces adjacent to hair shafts within hair follicles the distribution of apocrine sweat glands is limited to only a few regions of the surface of the body, primarily the axillae (armpits).

The composition of apocrine sweat gland secretions differs significantly from eccrine sweat compositions. Apocrine secretions have a high protein and carbohydrate content. Apocrine sweat combines with sebaceous gland secretions in hair shafts located in the axillae resulting in a cloudy viscous solution that clings to axillary hair and supports colonization by bacteria. Colonizing bacteria break down components of axillary sweat and these breakdown products are responsible for the characteristic odor associated with the axillary regions.

Abnormalities of the Integument

Notable abnormalities (pathologies) of the integument include **impetigo** - a superficial staphylococcal bacterial infection and **cellulitis** a deep bacterial infection that extends into the hypodermis. Superficial viral infections typically are caused by **papilloma virus** (warts) but many generalized viral infections produce surface viral-containing vesicles such as those associated with the herpes virus. Superficial tinea-species fungal infections cause the condition known as **athlete's feet**.

Generalized viral and other infections often produce immune related skin rashes and many drug hypersensitivities also produce skin rashes and mild temporary blistering in the form of **hives**. In more serious cases deep blistering and skin loss can occur with poison ivy reactions and severe drug sensitivity, infectious and autoimmune reactions. **Eczema** is a common hereditary hypersensitivity reaction of the skin. **Psoriasis** is an often severe and debilitating condition resulting from excessive rates of cell division in the epidermis. **Malignant melanoma** is a particularly deadly and common cancer of melanocytes usually related to excessive sun exposure. The resistance of the integument to infection in generally is impaired by high levels of **cortisol** - often associated with prolonged periods of psychological stress.

Bone

While the discussion of bones may seem to be a comparatively simple task it is much more complex than a one might imagine. An efficient means to begin the discussion is with the process of bone development.

Bone tissue cells are derived from **mesoderm**. The cells that produce the extracellular matrix of bone tissue are chondrocytes, fibroblasts and osteoblasts. Osteoblasts, fibroblasts and chondrocytes are all capable of independent motion and can migrate to sites of bone formation throughout the body. Osteoblasts are derived from **osteoprogenitor cells**. Osteoblasts secrete substances that form the first stage in the production of the extracellular matrix of mature bone tissue.

Membranous Bone Formation

During embryological and fetal development, bone formation occurs through one of two processes, either intramembranous formation or endochondral formation. Intramembranous bone formation occurs by the conversion of a region of **mesenchymal connective tissue** membrane into a bone. Membranous bone formation generally results in the creation of flat bones, including most of the bones of the skull.

Endochondral Bone Formation

Endochondral bone formation results in the creation of most other skeletal bones. The first stage of endochondral bone formation begins with the production of a **preliminary cartilaginous version of a particular bone.** This cartilage model of the future mature bone is constructed from substances secreted from fibroblasts and chondrocytes. These initial versions of bones have the same shapes as the mature bones that they will be converted to. This conversion process is called ossification.

Ossification

Endochondral Ossification begins with various physiological processes that progressively break down and reabsorb the cartilage version bone while osteoblasts simultaneously invade the collagen matrix. Osteoblasts synthesize and secrete the substances that in the extracellular space comingle to form a composite material called **osteoid.** Osteoid is a gelatinous substance that contains a high percentage of **collagen protein fibrils** and lesser amounts of ground substance. **Ground substance** is a homogenous aqueous solution of **proteoglycan molecules** such as **hyaluronic acid** and **chondroitin sulfate**. Osteoid progressively develops into a mature bone matrix.

Organic and Inorganic Components of Bone Matrix

The collagen fibrils contained in osteoid polymerize to form collagen strands. Collagen strands and ground substance comprise the organic component of the extracellular matrix of bone. This organic component has a composition of 90% collagen and 10% ground substance. The inorganic component of the extracellular bone matrix is composed of **calcium** and **phosphate** hydroxide salts. Most of these salts are in the form of **hydroxyapatite crystals**. Hydroxyapatite is a mineral with a chemical formula of $Ca10(PO_4)6(OH)_2$.

Deposition

During the next phase of bone formation - deposition - small hydroxyapatite crystals condense along the surfaces of collagen strands. These small crystals prompt further hydroxyapatite crystallization and the content of hydroxyapatite increases. In mature bone matrix 70% of the matrix consists of the inorganic component - hydroxyapatite and other mineral salts. The remaining 30% of the matrix is composed of the organic component of the matrix - collagen strands and ground substance. The combination of collagen strands and hydroxyapatite crystals give the extracellular matrix remarkably high tensile and compressional strength.

Further bone formation can proceed by one of two general pathways. One is the pathway to cortical bone formation and the other is the pathway towards trabecular bone formation.

Cortical Bone

Cortical bone forms the outer layers of nearly all bones. It is a dense structure with has a white, smooth-appearing surface. Cortical bone has a complex and high regular microscopic structure. The formation of this structure begins with the formation of concentric layers of bone that surround a central cavity. These formations are called osteons.

Osteons

Osteons are the structural subunits that form cortical bone. Osteons are cylindrical columns that are tightly packed together in parallel arrangement in cortical bone and often extend for the entire length of individual bones. The central cavity of an osteon is called a **Haversian canal**. Haversian canals contain blood vessels and nerves. **Volkmann's canals** are passageways between adjacent Haversian canals. Together, Haversian and Volkmann canals provide an interconnected network of passageways throughout cortical bone. This network provides pathways for the flow of oxygen and nutrients to all regions of the bone.

The width of the osteon increases as osteoclast form additional concentric layer of bone. The collagen strands within these layers are highly organized into overlapping parallel fibers that extend parallel to the course of the central Haversian canal and alternating with fiber layers that encircle the canal. The result is concentric layers of bone with collagen fibers that are arranged at right angles to adjacent concentric layers. This highly organized and compact structure of cortical bone results in a very high strength to weight ratio.

Osteocytes

During cortical bone formation, a small percentage of osteoclasts become trapped within the extracellular matrix. These **osteoclasts differentiate into osteocytes**. The osteocytes remain within the cortical bone is small spaces called **lacunae**. The osteocytes within these lacunae are extremely long-lived cells that continue to reabsorb old bone tissue and produce new bone tissue for the lifetime of the bone. This process helps to maintain the structural and functional integrity of the bone often for as long as an individual's entire lifespan. Due to these structural features, cortical bone is also classified **compact bone** (due to its high density), and as **lamellar bone** - bone consisting of layers or lamina containing collagen fibers that are arranged in parallel sheets. Cortical bone is also classified as **concentric bone** due to the concentric structure of the parallel osteon subunits of cortical bone.

Trabecular Bone

While the outer or superficial layers of most bones consist of very strong, very dense highly organized cortical bone, most bones also have adjacent underlying central regions composed of a different type of bone called trabecular bone. Trabecular bone is highly porous (filled with cavity spaces and passageways) with a fractal, coral-like structure that enormously increases the surface area of trabecular bone. Macroscopically a cross section of trabecular bone has a foamy appearance due to the myriad of spaces of varying sizes that are densely distributed throughout the bone matrix. Trabecular bone is also classified as **spongy** or **cancellous** (full of cavities) bone and as **medullary** (middle or centrally located) bone. Trabecular bone does not serve a significant structural function.

Hematopoiesis

The open architecture and high surface area of trabecular bone provide an ideal landscape for hematopoiesis. Hematopoiesis is the process that is required for **the production of the cellular components of blood** - red blood cells, **granulocytic** white blood cells (polymorphonuclear leucocytes (PMNLs) monocytes and macrophages, basophils, and eosinophils), **lymphocytic** white blood cells (B-cells and T-cells) and platelets. Hematopoietic (blood forming) tissue consists of **hematopoietic stem cells** and their lineage of cells that progressively differentiated into mature red blood cells, white blood cells **megakaryocytes**.

Fragments of megakaryocytes differentiate into platelets. **Platelets** circulate in large numbers in the bloodstream and are critical to **thrombogenesis** (clot formation) that is required for repair of leaks and tear in blood vessels. The hematopoietic function that occurs in the spaces within trabecular bone demonstrates that bone is much more than a connective tissue but is actually a complex organ that has other critical functions at least as important as the structural function. The substances within the cavities of trabecular bone is considered to be a particular type of connective tissue called **myeloid tissue**.

Bone Marrow

The cavities within trabecular bone contain all of the cells that participate in erythropoiesis and also contain adipocytes and the other mixture of cells and organic and inorganic molecules typical of a loose connective tissue extracellular matrix. In many bones - the large long bone of the arms and legs in particular - there is a central or medullary cavity surrounded by trabecular bone. This central cavity is filled with the loose connective matrix associated with trabecular bone. This material within the medullary cavity is called bone marrow. Bone marrow has hematopoietic activity and also has a high content of adipocytes. This allows bone to perform an additional function by providing a energy reserve in the form of fats that are stored within bone marrow adipocytes. Bone marrow is also referred to as a type of myeloid tissue.

Bone Membranes

In addition to an outer layer of cortical bone and an inner layer of trabecular bone, bones also have an outer membrane - the **periosteum** and a membrane located between the cortical and trabecular bone layers - the **endosteum**. The periosteum contains numerous nerve fibers -pain fibers in particular. Even slight injury to the periosteum causes excruciating pain that is a primary protective mechanism of the body.

Bone Remodeling

Bone is a dynamic organ that is undergoing a continuous process of renewal and adaptation to the changing demands of the external environment. The mechanical forces acting on bones cause continual damage in the form of **microfractures,** which must be repaired. Bone also responds to increased **mechanical stress** by increasing bone mass and **reconfiguring the shape of bone** to increase the bone's ability to function at higher levels of mechanical stress. Bone also serves as a crucial storage site of calcium and phosphate for all of the cells of the body. All of these functions -bone repair, growth and adaption to the mechanical demands of the external environment and the **uptake and release of calcium and phosphate** to and from the bloodstream and extracellular spaces within bone requires that there is a process to simultaneously break down bone matrix and create new bone matrix. This process is called bone remodeling. It occurs at the cortical surfaces of bones through the bone decomposing activities of cells called **osteoclasts** and the bone formation activities of osteoblasts.

It is not clear how the relative activity of osteoblasts and osteoclasts is regulated to precisely remodel a bone or a region of bone. There is some evidence that increased mechanical stress at a bone region generates small electrical currents that can be detected by osteoblasts and cause osteoblast activity to increase. Regardless of the precise manner in which remodeling is regulated, the overall process depends on the relative local activity of osteoblasts and osteoclasts. At regions where osteoblast activity exceeds osteoclast activity, the bone thickens, and where the reverse is true, bone is reabsorbed and the bone thins.

Metabolic Functions of Bone - Calcium and Phosphate Ion Levels

In addition to the production of osteoid, osteoblast also secrete an enzyme called alkaline phosphatase that promotes the mineralization of osteoid. This process removes calcium and phosphate ions from the blood and extracellular space and deposits the ions in newly formed bone in the form of hydroxyapatite crystals. The increased osteoblast activity therefore tends to decrease the levels of free calcium and phosphate ions in the body. Osteoclasts - which are derived from macrophages - have the capability to dissolve hydroxyapatite and disrupt collagen fibers in bone matrix. This activity releases calcium and phosphate ions into the circulation; therefore, increased osteoclast activity tends to increase the levels of free calcium and phosphate ions in the body.

In order for bone to function in its role of releasing or absorbing calcium and phosphate ions to maintain optimum levels of body calcium and phosphate ion levels, osteoclasts and osteoblast have to be responsive to the hormones that are designed to regulate these levels. There are numerous factors that influence calcium and phosphate levels in the body and numerous methods of monitoring these levels and numerous hormones that form a network of activities that influence these levels.

When the overall activity of osteoblasts exceeds the overall activity of osteoclasts, the overall bone mass of the body increases and the levels of calcium and phosphate in the body decreases. The reverse is true when overall osteoclast activity exceeds overall osteoblast activity. Ultimately the hormones that directly determine the relative activity of osteoblasts and osteoclasts are the thyroid hormone **calcitonin** and **parathyroid hormone** (PTH). Calcitonin binds to membrane receptors and osteoclasts resulting in inhibition of osteoclast activity. Calcitonin therefore tends to increase levels of body calcium ion. Parathyroid hormone stimulates the activity of osteoblasts, resulting in decreased levels of body calcium ion.

Osteoblasts can also be stimulated growth hormone by the pituitary, thyroid hormone (T3 and T4), the sex hormones testosterone and estrogen and by Vitamin D. The result is an overall increase in the bodies total bone mass.

Structural Functions of Bone

In the musculoskeletal system, bone acts as the primary structural component of the system, acting as anchoring points for skeletal muscles and as pivot points for body movement at bony joints. Moveable bony joints are articulations (meeting points) of the two bones that allow a variable range of motion depending on the type of joint.

Synovial Joints

There are 206 major bones in the adult human body and many other smaller bones called sesamoid bones. Nearly all of the major bones form articulations with adjacent bones (the patellae and the hyoid bone are notable exceptions). The widest range of motion occurs at synovial joints which consist of a fibrous joint capsule that encloses the ends of two articulating bones. Ligaments between the articulating bone ends surround the exterior of the fibrous capsule and bind the joint together. The ends of the bones within the joint capsule are covered by pads of cartilage called articular cartilage which provide mechanical protection to the ends of the bone and also are slippery, allowing ease of movement of the bones within the synovial capsule.

Synovial Fluid

The interior surfaces of the synovial capsule are covered with specialized connective tissue that forms a synovial membrane. Fibroblasts within the synovial membrane secrete components of synovial fluid. These contributions to synovial fluid consist of long chain sugar polymer molecules called **hyaluronic acid** and another molecule called **lubrin**. Both hyaluronic acid and lubrin provide lubrication to the joint structures within the synovial capsule Additional elements of synovial fluid include water and dissolved oxygen and nutrients that diffuse out of capillaries within the synovial capsule.

Types of Synovial Joints

The synovial joints with the greatest range of motion are the **ball and socket** joint of the pelvic girdle and the shoulders (glenohumeral joints). **Hinge joints** -such as those found at the elbow and knee allow a range of motion limited to primarily one plane or one axis motions of this type are usually the flexion-extension and abduction adduction movements. Most synovial hinge joints are pure hinge joints but are **compound or modified joints** that allow limited additional ranges of motion such as pronation and supination.

Ellipsoid or condylar joints - such as those found in the wrist and ankles have greater range of motion than hinge joints and less range of motion than ball and socket joints These allowed motions include two-axis - both flexion/extension and abduction/adduction. Simultaneous motions in both axes can generate circular motions or circumduction at the ankle and wrist. **Gliding or plane joints** allow only gliding or sliding movements of the articulating bone surfaces. Gliding joints are located in the carpals of the wrist and between spinal vertebral articulations. **Pivot joints** allow one bone to rotate around another bone on an axis at the articulation of the bones. The radioulnar joints and the atlantoaxial (first and second cervical vertebrae) joints are pivot joints. **Saddle joints** are saddle-shaped and allow the same types of motion as ellipsoid joint but with a greater range of motion. The thumb joint and the sternoclavicular joint are saddle joints.

Fibrous Joints and Sutures

Fibrous joints are much simpler in structure compared to synovial joints. Fibrous joints consist of varying proportions of cartilage and or collagen and elastic fibers and allow very limited mobility. Fibrous joints are typically located between the edges of two adjacent bones, forming a seam between the bone borders similar to the mortar between bricks or masonry stones. Joint movement is limited to hinge-like flexion and extension at the fibrous seam between adjacent bone edges. The **sternomanubrial joint** and the **sacroiliac joints** are fibrous joints that have a moderated amount of flexibility. Suture joints have very little fibrous content and almost not range of motion. They are the strongest joints and are analogous to seam welds between adjacent bone edges. The **bones of the skull** (except for the mandible) articulate with **suture joints**.

Bone Classification by Shape

The bones of the human body can be classified by shape into one of five general categories - long bones, short bones, flat bones, irregular bones and sesamoid bones.

Long Bones

Long bones possess a tubular shape with a long axis several times greater than cross-sectional diameter. The longest section of long bones is the bone shaft or diaphysis. The ends of long bones are called **epiphyses**. They are located at either end of the shaft (diaphysis) and have expanded and often complex geometries that are beautifully designed to allow the particular types of motion that occur with their articulations with adjacent epiphyses of within a synovial joint. The major bones of the upper and lower arms and legs - the **humerus, femur, radius, ulna, tibia and fibula** are long bones. The **phalanges** (finger and toe bones) and the **clavicles** (collar bones) are also long bones. Most long bones have medullary cavities and are a major site of erythropoiesis.

Epiphyseal Plates

The cartilaginous epiphyseal plates of the upper and lower extremities are a primary site for growth resulting in increased bone length. The adult height of an individual is determined by the amount of growth that occurs at the epiphyseal plates of these long bones and in the vertebrae of the spine. When the cartilage of the epiphyseal plates of long bones and vertebrae become fully mineralized into bone, no further increase in height can occur in an individual. The closure of these epiphyseal plates is a primary indication that an individual has reach adulthood.

Short Bones

Short bones have variable shapes, often cuboidal with dimensions of length width and height that are roughly equivalent.

The Wrist and Ankle Bones

The bones of the wrists and ankles **metacarpals** and the **metatarsals** and the middle bones of the hands and feet - the **carpals** and **tarsals** are short bones. There are eight carpal bones per hand and seven tarsal bones per foot. These bones are closely packed and have multiple interfaces with adjacent carpals or tarsals, At the ankle and wrist with some tarsal or carpal bones articulate with metacarpals or metatarsals. Metacarpals and metatarsals also articulate with adjacent long bone epiphyses of the radius and ulna or the tibia and fibula. Some tarsal and carpals also articulate or with epiphyses of phalanges. In the hands, these are the "knuckle" joints.

Due to their multiple articulations with adjacent bones

carpal and metacarpal and tarsals and metatarsal have a complex surface geometry and a somewhat irregular overall three-dimensional shape. These bones are designed to function as a group of subunits that allow very complex and subtle rearrangements of the contours of the palms of the hands and soles of the feet. These continuous alterations in the contours of the palms and soles are required particularly when walking on uneven surfaces or when grasping and manipulating objects.

While these multi bone systems allow remarkable adaptability during walking and running activities and exceptional dexterity of the hands, even seemingly minor injuries to an individual ankle or wrist bone can destabilize the entire wrist or ankle system leading to severe impairment of function.

Irregular Bones

Irregular bones as a general category have complex three dimensional geometries. the range of irregularity varies greatly. By far the most irregular bones are two of the bones of the skull - the **vomer** and the **sphenoid** bones. These bones have complex three dimensional overall and local structures consisting of bony walls, partitions, shelves, protuberances, compartments, passageways and openings that accommodate a variety of contents.

The sphenoid in particular is designed for a broad range of structural and functional purposes. Many anatomists have opined that the sphenoid is "a bone whose structure is so complex that it defies description". Several other bones of the cranium and the face are irregular bones or have regions that are irregular. These include the **ethmoid, mastoid and maxillary bones**. The bones of the **pelvis** - the ilium, ischium pubis and sacroiliac bones are irregular bones.

The **bones of the middle ear** - the **incus, malleus and stapes** (anvil, hammer and stirrup) are irregular in the sense that they do not have a simple shape, but they each have a very specific shape which allows them to function together as a unit. These three middle-ear bones form a linked, bony, mechanical system that transduces sound waves arriving at the tympanum (eardrum) in the outer ear canal to fluid waves within the canals of the inner ear.

The Spinal Vertebrae

The individual vertebrae of the spine are classified as irregular bones but they are comparable in structure and in their articulations with adjacent vertebrae to the short bones of the ankle and wrists. Their "irregularity" consists of their vertebral **foramen**, left and right **transverse processes** and dorsal midline single **spinous processes**.

The central canal of a vertebra is a tubular passage that aligns with the vertebral foramen of adjacent vertebrae. In the spine, these central canals form a continuous tube called the **spinal canal**. The spinal cord is contained within the spinal canal. The dorsal spinous process of a vertebra is a single long projection of the dorsal surface of a vertebra. The tips of spinous processes can as a group be seen and felt as the longitudinal arrangement of bumps that define the location of spine underlying the skin in the midline of the dorsal surface of the torso.

These additional features of a vertebrae are actually very regular and differ slightly but regularly between vertebrae primarily in the length and thickness of the spinous processes in the cervical, thoracic and lumbar sections of the spine and in the mass of the main body of the vertebrae from smallest at the first cervical vertebrae (C1 and C2) to largest at the most caudal lumbar vertebrae (L4 and L5). The vertebrae function as subunits of the overall spine.

Although the range of motion between adjacent vertebrae is limited, when these motions are coordinated along the entire length of the spine, they cumulatively can produce a remarkable range of bending and twisting spinal movements. As a result, the human body can adopt a vast number of specific postures in three dimensions and can coordinate changing postures to create extremely complex dynamic choreographies of continuous body movements.

Intervertebral Discs

A unique feature of the spinal vertebrae is the intervertebral disc. These are shock-absorbing structures consisting of a tough outer fibrous capsule that encases a gel-like substance called the nucleus pulposus. The discs act as a fibrocartilaginous joint between adjacent vertebrae.

Flat Bones and Sesamoid Bones

Flat bones are thin with a high surface area. They have an outer layer of cortical bone and a thin central layer of trabecular bone. Most of the **bones of the cranium** are flat bones. flat bones have a primary protective function - protection of the brain in particular- and have little if any role in erythropoiesis. Sesamoid bones are formed with muscle tendons. They have a mechanical function related to the amount of leverage that a muscle can generate on an attached bone. Most sesamoid bones are relatively small, a notable exception is **patella** which is located anterior to the synovial joint of the knee.

Bone and Joint Disorders

There are a number of diseases and other pathological conditions of bones and joints that are notable for their frequency and/ or severity in humans. Joint disorders are so common there is a medical specialty - rheumatology - that focuses exclusively on the diagnosis and treatment of these conditions.

Disorders of the Synovial Joints

The two most important synovial joint disorders are **rheumatoid arthritis** and **osteoarthritis**. Rheumatoid arthritis is an autoimmune disorder that attacks synovial joints, resulting in progressive, painful disfigurement and loss of function of joints throughout the body. Modern treatment involves monoclonal antibody and other immunological therapies that can prevent the progression of the disease if the condition is diagnosed in its early stages.

Osteoarthritis is a result of the wear and tear damage to articular cartilage in synovial joints. The mechanical forces acting on joints over decades of physical activity eventually wear away the cartilage in synovial joints resulting in the loss of the protection the cartilage provides to underlying bone. The unprotected articulating bones grind against each other and cause severe pain and eventually loss of function. Most middle-aged to elderly males have some degree of osteoarthritis. The condition is most serious when the knee and hip joints are involved. Damage due to osteoarthritis is the number one reason for hip and knee replacements in the U.S.

Infection, Inflammation and Physical Injury
Synovial fluid is susceptible to accumulations of **uric acid crystals** resulting in the excruciatingly painful inflammatory condition known as **gout**. Bacteria that enter the bloodstream often settle in synovial joints causing infection or **septic arthritis**. Many viral and **autoimmune diseases** also attack synovial joints and causing a sterile or **aseptic arthritis**. The joints are common sites of severe physical injuries including ligament and tendon tears and ruptures and joint sprains and dislocations. The **deep tendon reflexes** are a specialized local neuromuscular reflex that has evolved to limit these types of injuries.

A particularly significant class of joint disorders are those of the intervertebral discs. **herniated vertebral discs** usually occur due to awkward and or strenuous lifting and twisting activities. **Degenerative disc disease (DJD)** is a progressive deterioration of the intervertebral discs. Both conditions are very common - in fact, lower back pain associated with these disorders is the number one reason for persons to seek medical attention.

Disorders of the Bone
Osteoporosis is the most common serious bone disorder and most commonly occurs in **postmenopausal women**. The condition is a **loss of bone density** and disruption of bone structure primarily due to **inadequate calcium content**. Persons with osteoporosis are at greatly increased risk of bone fractures, most seriously fractures of pelvic bones or the femur. **Estrogen replacement therapy** in postmenopausal women can greatly reduce the incidence of osteoporosis but this form of treatment must be balanced against the risks of such replacement therapy including increased risk of cardiovascular disease. **Regular physical activity** and weight bearing exercise reduces the risk of osteoporosis.

Although rare in developed countries, **rickets** is a common bone disorder elsewhere. It is caused by **vitamin D deficiency**. Untreated, rickets results in deterioration of bone tissue, bones become increasingly brittle and fracture easily. **Osteomalacia** (vitamin D resistant rickets) causes disease similar to rickets including bone weakness, but also abnormal bone formation. The condition is the result of a defect in **vitamin D metabolism**.

Paget's disease is characterized by abnormal structural development including enlargement and thickening of bones that are brittle and easily broken. The condition results from abnormalities of osteoblast and osteoclast functions. **Perthes' Disease** occurs primarily in children. It is a disorder of the femoral head of the tibia at the ball-and socket joint of the hip. The condition is caused by inadequate blood supply to the femoral head and results in pain an impaired ability to walk or run.

Osteogenesis Imperfecta (brittle bone disease) is an autosomal dominant genetic disorder caused by defects in the enzymes involved in collagen production. The result is brittle bones that fracture easily. **Acromegaly** is condition caused by excess of growth hormone and continued growth hormone production after individuals have completed puberty. Most commonly the abnormal growth hormone production is due to a benign tumor of the pituitary gland. Untreated, acromegaly results in progressive enlargement of facial bones and of the bones of the hands and feet. This process can continue over the entire li8fe of an individual.

Bone Marrow Disorders
Bone marrow suppression and **bone marrow failure** is often a life-threatening condition that is relatively common. The hematopoietic cells of bone marrow are particularly sensitive to a wide variety of **drugs** - antibiotics, anti-inflammatories and anti-cancer and many other commonly used drugs. Bone marrow cells are also easily damaged by **environmental toxins** - such as cleaning agents, heavy metals and insecticides and herbicides. Bone marrow is also very vulnerable to radiation induced injuries from medical and dental X-ray imagery and from artificial and naturally occurring radioactive compounds in the environment.

As these conditions worsen and persist, the granulocytes and lymphocyte cell production drops or even ceases resulting in profound **impairment of the immune system**. Impaired red cell production results in severe anemia and impaired platelet production results in spontaneous hemorrhages. All of these effects can be rapidly fatal if not corrected promptly. Most blood cancers - **leukemias** and **lymphomas** originate from abnormal cells in the bone marrow.

Integument and the Aerodigestive Tract

The outer surfaces of the body are nearly completely covered by a protective layer of skin and associated cells and tissues known as the integument. The aerodigestive tract begins at the entryways of the mouth and nose. This tract is a complexly branching and diversely specialized tube that passes through the neck, thorax and abdomen/pelvic cavities and exits at the anal sphincter. Air, solid food, water and other ingested liquids enter the tract at the nose (hopefully air only) and mouth then begin a passage through the tract beginning at the common continuation of the oral and nasal cavities known as the pharynx. Lymphoid tissues - the tonsils and adenoids - ring the entry to the pharynx within the pharyngeal walls. The pharynx, as it begins to descend through the neck, bifurcates (branches into two pathways) into the respiratory and digestive tracts.

The Respiratory System

The Respiratory Tract

The initial segment of the respiratory tract is the trachea. The initial segment of the digestive tract is the esophagus. A specialized hinged plate structure - the epiglottis- can drop across the top of the trachea during swallowing. This prevents ingested solids and liquids from entering the trachea. The tracheal tube consisting of rings of cartilage and descends through the anterior region of the neck (the trachea can be felt with one's fingers beneath the surface of the anterior neck). At the midpoint of the neck, a specialized region of the trachea - the larynx - can be seen as the Adam's apple. The larynx contains the vocal cords and associated structures involved in the production of speech.

The trachea continues to the base of the neck where it enters the thoracic cavity. At about the mid-sternum level, the trachea bifurcates into a left and right main-stem bronchus. The right and left main-stem bronchi then enter their respective right and left lungs. The main-stem bronchi undergo numerous subsequent branchings into smaller and smaller and increasingly numerous air passages. This results in a dense tree-like network of airways that infiltrate the entirety of the lung tissues. The thinnest terminal branches of this respiratory airway tree are called bronchioles. At the terminal ends of the bronchioles, grape-like clusters of spherical air sacs called alveoli serve as the site of oxygen and carbon dioxide exchange between the blood contained in capillaries that encircle the alveoli and inspired air in the alveoli.

The Respiratory System

Along with the respiratory tract anatomy that has already been described, the respiratory system is composed of the lungs, internal spaces of the thoracic cavity and the muscular diaphragm that forms the floor of the thoracic cavity. The lungs are composed of separate lobes, three on the left and two on the right. The heart is positioned between the left and right lungs and is directly adjacent to the medial surfaces of the lower lobe of the left lung. Individual secondary bronchi branch off of the main-stem bronchi and enter the lobes of the lung. The diaphragm is a dome shaped muscle that is convex into the thoracic cavity. The superior surface of the diaphragm is adjacent to the inferior surfaces of the left and right lower lobes of the lungs. Importantly, the left and right phrenic nerves pass from the cervical spine through the center of the thoracic cavity and innervate the diaphragm. Damage to these nerves can paralyze the diaphragm, making the act of breathing impossible. The nasal sinuses also serve a role in the respiratory system. These are located in cavities within the facial and occipital bones of the skull.

Respiratory Physiology

The primary functions of the respiratory system are to deliver oxygen from the air to the bloodstream and to remove carbon dioxide from the bloodstream into air in the lungs and then out of the body during expiration (exhalation). The primary tissues and structures of the respiratory system are the respiratory airway - trachea, bronchi and alveoli, the lung tissue and the diaphragm. Breathing is usually involuntary, but can be under voluntary control for short periods of time.

Nervous System Control of Respiration

The basal breathing rate is driven by the medulla oblongata. Peripheral sensory receptors in major arteries and veins and within the brain itself monitor oxygen and pH levels and report this information to the hypothalamus and the medulla. Breathing depth and rate is modified as necessary to maintain optimum levels of oxygen and blood pH.

The smooth muscle cells in bronchial airways are also innervated by the sympathetic and parasympathetic nervous system Sympathetic signals cause relaxation of bronchial smooth muscle and this results in dilation of the bronchial airways. Parasympathetic signals have the opposite effect.

There is also a protective gag reflex that functions at the epiglottic region to prevent inhalation of solids or liquids.

Cilia

The epithelial cells lining the bronchial airways secrete mucous and also have numerous densely packed cilia on their membranes that are in constant coordinated motion to propel mucus and inhaled particulate matter out of the lungs through the trachea.

Breathing Mechanics

When the epiglottis is open, the respiratory airways are continuous with the outside air. The flow of air is determined by the relative air pressures inside of the airway and the outside air. When the diaphragm contracts, the convex surface of the diaphragm within the thoracic cavity flattens; this increases the volume of the thoracic cavity surrounding the lungs. This causes a drop of pressure inside the thoracic cavity below that of the outside air. The resulting pressure differential between the airways within the lung and the outside air drives air from the outside through the respiratory airways and ultimately to the alveolar air sacs.

Inspiration

Lung tissue expands during the inspiratory phase of the breathing cycle. Lung tissue is elastic and the expansion that occurs during inspiration dynamically stretches lung tissue. This process requires energy in the form of muscular work that is done by the diaphragm to increase the volume of the thoracic cavity and to decrease the pressure in the thoracic cavity.

Expiration

When the diaphragm relaxes, the elastic tissue in the lung relaxes to its normal level of relaxation. Air pressure within the lung then increases and exceeds that of the outside air. Air within the airways is then driven out of the lungs by the differences in pressure inside and outside of the lung. This term for this portion of the breathing cycle is expiration. Expiration - in contrast to inspiration - is a passive process that does not require energy utilization by the body.

Gas Exchange - Diffusion

At the microscopic level, gas exchange between the bloodstream and the alveolar air is driven by diffusion. Diffusion is movement of particles from one region to another region that is driven by difference in the concentration of particle in one region compared to the other region. The blood arriving at the capillaries surrounding the alveoli is pulmonary arterial blood - which is deoxygenated blood. The oxygen concentrations in this blood are much lower and the carbon dioxide concentrations are much higher in this capillary blood than the air contained in nearby alveolar air sacs.

Microscopic Physiology

The microscopic physiology of the capillary/alveolar region provides the optimum possible conditions for diffusion to occur - very short diffusion distances with a minimum of physical barriers to the diffusion movements. Oxygen molecules must diffuse through a one-cell-layer thick alveolar wall then through a one-cell-layer-thick capillary wall and then through a cell membrane of a red blood cell. The reverse is true for carbon dioxide molecules, which are diffusing in the opposite direction - from the blood and into the alveolar air sacs. In the red blood cell, oxygen molecules bind to hemoglobin molecules.

This process re-oxygenates the capillary blood and rids the blood of carbon dioxide. This blood is then delivered back to the heart for recirculation throughout the body.

The Digestive System

The Digestive Tract

The digestive tract, beginning as the esophagus, follows along the same path as the trachea, immediately posterior or dorsal to the trachea. At the bifurcation of the trachea, the esophagus continues inferiorly to the base of the thoracic cavity, where it passes through an opening in the muscular diaphragm and enters the abdomen. Just after entering the abdomen, the esophagus connects to the stomach. A muscular sphincter - the gastroesophageal (GE) sphincter - seals the passage of the digestive tract at the junction of the esophagus and the stomach. The GE sphincter opens only during the passage of ingested material from the esophagus into the stomach.

At the distal end of the stomach the digestive tract continues as the small intestine. The region of the small intestine that accepts the contents of the stomach is the duodenum. Another muscular sphincter - the pyloric sphincter - seals the passageway between the stomach and the duodenum. The sphincter will open at appropriate intervals to allow stomach contents to pass into the duodenum. Also, substances produced by the liver and the pancreas that are involved in the digestive process are secreted into the duodenum through the common bile duct. The digestive process continues as nutrients and water continue through the small intestine, beginning at the duodenum then through two subsequent segments of the small intestines, the jejunum and then the ileum. The ileum connects to the first segment of the large intestine - the cecum.

At this point, all of the nutrients and most of the water passing through the digestive tract have been absorbed. Indigestible bulk material continues to pass through the sequential segments of the large intestine, beginning with the cecum, and next the ascending, then the transverse and then the descending colon. Most of the remaining water in the material within the large intestine is absorbed and feces are formed during this stage of the journey through the digestive tract. The feces pass into the terminal segments of the large intestine - the sigmoid colon and the rectum - and then pass out of the body via defection through the anal sphincter.

The Digestive System

Along with the digestive tract anatomy that has already been described, the digestive system also consists of salivary glands, the liver, the gallbladder, the pancreas and a specialized regional venous circulatory system - the hepatic portal circulatory system - that carries blood from capillary beds in the intestines to capillary beds located in the liver. The salivary glands are located in the oral cavity. The liver is located on the right upper quadrant of the abdominal cavity, directly below the inferior surface of the diaphragm.

The gallbladder is connected to the liver and is nestled between liver lobes at the inferior surface of the liver. The pancreas is located in the left upper quadrant of the abdomen. Partially retroperitoneal (buried) in the dorsal abdominal wall. The pancreatic duct and the gallbladder duct merge to form the common bile duct. Recall that common bile duct connects with the duodenum. An additional important anatomical relationship is that the stomach is anterior to the pancreas and inferior and to the left of the liver.

Digestive System Physiology

The function of the digestive system is to bring macronutrients, micronutrients, electrolytes and water into the body. The macronutrients are carbohydrates, fats and proteins. Electrolytes, when they are dissolved in body fluids, are the elemental ions $Na+$, $K+$, $Ca++$, $Mg++$ and $Cl-$ The micronutrients are vitamins and trace minerals. The digestive system also functions best when the diet includes indigestible plant fiber, which is composed primarily of cellulose.

An often unappreciated fact regarding the digestive system is that, although the lumen (or canal) of the digestive tract is surrounded by the tissues and organs of the thorax and abdomen, the contents within the lumen of the digestive tract are literally outside of the body. Nothing that has been consumed orally and that is subsequently within the digestive lumen has been either absorbed by a cell of the body, nor has it passed through a surface epithelial cell layer into internal body regions.

The nutritional requirements of the body are the solid

and liquid substances that must be consumed and then absorbed into the body. These are water, macronutrients and micronutrients.

Macronutrients

Proteins

Proteins are composed of one or more chains of amino acids. The human body requires 22 specific amino acids in order to assemble the tens of thousands of different proteins that the body uses for a myriad of structural and enzymatic functions. Seven of these amino acids are classified as essential amino acids because they cannot be synthesized from other molecular compounds by biochemical processes that occur within the body. In a typical American diet, most protein is acquired by eating meat, but all amino acid requirements can be supplied by a properly selected vegetarian diet. Excess dietary proteins can be converted to fat by the body. Inadequate protein intake during early childhood development can result in the starvation state known as kwashiorkor.

Carbohydrates

Carbohydrates are sugars or starches (polysaccharides). Starches are polymer sugar molecules. The primary role of carbohydrates in the body is to serve as a source of chemical energy. The product of these energy extraction reactions is the molecule ATP and a few other molecules (NADH and NADPH). These molecules are used primarily in anabolic biochemical reactions.

Aerobic Metabolism

Anabolic metabolism is the construction of larger and more complex molecules such as proteins, from smaller and simpler molecules. Anabolic chemical processes by themselves are energetically unfavorable. When ATP molecules are coupled with (participate in) these reactions, the overall reaction is energetically favorable and therefore these anabolic reactions tend to proceed spontaneously.

Anaerobic Metabolism

In aerobic (where oxygen participates) cellular respiration, carbohydrates in the form of the sugar glucose and oxygen are converted to carbon dioxide, water and ATP molecules. This type of respiration is also known as oxidative phosphorylation. The body can also extract chemical energy from carbohydrates by anaerobic (Where no oxygen participates) respiration. In humans, when insufficient oxygen is available for oxidative phosphorylation, anaerobic metabolic chemical reactions convert glucose to lactic acid and ATP. This occurs primarily in skeletal muscle cells during intense physical activity.

Structural Roles of Carbohydrates

Sugars also are used in the synthesis of various complex molecules, including glycoproteins and glycolipids. The sugars ribose and deoxyribose are critical structural components of DNA and RNA molecules. Wheat flour products and refined sugars - sucrose and fructose - are the primary source of carbohydrates in American diets. A diet of fruits and vegetables can provide all carbohydrate needs of the body.

A limited amount of excess dietary carbohydrates can be converted to glycogen - a glucose polymer molecule that is stored in the liver. Alternatively, carbohydrates can be converted to fats that are subsequently stored in adipose (fat) cells.

Fats

Dietary fat consists of long chain fatty acid molecules. The fatty-acid molecule structure is primarily a hydrocarbon chain. Fats are essential structural elements in cell membranes and are components of many other important biological molecules. Fats are readily convertible to glucose in the body and stored fat in adipocytes (fat cells) serves as the major reserve of stored energy in the body.

Saturated and Unsaturated Fats

A fat is a saturated fat if all of the carbon-carbon bonds of the hydrocarbon portion of the fatty acid molecule are single bonds; the fat is an unsaturated fat if the hydrocarbon portion of the molecule contains one or more carbon-carbon double bonds. Most animal fats are saturated fats. Most vegetable fats are unsaturated fats.

Triglycerides and Cholesterol

Triglycerides are a form of fat consisting of three fatty

acids bonded to a small molecule called glycerol. Cholesterol is a 4-ring-structure derivative of fatty acids. Cholesterol is also an important component of cell membranes and it is also the molecule that is used by the body to synthesize the steroid hormones.

HDL and LDL Cholesterol

Cholesterol that is circulating in the bloodstream is bound with various proteins into lipoprotein particles. The most significant of these are the high-density lipoprotein (HDL) and low-density lipoprotein (LDL) particles.

High levels of LDL cholesterol in the bloodstream are associated with increased risk for the atherosclerosis related diseases - coronary artery disease (CAD) and stroke. High levels of HDL cholesterol in the bloodstream are associated with a decreased risk for CAD and stroke. In humans, the most desirable blood cholesterol profile in terms of an associated lowest risk for cholesterol associated disease is a high HDL: LDL blood cholesterol ratio, conversely the greatest risk for cholesterol associated disease is a low HDL: LDL blood cholesterol ratio.

Vitamins

Vitamins are small molecules that are critical participants is a wide variety of biochemical processes, usually as cofactors for various enzymes. Although they are required is relatively small amounts, they cannot be synthesized by the body and therefore must be obtained through the diet. Most vitamins are water-soluble, but the vitamins A, D, E and K are fat soluble.

Vitamin Deficiencies

Vitamin D is essential for the absorption of calcium from the digestive tract. Vitamin D deficiency results in osteoporosis - brittle bones that are prone to fracture under minor stress. Vitamin C is critical to maintaining the strength of collagen - the major connective structural protein in the body. Vitamin C deficiency results in scurvy, a condition that leads to tooth loss, visual impairment, and easy bruisability. When uncorrected by increased vitamin C intake, scurvy is eventually fatal. Vitamin B12 is essential for cell growth and maturation. Vitamin B12 deficiency results in anemia- a deficiency of red blood cells.

Minerals

Minerals are required for a vast array of body functions. They include the elements sodium potassium, magnesium, chlorine, calcium, phosphorus, sulfur and iron. Relative to vitamin requirements, most of the minerals are required in significantly larger amounts - calcium and phosphorus in particular. Zinc, selenium, copper and a few other elements are also required but in relatively tiny amounts. For this reason, they are often called the" trace" dietary elements.

Osteoporosis and Iron Deficiency Anemia

Calcium and phosphorus are major components of bone. Deficiency of calcium and phosphorous results in osteoporosis and impairment of muscle and nervous system functions. Iron is an essential component of hemoglobin - the molecule that binds oxygen in red blood cells. Iron deficiency results in anemia.

Digestion

Macronutrients must be broken down (digested) into individual small molecules before they can be absorbed from the digestive tract by intestinal epithelial cells. Starches and other polysaccharides must be broken down into simple 5 or 6 carbon sugars - primarily the sugars glucose and fructose.

Proteins must be broken down into individual amino acids. Fatty acids can be absorbed directly, but they need to be emulsified (separated into tiny droplets) prior to absorption. A variety of enzymes are required for the breakdown of polysaccharides and proteins. These enzymes are synthesized by cells located in the digestive system.

The digestive process begins in the mouth with the mechanical pulping of solids through the act of chewing. During this process, the enzyme salivary amylase - which is synthesized by cells of the salivary glands - is mixed into the food mass where it begins to break down any starches that may be present in the food mass.

Peristaltic Motion

During swallowing, in the pharynx, the pulped food mass is compressed into a doughy consistency food-ball called a bolus. The bolus then passes into the esophagus. Beginning at the esophagus - and for the remainder of the journey through the digestive tract - the solid material in the food bolus will be propelled along by rhythmic contractions of the digestive tract called peristalsis. This peristaltic motion is produced by smooth muscle cells located in the walls of the digestive tract (esophagus, stomach, small intestines and large intestines).

Intraluminal Barriers - the GE and Pyloric Sphincters

At the terminal (distal) portion of the esophagus, the food bolus must pass through a muscular sphincter. In biology, sphincters are rings of muscle tissue that can contract - as the iris of the eye contracts - and thereby seals off a lumen (passageway) such as the lumen of the digestive tract. This process is called constriction, the relaxation of the sphincter reverses this action and opens the pathway - this process is called dilation.

Normally, except when a food bolus is passing from the esophagus into the stomach, this sphincter - the gastroesophageal (GE) sphincter - is tightly constricted. This is because the contents of the stomach are strongly acidic - roughly equivalent to the pH of battery acid. This stomach fluid will cause severe damage to any unprotected body tissues. Heartburn occurs when stomach contents leak through the GE sphincter. A second muscular sphincter - the pyloric sphincter - is located at the distal end of the stomach cavity, where it where it seals off the entryway to the initial segment of the small intestinal tract - the duodenum.

The Stomach

The stomach protects its inner wall lining from acidic injury by secreting large amounts of mucous onto the inner surface of the gastric lumen. The stomach creates this acidic environment by synthesizing and secreting hydrochloric acid. This highly acidic fluid by itself causes widespread chemical breakdown of proteins and carbohydrates, but the stomach also synthesizes and secretes a powerful proteolytic (protein cutting) enzyme called pepsin. Pepsin is the first enzyme that engages in the enzymatic breakdown of all proteins.

Chyme

The stomach also engages is a considerable amount of mechanical digestion. The Stomach walls are thick and constructed of several heavy muscle layers. This allows the stomach to generate powerful contractions that reduce food boluses into slurry of water and partially digested lipids, proteins and carbohydrates referred to as chyme.

Intrinsic Factor

Another notable substance secreted by the stomach is intrinsic factor. Intrinsic factor is a substance that the small intestinal epithelial cells require for the absorption of vitamin B12.

The Small Intestine

At a time determined by the demands of the body, the stomach will release its contents into the adjacent distal segment of the digestive tract, the duodenum of the small intestine. The duodenum is the first of three continuous segments of the small intestine. The second segment is the jejunum and the third and final segment is the ileum.

The Duodenum

The duodenum contains cells that synthesize and secrete the hormones secretin and cholecystokinin (CCK). Prior to the release of the stomach contents into the duodenum, these hormones are secreted into the bloodstream. The absorption of dietary iron occurs exclusively in the duodenum.

Bile

When CCK arrives at the gallbladder, it stimulates the release of bile that is stored in the gallbladder into the gallbladder duct. The gallbladder duct connects to the common bile duct; Bile travels from the gall bladder duct into the common bile duct and then empties into the lumen of the duodenum. Bile that enters the duodenum will be used to emulsify fats that are present in the digestive contents of the stomach once these contents are delivered into the duodenum.

Pancreatic Enzymes and Bicarbonate Ion

Secretin stimulates the pancreas to release a volume of bicarbonate-ion-rich solution into the lumen of the duodenum. The bicarbonate solution is a moderately-strong basic solution which serves a critical role in the digestive tract, namely the neutralization of the highly acidic stomach contents as they are delivered into the duodenum. The pancreas also secretes a number of other digestive enzymes into the duodenum. For the HESI, the only specific digestive pancreatic enzyme that one need be aware of is the proteolytic enzyme trypsin.

Absorption of Water and Nutrients

The absorption of water and nutrients begins in the small intestine. Whether through simple diffusion or facilitated or active transport, the rate of the absorption of substances is primarily dependent on the surface area through which absorption occurs. This is true for all diffusion based transport. The transport of gases across the body -airway interface in the lungs is greatly increased by segmentally increasing the surface area of the airways - at the level of alveoli; the diffusional surface area is approximately the area of a tennis court.

Villi, Microvilli and the Brush Border

The total surface area of the small intestine is approximately 250 square meters (interestingly, this is about the same area as the surface area of the alveoli in the lungs).

In the small intestines, surface area is increased first by the intestinal villi - finger like projections of the inner surface of the intestines into the intestinal lumen. Next, the outer surfaces of villi are covered in microscopic finger-like extensions called microvilli. The microvilli layer forms the brush-border of the intestinal epithelial cell lining. The brush border is where the absorption of water and nutrients from the intestinal lumen and into the body occurs.

Anatomical Sites and Details of Absorption

Amino acids from the enzymatic breakdown of proteins, and fats that have been reduced to fatty acids are absorbed through the brush borders of intestinal epithelial cells. The sugars present in the intestine often require further breakdown by enzymes (disaccharidases) located in the brush border prior to absorption. Amino Acids and sugars are transported out of the epithelial cell and are absorbed by nearby capillaries. Absorbed fatty acids within the epithelial cells are processed into specialized particles and are then transported out of the cell and into lacteals - lymphatic vessel structures located in the core of villi. Water is absorbed from the intestine by passive diffusion.

The majority of nutrients are absorbed through the jejunum. Vitamin B12 and bile salts - components of bile - are absorbed in the terminal ileum. 80 percent of ingested water is absorbed in the small intestine.

The remainder of intestinal water is absorbed through the large intestine. There are no other significant digestive events other than fecal formation and defecation through the anal sphincter that occur in the large intestine.

The Liver

The liver serves numerous vital roles in the body and although considered an organ of the digestive system, has roles in other organ systems at least as important (if not more) than the digestive role.

Detoxification and Drug Metabolism

The liver receives the venous blood that from the intestines via the hepatic portal circulatory system liver cells are capable of carrying out thousands of complex chemical reactions are responsible for the majority of the catabolic chemical functions of the body. This includes the detoxification of harmful molecules in the bloodstream, the processing of drugs that are present on the bloodstream and conversion of waste products produced by the turnover of cells -red blood cells in particular - and other organic debris that is generated by the continual metabolic activities of the cells of the body. All of the cells in the body are subject to damage and lethal injury and all of the cells of the body are generating waste products from the metabolic activities that are occurring within the cells on a continual basis.

In particular, the lifespan of red blood cells is 120 days, so the entire volume of red blood cells in the body must be recycled every four months. These waste products include large amounts of fragmented cell membrane, DNA, RNA hemoglobin and products resulting from chemically degradation of hemoglobin, and other cell proteins.

Cholesterol Metabolism

The degradation of cholesterol and related molecules is accomplished by the liver through the conversion of these molecules into bile acids. These are further processed into bile and secreted to the gall bladder and then to the duodenum. In addition to emulsification of fat, bile is also required for the uptake of the fat-soluble vitamins A, D, E and K. Excess body cholesterol is removed from the body in bile acids that remain in the feces.

Nitrogenous Wastes and Production of Urea

Of particular significance are the nitrogen containing (nitrogenous) waste products resulting from protein and nucleic acid degradation. These waste products are highly toxic to cells and the liver converts these nitrogenous waste products into the molecule urea, which is a small, highly water-soluble, nontoxic nitrogen-containing molecule. Urea is easily filtered out of the bloodstream and transferred into urine by the kidneys. Urine is subsequently excreted from the body during urination.

Carbohydrate Metabolism

The liver regulates glucose levels in the blood by absorbing excess glucose from the bloodstream and then converting this excess glucose into long highly branched molecular chains of glucose. This glucose polymer molecule is call glycogen. Glycogen is stored in liver cells. If the level of glucose in the bloodstream falls below normal levels the liver cells can rapidly convert glycogen back into glucose and release this glucose into the bloodstream thereby restoring low blood glucose levels to normal levels. When glycogen reserves are exhausted, the liver can synthesize new glucose molecules from proteins and lipids. This process is termed gluconeogenesis.

Lipoprotein Synthesis

Liver cells also receive fats and cholesterol absorbed through the small intestine and process these fats and cholesterol molecules into lipoprotein particles, most notably the HDL and LDL lipoprotein-cholesterol complex particles. These particles are then released into the bloodstream by the liver cells.

Water Distribution

An additional important role of the liver is the production of the protein albumin. This protein is synthesized by liver cells and subsequently secreted into the bloodstream. Albumin molecules remain in the bloodstream and act as osmotic particles that favor retention of water within the bloodstream. This is a critical role that maintains the proper balance of water distribution between the intravascular spaces and the extravascular compartment of the body.

The Nervous System

The nervous system can be anatomically divided into the central nervous system and the peripheral nervous systems.

The Central Nervous System

The central nervous system, as previously noted, consists of the brain - located in the cranial cavity and the spinal cord - located in the vertebral canal of the spine. Also mentioned was that the outermost or most superficial region of the terminal end of the brain, the cerebral cortex, consists of five regions or lobes. The frontal, parietal temporal and occipital lobes that underlie the cranial bones of the corresponding designations. The cerebral cortex is divided into two hemispheres, right and left, that are connected by large nerve tracts. The largest of these tracts is the corpus callosum. Each hemisphere consists of the five cerebral cortical lobes - thus there are right and left frontal, parietal temporal and occipital lobes.

The regions of the brain between the cerebral cortex and the spinal cord include the midbrain, the cerebellum and the brainstem. The brainstem is the brain region that is continuous with the spinal cord as it enters the brain at the base of the skull. More specific notable brain regions include the medulla oblongata, located in the brainstem and the hypothalamus, located in the midbrain at the base of the skull. The pituitary gland is an important endocrine structure that is located adjacent to and inferior to the hypothalamus.

The spinal cord is the distal continuation of the brain stem and is contained within the vertebral canal. Beginning at the base of the occipital region of the skull, the spinal cord continues to its terminus at the junction of the first and second lumbar vertebrae. The spinal cord has relatively few neuron cell bodies; it consists mainly of nerves that relay information between the brain and neurons of the peripheral nervous system. The 31 pairs of spinal nerves exit the spinal cord at the interspaces between adjoining vertebrae - one pair per intervertebral junction.

The 12 pairs of cranial nerves and 31 pairs of spinal nerves become important elements of the peripheral nervous system once they have exited from the cranial or vertebral cavities.

The Peripheral Nervous System

All elements of the nervous system - neurons, nerves (axons of neurons), sensory cells, effector cells (muscle cells and glands) and supporting cells and structures - that are not located either inside of the skull or the spinal column - are classified as elements of the peripheral nervous system.

It is very important to understand that this is a purely anatomical definition. All of the neurological activity in the body is ultimately under the control of central nervous system and all of the neurons in the peripheral nervous system have nerve pathways that connect to the brain.

There are two broad divisions of the peripheral nervous system; 1) the voluntary or somatic nervous system, and 2) the involuntary or autonomic nervous system.

The Somatic (Voluntary) Nervous System

The somatic nervous system, as previously mentioned, consists of 12 pairs of cranial nerves and 31 pairs of spinal nerves. These nerves carry sensory information from sensory receptor cells located throughout the body to the brain, and carry instructions - in the form of electrical impulses - from to brain to effector cells located throughout the body. In most cases the effector cells are skeletal muscle cells or glands - endocrine glands and exocrine glands.

The sensory information provided by the peripheral nervous system is integrated with other conscious thought processes and allow one to make a voluntary decision to carry out physical actions. These decisions are translated into actions beginning with the generation and transmission of electrical signals through the somatic nerves to skeletal muscles. Skeletal muscles relax and contract in a fashion that results in the desired body movements. Very often these highly complex movements occur in the muscles of the vocal cords to produce speech.

Somatic Ganglia

An important anatomical feature of the somatic nervous system is that the spinal peripheral nerves originate from collections of neuron cell bodies located in discrete regions of the vertebrae but outside of the vertebral canal. Collections of neuron cell bodies not located in the central nervous system are classified as "ganglia" The sensory ganglia are in dorsal regions of vertebrae and are called dorsal root ganglia. Neurons in the dorsal ganglia contribute the sensory nerve fibers to spinal nerves. In ventral regions of the vertebrae, ventral root ganglia neurons contribute the nerve fibers that send signals to effector cells. These types of nerves are called motor nerves.

The Autonomic (Involuntary) Nervous System

Most of the neural regulatory activity of the body is not under voluntary control. The central nervous system regulates the majority of the body's functions through the involuntary or autonomic nervous system. The two divisions of the autonomic nervous system are the sympathetic and the parasympathetic nervous systems. These are commonly described as - for the sympathetic division - the "fight or flight" nervous system and - for the parasympathetic division - as the "rest and digest" nervous system. Again, it is important to realize that both systems are directly connected to specific regions of the brain. They are not an independent peripheral nervous system, rather they have an extensive peripheral component and they have a highly complex central component as well.

One general anatomical feature of note is that the autonomic nerve fibers are usually not organized into separate specific nerves, but often are nerve fibers that that follow the course of and may even be adherent to blood vessels or somatic nerves.

The Sympathetic Nervous System

The peripheral component of the sympathetic nervous system begins with the neuron cell bodies located in the sympathetic ganglia. Most of these ganglia are located in pairs just lateral to the spinal cord and are therefore often referred to as the sympathetic "chain" ganglia.

These ganglia send nerve fibers throughout the body, in particular to the organs, glands and blood vessels of the body.

The Parasympathetic Nervous System

The peripheral component of the parasympathetic nervous system begins with the neuron cell bodies located in the parasympathetic ganglia. In contrast to the sympathetic ganglia, the parasympathetic ganglia are usually located close to the organs and local anatomic regions that they innervate (supply nerves to). The Vagus nerve or tenth (X) cranial nerve is of particular importance in the parasympathetic nervous system. This nerve carries parasympathetic nerve fibers to most of the major organs of the body, including the heart, lungs and much of the digestive system.

Neurophysiology

Neurons

At the cellular level the production, transmission and processing or integration of information in the form of electrical impulses is carried out by neurons. Neurons are electrically excitable cells (muscle cells are also electrically excitable cells). All cells in the body maintain concentration levels of ions inside of the cell - Na+, K+ and Na+ and Cl- in particular, that are different than the ion concentrations outside of the cell. This causes a voltage difference across the cell membrane. Electrically excitable cells have specialized membrane pores and ion pumps that can use this voltage difference to generate a voltage spike called an action potential that travels along the cell membrane.

Axons, Dendrites and Synapses

The neuron has in, most cases, a very long membrane extension that looks like a tail called the axon. The nerves of the body are composed of these neuron axons. The sciatic nerve, which extends from the spine to the toes, can consist of numerous individual neuron axons that are each several feet in length. Action potentials generated by the neuron at the base of the axon travel along the axon to its terminal end.

At the end of the axon there is usually a dendrite - a branch like extension of another neuron. The action potential in the first neuron axon causes the release of neurotransmitters - small molecules that diffuse across the gap between the axon and the dendrite of the second neuron. The neurotransmitter molecules bind to receptors on the second neuron's dendritic membrane. This can cause the second neuron to generate its own action potential which again travels down the second neuron's axon.

By this method electrical impulses can be transmitted from one neuron to another. The location where the diffusion of neurotransmitters between two neurons occurs is called a synapse. There are estimated to be over 100 trillion synapses in the human brain.

General Functions of the Nervous System

Sensory Functions

The function of the nervous system is to monitor, regulate and coordinate all other body functions and to adapt to the external environment as needed. The nervous system attempts to maintain the optimum internal and external environment for the survival of the organism. In humans, these include uniquely high-level thinking abilities that allow us to exert unprecedented levels of voluntary control over our environment. This begins with the sensory functions of the nervous system.

The nervous system collects an enormous amount of information about the internal conditions of the body and about the outside environment. This collection process begins with sensory receptor cells. Sensory receptor cells are specialized to detect many types of stimuli. When they detect the things they were designed to detect, they report this information to the brain through electrical signals that they generate and then transmit to the brain via sensory nerves.

The Visual System

The eyes are sensory organs designed to collect visual wavelength photons. In the retina of the eye, rods and cones - the visual sensory receptor cells - absorb photons that enter the eye. The rod and cone cells generated electrical signals that are sent through the optic nerve. The optic nerves are the cranial nerve II (2) pair of the 12 pairs of cranial nerves of the somatic nervous system. This information is processed at many areas in the brain. Final processing of visual information occurs in the occipital lobes of the cerebral cortex for this reason the occipital cortex is also called the visual cortex). Presumably this is where the conscious visual perception of the world is generated.

The Auditory and Vestibular System

Sound waves generated by movements in the environment around us are received at the ear and are converted to electrical signals by hair cells located in the cochlea of the inner ear. These signals are transmitted to the brain via the acoustic nerves - cranial nerves XIII (8) of the somatic nervous system. These signals are also widely processed throughout the brain and ultimately are integrated into a conscious perception of sound in the temporal lobes of the cerebral cortex - also known as the auditory cortex.

The vestibular sense is the set of sensations perceived when one's body is it is undergoing acceleration. The accelerations in all three translational dimensions - back-forward, up-down and side to side are detected by vestibular sensory cells. Rotation (which is always an acceleration) in any of the three rotational axes is also detected by vestibular sensory cells. Vestibular sensory cells are located in the semicircular canals. The semicircular canals are located in the cochlea of the inner ears. Vestibular information also travels through the acoustic nerve. Much of the processing of vestibular information occurs in the cerebellum of the brain.

The Somatosensory System

The sense of touch actually consists of many types of sensory information light touch, pressure vibrations heat, cold and pain and a sense of body posture and relative positions of the parts of the body. These sensations are collectively classified as somatosensory information. Various types of sensory receptors located primarily near the surface of skin but also in deep structures of the body transmit somatosensory information via the cranial and spinal somatic nerves to a sub-region of the parietal lobes of the cerebral cortex. This region is designated as the sensory division of the somatic cortex. This is where the conscious perceptions of touch, heat, cold and pain are generated.

The Olfactory and Gustatory Systems

The sense of taste (olfaction) begins with the detection - by taste buds located in tongue - of molecules contained in the foods and beverages that are dissolved in saliva in the mouth. The types of taste we can detect are; salty, sweet, sour, bitter and umami. Umami is a recently identified taste category that is - no kidding - defined as the "delicious" taste.

For the sense of smell, the odor receptors in the nose are capable of detecting thousands and perhaps millions of different odors corresponding to molecules that are present in the air that we breathe. No further level of detail is required by the HESI for the neurophysiology of the taste and smell sensations.

Motor Functions

The somatic sensory cortex is adjacent and lateral to the somatic motor division of the somatic cortex. When a conscious decision is made to carry out voluntary movements, the electrical signal to do so are first generated by neurons in the somatic motor cortex. These signals are then transmitted ultimately to voluntary skeletal muscles via the peripheral somatic nerves.

Notice that the peripheral somatic nerves transmit sensory information to the brain and instructions in the form of electrical signals from the brain to the muscles of the body. They are not purely sensory nerves or purely motor nerves; they are therefore designated as "mixed nerves".

The motor cortex signals to initiate movement and the myriad of involuntary movements that occur continuously in the body require huge amounts of processing at lower brain levels before they can be expressed as actual signals to the muscles. Most notably, precise and complex movements and maintenance of balance and body posture in particular are heavily dependent on processing that occurs in the cerebellum. The basal ganglia and substantia nigra are also crucial in the generation of movement. Degeneration of the substantia nigra results in the progressive movement disorder Parkinson's disease.

Integrative Functions

Overall the nervous system functions as an information processing system of incredible complexity. The functions can be generalized as sensory functions, motor functions and integrative functions. The somatic systems sensory and motor functions are described above, but there is an integrative function that bridges the sensory and motor functions. These integrative functions involve cognitive awareness and intellectual and emotional thought processes that generate organized strategies of actions and complex behaviors that when operating properly enhance one's ability to survive in a complex society.

These integrative processes are deeply connected to processing that occurs in the frontal cortices and also depend on continuous input from regions of the brain crucial to maintaining homeostasis, and to regions that are central in memory processing and those involved in generating primitive drives such as hunger, thirst and nurturing behaviors and basic emotions such as anger, fear and happiness.

Homeostasis and Vital Baseline Body Functions

At the most vital and fundamental needs level; the nervous system must strive to maintain the minimum levels of oxygen and glucose for cell survival. Equally important is the maintenance of the proper pH levels of fluids, and the proper concentrations of electrolytes in body fluids. Finally, survival is critically dependent on maintaining a proper core body temperature.

The nervous system accomplishes this by establishing set points for blood pressure, oxygen, pH, glucose, osmolality (electrolyte concentration) and temperature. Levels that diverge from these set point values can be fatal within minutes to hours. Specialized detector cells in the peripheral body and also in the hypothalamus are able to determine the real-time values for all of these set point criteria. The maintenance of these key chemical and physiological parameters represents homeostasis at the level of the entire human body with respect to the external environment.

Blood Pressure and Oxygen Levels

A continuous supply of oxygen and nutrients requires a continuous breathing and heart rate and an adequate blood pressure to drive the circulation of oxygen and nutrients to all cells in the body. When the nervous system detects inadequate blood pressure or oxygen levels it sends signals to increase breathing rate and breathing volume, increase the output of blood by increasing the force and rate of heart contractions and by adjusting the resistance of blood vessel by constriction or relaxation of smooth muscle cells in blood vessel walls.

Osmolality

Inadequate blood pressure and unacceptably high osmolality triggers thirst leading to single-minded activities devoted to the acquisition of drinkable water. The nervous system also triggers the endocrine system to signal the kidney to retain water and to concentrate the urine and to secrete electrolytes to lower osmolality. Low osmolality when detected results in nervous signals and hormone level adjustments to cause the kidneys to remove water by producing dilute urine and to reabsorb electrolytes to increase osmolality.

Glucose

Low glucose levels trigger signals that directly or through hormonal effect increase the production of glucose and the delivery of glucose to the circulation. High glucose levels are similarly readjusted most notably by adjustments of level of the hormone cortisol. Low glucose also triggers the drive state sensation of intense hunger, leading to behaviors devoted to the acquisition of food.

Core Body Temperature

Temperature adjustments are generated by signals to the blood vessels in the skin to constrict or dilate and thereby either decrease or increase blood flow to the skin. Increased blood flow to the skin results in transferal of internal heat from the blood to the body exterior. Blood vessel constriction has the opposite effect. The primitive drive state sensations of excessive heat or cold generate voluntary actions to seek warmth and shelter or find cooler local environments.

pH

There are no particular drive state sensations associated with excessively high or low blood pH, but the nervous system carefully monitors and adjusts pH to maintain an optimum pH level between 7.35 and 7.45. The primary means of compensation for low pH is signals to release hormones that cause the kidney to secrete hydrogen ion. Chemically this results in the production of bicarbonate ion by the kidney that then enters the bloodstream. Hydrogen ion is excreted in the form of carbonic acid and free hydrogen ion.

The respiratory system can increase blood pH by increasing breathing rate and thereby decrease the levels of CO_2 in the blood. This lowers the levels of blood carbonic acid and increases the levels of blood bicarbonate ion. This increased breathing rate is also generated by the nervous system in response to excessively low blood pH.

The Medulla Oblongata

The medulla oblongata is among the most ancient regions of the brain. It is located in the brainstem adjacent to the spinal cord. The medulla is responsible for maintaining heart rate, breathing rate and blood pressure and plays other key roles in homeostatic control of all body systems.

The Hypothalamus

The hypothalamus is a midbrain structure located at the base of the skull. The hypothalamus is a critical region in homeostatic regulation. It either detects directly or indirectly blood pH and osmolality levels, oxygen levels and numerous other biochemical and physiological metrics. Most of the drive state sensations including hunger, thirst and excessive heat and cold are generated by the hypothalamus.

The hypothalamus is integrated with other brain regions to respond to homeostatic needs via activation of the sympathetic and parasympathetic nervous system and through the secretion of hypothalamic hormones that directly influence the activity all other endocrine glands throughout the body.

The Autonomic Nervous System

The autonomic nervous system, consisting of the sympathetic and parasympathetic nervous systems, is activated through complex processing at all levels of the central nervous system. The homeostatic control systems of the central nervous system often exert regulatory control over a wide variety of biochemical and physiological function through a combination of sympathetic and parasympathetic induced physiological and biochemical responses. The sympathetic response can be nearly instantaneous, particularly with the effects on the cardiovascular system.

The Sympathetic Nervous System

Sympathetic nerves release neurotransmitters to cardiac muscle and smooth muscle located in bronchial walls, intestinal tract walls, and the walls of blood vessels that generate rapid response to environmental circumstances that require aggressive and highly energetic responses (fight or flight responses). The sympathetic effects in such circumstances include increased force of heart contractions, increase heart rate, increased blood pressure, redirection of flow of blood from the intestines to the skeletal muscles, suppression of peristalsis and dilation of the bronchial airways.

The sympathetic system also innervates the adrenal medulla and can cause the release of epinephrine and norepinephrine into the bloodstream. This creates a maximal and persistent overall state of dynamic alertness and physiological readiness to engage in pursuit of prey, physical combat, or escape from life threatening situations.

The Parasympathetic Nervous System

The parasympathetic nervous system innervates most of the same glands, cardiac muscle and smooth muscle cells as the sympathetic system. The effects of the parasympathetic system are the opposite if the sympathetic effects in most cases. The parasympathetic system predominates during periods when the body requires rest and regeneration and digestion of food. Perhaps most importantly, the body requires a continuously adjusting balance between the sympathetic and parasympathetic states. This is referred to as the autonomic tone of the body and it is essential for the continuous optimal performance of all body systems.

Protective Reflexes

A very important class of specialized nervous system function is the protective-reflex class of functions. There are other primitive reflexes such as the Babinski reflex, the root reflex and others that are rather complex and beyond the scope of the HESI. The simple protective reflexes, most notably the deep tendon reflexes, are extremely simple two- or three-neuron circuits that are completely outside of the central nervous system.

These reflexes respond instantaneously to stimuli that represent potentially dangerous forces acting on the body. Examples include the instantaneous withdrawal of a body part from a hot surface. The deep tendon reflexes are usually the reflexes involved in this type of reflex, but they are also very important when the limbs and joints are experiencing possibly catastrophic mechanical forces. The deep tendon reflexes have mechanoreceptors that trigger impulses when a dangerous level of mechanical stress is detected. The mechanoreceptor signal travels through one or two neurons and synapses on a skeletal muscle that contracts to counteract the forces that are threatening injury at a bone or joint region. A specific example of a deep tendon reflex is the patellar tendon reflex that is elicited by tapping the patellar tendon of the knee with a reflex hammer.

The Endocrine System

The endocrine system is the system that synthesizes and secretes hormones in the body. Hormones exert a vast array of effects on the body. The endocrine system includes purely endocrine glands, whose sole function is the synthesis and secretion of hormones and also other tissues and organs that, in addition to their primary or co-functions, also synthesize and secrete hormones.

There is an important anatomical distinction between the two general types of glands, endocrine glands and exocrine glands. Exocrine glands do not necessarily secrete hormones; they can secrete many other substances. The anatomical distinction for exocrine glands is that all exocrine glands secrete substances through a duct. A duct is a tube that leads to an anatomical surface, such as the surface of the skin or the surface of the intestinal tract. The common bile duct is an example.

All endocrine glands secrete hormones and by anatomical definition, all endocrine glands secrete hormones directly into the bloodstream or the lymphatic system. Also by anatomical definition, no purely endocrine gland contains secretory ducts. This is why the endocrine glands are sometimes referred to as "ductless" glands.

The Hypothalamus and the Pituitary Gland

The hypothalamus and the pituitary gland are closely related anatomically. Together these two structures serve as master controllers of the endocrine system through the secretion of hormones that regulate the levels of other hormones. The hypothalamus is a region of the brain but it also synthesizes and secretes many critically important hormones. It is located in the inferior midbrain directly above the central region of the base of the cranial cavity.

The pituitary gland is attached to the inferior portion of the hypothalamus by a connective stalk. The pituitary gland occupies a small depression or crater in the base of the skull called the sella turcica. The pituitary secretes a wide variety of hormones. An Important anatomical feature of the pituitary gland is that the posterior pituitary synthesizes only two hormones - oxytocin and vasopressin - and all other pituitary hormones are synthesized by the anterior pituitary.

The Pineal Gland

The pineal gland is located within the midbrain and is essentially at the anatomical center of the brain. The pineal gland produces melatonin, which regulates sleep patterns and circadian rhythms.

The Thyroid and Parathyroid Glands

The thyroid glands are located superficial and to either side of the midline of the tracheal cartilage - Many anatomists classify the thyroid as a single gland with left and right lobes. The parathyroid glands are notable for being, in a sense, glands within glands. There are usually four parathyroid glands, buried deeply in the thyroid gland, usually two per lobe. The thyroid glands secrete thyroid hormones and calcitonin. The parathyroids secrete parathyroid hormone (PTH).

The Pancreas

The pancreas is not a purely endocrine gland, it also has

critical exocrine gland function as a part of the digestive system, but its endocrine function is even more important. The pancreas secretes the hormones glucagon and - most importantly - insulin. The pancreas as previously described, is located in the upper right quadrant of the abdomen, in a partially retroperitoneal position, immediately below the diaphragm and posterior to the stomach.

The Adrenal Glands

As we have discussed, the adrenal glands rest upon the superior surface of the kidneys, one gland per kidney. The anatomical structure of the adrenal gland is significant in that the adrenal cortex (the surrounding outer layer) synthesizes the corticosteroid hormones, including cortisol and aldosterone and the adrenal medulla (the central region) synthesizes epinephrine, norepinephrine and dopamine.

The Gonads

The gonads have two important co-functions; the production of male or female gametes and the synthesis of sex hormones. The gonads in males are the testicles and are located externally within the testicular pouches. They synthesize the male sex hormone testosterone. The gonads in females are the ovaries, which are located lateral to and at the level of the superior region of the uterus, one ovary one the left and one on the right. The distal entry into either the left or right fallopian tube is closely adjacent to the left or right ovary. The fallopian tubes provide a passageway into the uterine cavity. The uterus is a midline pelvic organ that is posterior to the urinary bladder and anterior to the rectum. The ovaries synthesize the female sex hormone estrogen.

Endocrine Physiology

While a large majority of the central nervous systems responses are rapid in the form of electrical signals and muscular responses. The nervous system also exerts profound control over all aspects of the body through its influences on the endocrine system. In contrast to direct nervous- signal-mediated control, which generally produce rapid but short-lived effects; hormonal effects are usually much slower in their actions and their effects are often cumulative over longer periods of time - in some cases years or even decades.

Many hormonal systems also function relatively independently of the central nervous system. Also, there are many other hormones or hormone-like molecules that are produced and secreted by virtually all tissues and organs of the body. For instance, the duodenum synthesizes and secretes the locally active hormones CCK and secretin.

The Hypothalamic Hormones

As we have discussed, the hypothalamus is a critical brain region for the maintenance of homeostasis within the body. A Primary mode of this regulation of homeostasis by the hypothalamus is through the release of hypothalamic hormones. Primary hormones secreted by the hypothalamus include:

Thyrotropin-releasing hormone (TRH) - This hormone acts on the anterior segment of the pituitary gland and stimulates the release of thyroid-stimulating hormone (TSH).

Corticotropin-releasing hormone - This hormone also acts on the anterior segment of the pituitary gland and stimulates the release of adrenocorticotropin hormone (ACTH).

Growth hormone-releasing hormone (GHRH) - This hormone stimulates the release of growth hormone (GH) from the anterior segment of the pituitary gland.

Gonadotropin-releasing hormone (GnRH) - This hormone stimulates the release of follicle-stimulating hormone (FSH) from the anterior segment of the pituitary gland.

Somatostatin (also known as growth-hormone-inhibiting hormone - GHIH) - This hormone inhibits the release of growth hormone (GH) and follicle-stimulating hormone from the anterior segment of the pituitary gland.

The Pituitary Gland Hormones

The pituitary gland is directly connected to the hypothalamus and the two structures together regulate nearly all body functions via hormonal control. The two major functional/anatomical regions of the pituitary gland are the posterior pituitary and the anterior pituitary.

The Posterior Pituitary Gland Hormones

Many authorities consider the posterior pituitary to be part of the hypothalamus. The posterior pituitary secretes two hormones; oxytocin and vasopressin (also known as antidiuretic hormone - ADH).

Oxytocin

Oxytocin triggers the milk letdown reflex in nursing mothers.

Vasopressin (or ADH)

Vasopressin is a very important hormone that regulates blood pressure and the fluid balance of the body. The blood pressure effects are partially accomplished by ADH effects on smooth muscle in the walls of blood vessels. ADH causes smooth muscle contraction in blood vessel walls which in turn constricts blood vessel passageways. This results in an increase in blood pressure.

The other actions of ADH are on the microscopic filtering units of the kidney - the nephrons. There are an estimated 1 million nephrons per human kidney. ADH decreases the loss of water from the body by causing the nephrons to reabsorb water from fluids that have been filtered out of the bloodstream and are in the process of passing out of the kidney filtering system and into the bladder. There are even more complex actions of ADH on the nephrons that result in adjustments to the body's levels of electrolytes and blood glucose levels. These are beyond the scope of the HESI.

Anterior Pituitary Gland Hormones

The hormones secreted by the anterior pituitary are described below.

Adrenocorticotropic Hormone (ACTH)

ACTH is secreted continuously but at increased levels when the body is under physical or psychological stress and when blood glucose is too low. ACTH stimulates the cortex of the adrenal gland to release of the corticosteroid hormone cortisol.

Thyroid-stimulating Hormone (TSH)

TSH stimulates the thyroid gland to release thyroid hormones. Thyroid hormones are the primary hormones that establish the overall metabolic rates of the body.

Luteinizing Hormone (LH) and Follicle-stimulating Hormone (FSH)

LH and FSH are critical in the differentiation of cells to produce both male and female gametes and are the primary regulators of the female menstrual cycle.

Prolactin (PRL)

Prolactin stimulates glandular growth of mammary glands and subsequent production of milk in breastfeeding females. It also has many other functions that are beyond the scope of the HESI.

Growth Hormone (GH)

The levels of GH during childhood determines the maximum lean body mass and height that individuals attain by the time they complete this type of growth. This completion of growth is the physiological definition of adulthood.

Melanocyte-stimulating Hormone (MSH)

The levels of MSH, particularly during prenatal (before birth) development determines the darkness of skin color and is the basis for racial differences in skin color.

The Thyroid Hormones

The thyroid gland produces and releases two types of thyroid hormone, thyroxine (T4) and triiodothyronine (T3) and the hormone calcitonin. Calcitonin is discussed together with parathyroid hormone since both are closely related in their function - the regulation of the concentration of calcium ion (Ca++) in the blood.

T3 and T4

Iodine atoms are included in the structure of the thyroid hormone and iodine deficiency leads to hypothyroidism and enlargement of the thyroid gland (this is called a goiter).

The release of thyroid hormone is triggered by the pituitary hormone TSH. T3 is more potent than T4 but both hormones have the same effects. Thyroid hormones directly affect nearly every cell in the body and the overall effect is to increase the basal (baseline) metabolic activity of the body.

Notable effects of thyroid hormone include increase in

rates of protein synthesis, regulation of fat, protein and carbohydrate metabolism, promotion of cell differentiation and enhancement of bone growth and regeneration. Excessively high or low levels of thyroid hormones can be fatal.

Calcitonin and Parathyroid Hormone (PTH)

PTH is synthesized and secreted by the parathyroid glands. PTH - along with the hormone calcitonin - is vitally important in the regulation of blood levels of calcium ion (Ca++). The activity of calcitonin and PTH is on cells that are involved in the breakdown and regeneration of the calcium rich mineral hydroxyapatite - the major mineral that forms the extracellular matrix of bone.

The Pancreatic Hormones -Glucagon and Insulin

In addition to its exocrine function in the synthesis and release of digestive hormones and bicarbonate ions, the pancreas in its endocrine gland role, synthesizes and releases two hormones, glucagon and insulin. Both hormones are vital to maintaining proper levels of blood glucose. Insulin also is essential to most cells for the uptake of glucose into the cell. Insulin is produced by pancreatic islet cells. In type 1 diabetes, islet cells are attacked and destroyed by the body's own immune system. A total lack of insulin is fatal within hours to days.

The Adrenal Cortical (Steroid) Hormones - Cortisol and Aldosterone

The adrenal cortical hormones are steroid hormone. Steroid hormones are molecules that are modified versions of the cholesterol molecule. Other hormones are either small water-soluble molecules or polypeptides - amino acid chains that are the same type of chains that are assembled from mRNA transcribed to form the protein products of genes.

Since the steroid hormones are based on a lipid type molecule -cholesterol-they are fat-soluble, rather than water-soluble. Steroid hormones are secreted into lymphatic vessels rather than blood vessels. The principle cortical hormones are the glucocorticoid steroid hormone cortisol and mineral corticosteroid hormone aldosterone. The adrenal cortex also produces the precursor molecules that are transformed by the gonads into the male hormone testosterone and the female sex hormone, estrogen.

Cortisol

Cortisol release is stimulated by the pituitary hormone ACTH. Cortisol has a wide range of actions including regulating the metabolism of fats, proteins and carbohydrates. Cortisol also plays an important role in the immune system -generally this involves suppression of the immune response. Cortisol also is involved in the regulation of glucose levels. Cortisol stimulates the liver to synthesize new glucose molecules by a process termed gluconeogenesis.

Baseline levels of cortisol are essential to life. An absence of cortisol is fatal within weeks to months.

Aldosterone

Aldosterone is a critical hormone in the regulation of blood pressure and electrolyte concentrations in the body. This regulation mechanism is highly complex and involves several other hormones in what is termed the renin-aldosterone-angiotensin hormone axis.

The Gonadal Hormones - Testosterone and Estrogen

The gonadal hormones - testosterone and estrogen - are synthesized in the testes in males and in the ovaries in females. The sex hormones are synthesized from cholesterol based precursors that are produced in the adrenal cortex. During the prenatal stage, testosterone is responsible for the development of male external genitalia. During adolescence, the sex hormones are responsible for the development of secondary sexual characteristics - pubic hair, testicular maturation, and breast development. Estrogen also appears to provide protection from coronary artery disease and osteoporosis in premenopausal females.

The Cardiovascular System

The anatomy of the cardiovascular circulatory system begins with the heart, which is located at the base of the thoracic cavity directly superior to the diaphragm and centered slightly to the left of the midline of the sternum. The lower lobes of the left and right lungs are immediately lateral to the lateral walls of the heart.

The heart consists of muscular walls that enclose four

chambers, the thin-walled right and left atria and the thick-walled right and left ventricles. The right and left ventricles share a common medial wall - the interventricular septum - as do the right and left atria - the interatrial septum. The right atrium is directly superior to the right ventricle and the left atrium is directly superior to the left ventricle. The atria and ventricles are separated by a common septum - the atrioventricular septum - which forms the bases or floors of the atria and the ceilings of each atrium's underling ventricles.

Cardiovascular Blood Flow

Deoxygenated blood from all other regions arrives at the heart from the body via veins. The smaller veins eventually pass blood through to either the superior or inferior vena cava - the largest veins of the body. The superior and inferior vena cavae empty into the right atrium. Blood then passes from the right atrium through a three-leaflet valve - the tricuspid valve- into the right ventricle. Subsequently, this blood is pumped out of the right ventricle through a two-leaflet valve - the pulmonic valve - into the main pulmonary artery. Blood in the main pulmonary artery continues to either the left or right pulmonary arteries, which then enter either the left or the right lung.

Pulmonary Blood Flow

The pulmonary arteries branch into increasingly smaller and more numerous arteries. The smallest terminal arterial branches are the arterioles. From the arterioles, blood passes into capillaries - one-cell-thick-walled vessels. Blood passing through these capillaries exchange oxygen from inspired air in alveolar airspaces. Carbon dioxide diffuses out of the blood in the capillaries and into the alveolar airspaces. This carbon dioxide it is then expelled from the body through respiratory airways during exhalation (expiration).

The capillary blood, now oxygenated, passes to venules, then to larger veins and finally returns to the heart via the main pulmonary veins. The main pulmonary veins (usually there are four of these) empty into the left atrium. Blood from the left atrium passes into the left ventricle through a two-leaflet valve - the mitral valve. The blood is then pumped out of the heart from the left ventricle through a two-leaflet valve - the aortic valve - into the aorta.

The aorta is the largest artery in the body. From the aorta, oxygenated blood is delivered through a network of branching arterial trees to all regions of the body. Oxygen and nutrients are transferred to tissues and carbon dioxide and other waste products are absorbed at capillary beds. Capillary blood, now deoxygenated, returns to the heart through networks of veins as already described.

Portal Vein Systems

An important anatomical concept in the cardiovascular system is that blood that is pumped out of the heart, either via the left or the right ventricle always first enters a main artery, then travels to sequentially smaller arteries then to the smallest arteries - arterioles and then into capillaries. From capillaries, this blood next travels to the smallest veins - venules and then to larger veins. Most of this blood travels to sequentially larger veins and directly back to the heart, but some of the blood is routed through a second set of capillary beds, most notably this occurs with venous blood travelling from capillary beds located in the intestines to capillary beds located in the liver. This type of circulatory anatomy is classified as a "portal system or portal circulation".

Cardiovascular (Circulatory) Physiology

The primary functions of the cardiovascular system are 1) to deliver oxygen from the lungs to all of the cells of the body along with water, electrolytes, glucose, and other essential substances. 2) To transport waste products to the organs responsible for detoxifying and excreting waste products from the body. Carbon dioxide is delivered to the lungs and other wastes are delivered either directly to the kidneys or indirectly to the kidneys through the liver. To accomplish these functions, the circulatory vessels must maintain a large, driving blood-pressure differential between the arterial side of the heart (the left heart) and the venous side of the heart (the right heart).

Mechanics of Cardiac Pressure and Blood Flow

The heart is a muscular organ composed primarily of cardiac muscle. The atria of the heart are thin-walled compared to the ventricles of the heart. This is because the atria receive low pressure venous blood from the body and do not need to generate high blood pressure to pump blood to the ventricles. The ventricles are comparatively thick-walled and are designed to generate high blood pressures that drive blood through the arterial vessels.

The direction of blood flow within the heart is accomplished by the arrangement of one-way valves within the heart and by the sequence in which various regions of the heart contract during a cardiac cycle.

Veins to Atria

Venous blood enters the atria through one way valves. When the atria are relaxing, pressures inside the atria are lower than venous pressures. This drives venous blood through the one-way valves and into the atria. When the atria begin to contract, pressure within the atria rises. When this pressure exceeds venous pressure blood attempt to flow back into the veins, but the one-way valves slam shut as this begins to occur, sealing of the blood route between atria and veins.

Atria to Ventricles

As the atria continue to contract, pressure continues to rise until the pressure exceeds the pressure in the underlying ventricles. This forces open the one-way valves between atria and ventricle. In the right side of the heart, this is the tricuspid valve; on the left side of the heart, this is the mitral valve. As blood is driven into the ventricles from the atria, the ventricles begin to contract. When ventricular pressures exceed atrial pressure the initial reversal of blood flow causes the tricuspid and mitral valves to slam shut, preventing blood flow from the ventricles back into the atria.

Ventricles to Arteries

The ventricles continue to contract and blood pressure rises until it exceeds blood pressure in the arterial outflow tracts of the ventricle - the main pulmonary artery for the right ventricle and the aorta for the left ventricle. The higher pressure inside the ventricles force open the one-way valves between the ventricles and the arterial outflow tracts. These valves are the pulmonic valve of the right ventricle and the aortic valve of the left ventricle. The ventricles continue to contract and drive all of the blood within the ventricular chambers past the one-way valves and into the arterial circulation.

This pressure corresponds to the highest blood pressures that the heart produces and this pressure is sufficient to drive blood through the entire circulatory pathway back to the atria, where the cardiac cycle repeats. As the ventricles relax, pressure within the ventricle drops below the arterial outflow tract pressure. The reversal of blood flow from the arteries back into the ventricles is prevented when this backflow causes the pulmonic and aortic valves to slam shut, sealing off the arterial-ventricular blood flow routes.

The Electrical Activity of the Heart

Cardiac muscle cells do not require nervous impulses to trigger contraction. An isolated cardiac muscle cell will rhythmically contract on its own. In the heart, cardiac muscle cells have open connections with adjacent cardiac muscle cells that allow the cell cytoplasm to flow between cells. This type of cellular organization is called a syncytium. This syncytium arrangement of cardiac muscle cells allows electrical signals to freely pass from one cell to another.

The Sinoatrial (SA) Node

The heart must contract in a precisely synchronized fashion to cause blood to be pumped in the proper manner and direction throughout the circulatory system. The atria must begin to contract from top to the base of the atrioventricular septum. This squeezes blood toward the tricuspid and atrial valves. Next the ventricles must contract beginning at the base of the ventricles and progressing toward the pulmonic and aortic valves.

This coordinated contraction pattern begins with the sinoatrial node tissue located in the wall of the right ventricle. This tissue has an intrinsic (inbuilt) ability to generate electrical signal at a rate on average of 60-80 signals per minute. For this reason, the sinoatrial node is referred to as the "pacemaker" of the heart. The electrical signals generated at the SA node are conducted through the cardiac muscle of the atria with a geometrical progression that automatically produces the desired contraction pattern of the atria.

The Atrioventricular (AV) Node and Purkinje Fibers

The electrical signals in the atria are blocked from progressing to the ventricles by the atrioventricular

(AV) septum, which is constructed from non-conducting tissue. The atrioventricular node - located just above the AV septum - conducts electrical signals from the atria through the AV septum and into large conductive fibers called purkinje fibers located in the walls of the ventricles. These fibers rapidly transmit electrical signals throughout the ventricular cardiac muscle walls. The specific arrangement of the purkinje fibers results in the desired contraction pattern of the ventricles.

Arteries

Arteries are designed to withstand the high pressure generated by the ventricles of the heart. Arteries also must to be able to stretch when blood flow volumes increase greatly during ventricular contractions and to contract to maintain adequate blood pressures in the intervals between ventricular contractions. This requires that thick arterial walls that contain elastic protein fibers and a layer of smooth muscle cells.

Arterioles

As the arterial vasculature progresses from the heart, large arteries undergo numerous branchings into smaller diameter arteries. The final arterial branches are the arterioles. Arterioles are the smallest diameter arteries and they connect to capillaries. The arteriole walls contain smooth muscles that can relax or contract in response to numerous types of stimuli, some local and some in the form of hormonal or electrical to signals from the nervous system. Arteriolar contraction can completely close off blood flow to capillary beds and arteriolar relaxation increases blood flow to capillary beds. It is at this level that many systems of the body regulate blood distribution and organ function based on the needs of the body at any given time.

Capillaries

Capillaries are designed to maximize the diffusion of substances into and out of the circulatory system. This is accomplished by minimizing the structures and distances that substances must cross when passing through capillary walls. This is the reason that capillaries are only one-cell layer in thickness.

Fluid Compartments of the Body

There are three major fluid compartments of the body - the intravascular space - inside of blood vessels and the heart; the extracellular space - the space outside of the blood vessel, heart and all cells of the body; and the intracellular space - the total space within all the cells of the body. Oxygen, nutrients water and waste products and all other water-soluble biological substances diffuse between the intravascular space and the extracellular space and between the extracellular space and the intracellular space.

Water diffuses freely between all three spaces; the distribution of water is determined by the osmolality of the fluid compartments. The major osmotic particles in fluid compartments are proteins - which do not diffuse across cell membranes that separate fluid compartments (except by active transport processes).

When the arterioles feeding capillaries are open, the blood pressure within capillaries is higher than the fluid pressure in the extracellular compartment; this drives water out of the capillaries. The proteins in blood inside of capillaries limit the water loss from the intravascular space by osmotic pressure effects. Oxygen, nutrients and other essential biological substances diffuse down concentration gradients out of the capillaries and into the extravascular space. The reverse process occurs for waste products in the extracellular space.

Veins

Excess water is reabsorbed by lymphatic vessels and by the venules - the venous vessels at the other end of capillaries. These are the terminal branches of the venous side of the circulatory system. Veins return blood to the heart (except in portal systems). Venules converge on large veins and these to still larger veins, eventually converging into the superior and inferior vena cava.

The blood pressure in veins is much lower than on the arterial side, consequently veins are thin-walled since they are not subject to high arterial pressure. Venous blood flow from the extremities is greatly aided by skeletal muscle contractions and associated limb movements. Veins also have internal one-way valves that allow blood to flow freely towards the heart but prevent blood flow in the opposite direction (backflow).

Autonomic Effects on the Heart and Blood Vessels

The activation of the sympathetic nervous system can have profound effects on the circulatory system Cardiac muscle cells responds with increased force of contractions which increases blood pressure, the sinoatrial node responds with increased electrical impulse rate resulting in increased heart rate. Major arteries constrict resulting in higher blood pressures and other arteries and arterioles relax or constrict so that blood flow is directed away from the digestive system, away from the skin (to reduce bleeding that may occur during strenuous activity) and toward the skeletal muscles. The actions of the parasympathetic nervous system generally have the opposite of theses sympathetic effects.

The Urinary System

The urinary system consists of the kidneys, renal arteries and veins (renal is an adjective meaning "related to the kidney" or "of the kidney"), ureters, urinary bladder and urethra. The kidneys are bean-shaped and are located, as previously mentioned, within the walls of the abdomen in a dorsolateral position on either side of the lumbar spine. This "buried in abdominal wall tissue" location is referred to as a retroperitoneal position, (The pancreas is also in a partial retroperitoneal position).

The renal arteries carry blood to the kidney where it eventually arrives at capillaries surrounding microscopic filtering units called nephrons. Blood filtration occurs at these sites. Filtered blood from nephrons moves through venous networks and emerges from the kidneys within the renal vein. Filtered products from the nephrons pass through tubules that empty into a central collecting cavity in the kidney known as the renal pelvis.

The ureters (one per kidney) are thin tubes connecting the renal pelvis to the urinary bladder. The ureters transport the kidney's' filtered liquid wastes - urine - from the renal pelvis to the urinary bladder. The urinary bladder is a distensible (inflatable) bag-like structure which is located in the central anterior pelvic region of the abdominal/pelvic cavity. The bladder stores urine until it is released through another tube - the urethra.

The urethra carries the urine outside of the body, exiting at the meatus (outer opening) of the glans penis in males and immediately anterior the entrance of the vagina in women. An additional important anatomical relationship of the urinary system is that the adrenal glands, which secrete many essential hormones as part of the endocrine system, are located directly adjacent to the superior surfaces of the kidneys - one adrenal gland per kidney.

The Kidneys

The Kidneys have several critical functions in the human body. Obviously, the kidneys produce urine but this is only the final stage of kidney function. The production of urine and its transport to the urinary bladder is the excretory function of the kidneys. This excretory function reflects the other functions of the kidney which include maintaining an optimum volume of total body water and optimum concentrations of electrolytes within the fluid compartments of the body.

Additionally, the kidneys play a crucial role in maintaining an optimal pH of body fluids and in maintaining an optimum blood pressure. The kidney removes soluble waste products from the body, most notably urea, bilirubin, organic acids including uric acid and ammonia. The kidney also has direct endocrine functions. These are the production of the hormones renin, erythropoietin and calcitriol.

Gross Anatomy

There are two kidneys, each located to anterior and laterally - either the left or right - of the spine in a retroperitoneal (buried in abdominal wall) position in the posterior wall of the abdominal cavity. Both kidneys are immediately inferior to the diaphragm. The left kidney is adjacent to and posterior to the spleen. The right kidney is adjacent to and posterior to the liver.

The adult human kidneys are bean-shaped organs with an average size of about 10 to 13 cm in length, 5 to 7.5 cm in width and 2 to 2.5 cm in thickness. The long axis of the kidney parallels the long axis of the body.

HESI A² - Spire Study System

The lateral surfaces of the kidneys have a convex curvature and the medial surfaces have a concave curvature The upper region of the kidney is called the superior pole and the lower region is called the inferior pole, An adrenal gland is located adherent to the superior pole of each kidney.

Each kidney's outer surface is enclosed by a tough fibrous layer of tissue called the renal capsule. A layer of fat called the perinephric fat surrounds the renal capsule. The perinephric fat is surrounded by a connective tissue membrane called the renal fascia. The renal fascia is surround by a second layer of fat - the paranephric fat layer. The renal hilum is a recessed region in the center of the medial surface of the kidney. The hilum contains the major blood vessels that supply the kidney - the renal artery and two renal veins -and the proximal end of the ureter.

The solid tissue of the kidneys is divided into two anatomical regions. The outer region is the **renal cortex**, and the inner region is the **renal medulla**. The kidney is also subdivided into ten to fifteen **renal lobes**. The lobes are arranged sequentially as the wedges of an orange to produce the overall kidney structure. Each lobe consists of an upper or outer layer of renal cortex and a medial or deep cone-shaped region of renal medulla called a **renal pyramid**.

The apex of each renal pyramid is called a papilla. Several adjacent renal papillae project into a cavity called a **minor calyx**. Several adjacent minor calyxes fuse medially into a larger cavity called a **major calyx**. The major calyces empty into a central cavity called the **renal pelvis**. The renal pelvis narrows into a tube that becomes the **ureter**. The ureter exits the kidney through the renal hilum and continues inferiorly to merge with the urinary bladder. The renal pelvis and the major and minor calyxes together form a continuous cavity called the **renal sinus**.

Microscopic Anatomy
The functional unit of the kidney is a microscopic structure called a nephron. There are approximately one million nephrons in the human kidney. The nephron consists of two subunits - a tuft or tangled cluster of capillary loops called a **glomerulus**, and a one-

to-two cell - thick-walled **renal tubule.** The renal tubule consists of four segments. These are **Bowman's capsule**, the **proximal convoluted renal tubule**, the **loop of Henle** and the **distal convoluted renal tubule**.

Bowman's capsule forms the distal end of the renal tubule. It is a balloon -like expansion of the tubule contains a deep invagination that is occupied by a single glomerulus. The glomerulus and the Bowman's capsule that surrounds the glomerulus together are referred to as a **renal corpuscle**. The renal corpuscle appears as a small tangled ball of yarn - the glomerulus - that is tightly positioned as an object within a vase that has a spherical body and a very short narrow neck - Bowman's capsule. The body of the capsule encloses the entire glomerulus except for the stalk of the glomerulus which consists of the afferent and efferent stems of the glomerular capillary.

General Anatomy of Renal Blood Vessels, Renal Tubules and Collecting Tubules
The afferent capillary stem connects the glomerulus to an arteriole supplied by blood from an **interlobular artery**. The interlobular arteries are branches of **arcuate arteries**. Arcuate arteries are located in the boundary region between the renal medulla and the renal cortex. Arcuate arteries are branches of **interlobar arteries** that are located between renal pyramids. Interlobar arteries are branches of **segmental arteries** and segmental arteries are branches of the **main renal artery**. the arcuate artery.

The efferent stem of the capillary continues to follow a course alongside the remainder of the renal tubule. The efferent capillaries form numerous loops that encircle the renal tubule along its course. These sections of capillaries are called **peritubular capillaries**. The peritubular capillary finally connects to a venule located in the renal cortex near the boundary of the renal cortex and the renal medulla.

The course of the renal tubule continues from Bowman's capsule- within the renal cortex - as the proximal convoluted tubule. The distal end of the proximal tubule then forms a sharp bend and dives deep into the renal medulla. At the apex of the renal pyramid, near the boundary with the renal pelvis, the tubule forms a tight 180-degree U-turn and reverses its course, continuing very closely alongside the descending portion of the tubule. This **long, thin u-shaped portion of the renal tubule** is called the loop of Henle.

Adjacent peritubular capillaries form a netlike structure that surround the loop of Henle called the **vasa recta**. The distal segment of the loop of Henle reenters the cortex and continues within the cortex as the distal convoluted tubule. The distal tubule terminates at a **renal collecting tubule**. Numerous other distal tubules from adjacent nephrons also connect with the collecting tubule. Collecting tubules dive directly through the renal medulla and terminate into minor renal calices.

Microscopic Structure of the Renal Corpuscles

The capillary walls of glomeruli in renal corpuscles have small gaps in the junctions of adjacent endothelial cells called **fenestrations**. This feature is a major difference in structure compared to most other capillaries. In the majority of capillaries, the endothelial cells that form the capillary walls have very tight intercellular junctions.

Water, nutrients, electrolytes, oxygen, carbon dioxide and cellular waste products must diffuse through the endothelial cell bodies to move between the intravascular space of the capillaries and the extravascular space surrounding the capillaries. between endothelial cells, as a result the walls of the capillary tufts are uncharacteristically permeable to water and dissolved solutes such as electrolytes, glucose amino acids urea, uric acid and other substances.

The fenestrations are essentially tiny pores in the glomerular capillary wall. Consequently, glomerular capillary walls are very leaky, and their intravascular fluid contents readily pass through these fenestrations. Substances which are usually not able to pass from the capillary through fenestrations are macromolecules such as proteins and other polypeptides, lipid molecules - triglycerides and free fatty acids, and the cellular components of blood - red and white blood cells and platelets.

The glomerular capillary walls are pressed tightly against an adjacent section of the glomerular membrane wall. The membrane of Bowman's capsule separates the interstitial spaces of the renal tissues from the internal lumen of the capsule. This membrane consists of a single-cell-thick parietal outer layer of very thin squamous epithelial cells and an underlying single-cell-thick visceral layer of cuboidal epithelial cells called **podocytes**.

A basement membrane separates the capillary endothelium from the squamous epithelium of Bowman's capsule. The podocytes have extended segments called **foot processes** or **pedicels** that press tightly against the internal surface of the outer layer of squamous epithelial cells. There is a small gap between adjacent foot processes. These gaps are called **filtration slits or filtration diaphragms** and consist of two layers of podocyte cell membrane separated by a very thin layer of cytoplasm.

Consequently, at the interface between glomerular capillary walls and the wall of Bowman's capsule there is a very small distance separating the lumen of the capillary from the lumen of Bowman's capsule. There are also very few physical barriers separating the intravascular contents of glomerular capillary and the lumen of Bowman's capsule.

Blood Pressure and Renal Filtration

Most non-cellular Contents within the capillaries can pass freely through the capillary fenestration then can diffuse a short distance across the basement membrane. These diffusing contents then pass through the very thin outer squamous epithelial cells of Bowman's capsule, across an adjacent filtration slit between podocyte foot process and finally into the lumen of Bowman's capsule. This fluid is now called a **renal filtrate**.

As the filtrate continues through the renal tubule and the renal collecting tubule it will be continuously processed by active and passive **reabsorption** of water, electrolytes, glucose, bicarbonate ions and amino acids and small polypeptide (oligopeptides) from the tubule and into the interstitial spaces of the kidney and from there reabsorbed into the peritubular capillaries. A few substances will be actively **secreted** from the interstitial spaces of the kidney into the renal and collecting tubules.

While a major force that drives fluid components of capillaries into the surrounding extravascular space in most capillaries is osmotic pressure - the movement of water and dissolved particles from regions of high concentration to regions of lower concentration, another critical driving force is the pressure gradient between the fluid within capillaries and the fluid is the extracellular space surrounding capillaries.

The higher the differential pressure gradient the greater to driving force in the direction of high pressure to low pressure, In most regions of the body the pressure differential favors the movement of fluids from capillaries into the interstitial space for the first half of the length of the capillary - that originating from an arteriole, and favors the movement of fluid from the extracellular space into capillaries and the remaining half-length of the capillary - the segment that connects to a venule. The balance between these two processes determines how much fluid volume occupies the extracellular space. Increasing blood pressure tends to drive this balance toward the extracellular space and increases extracellular fluid volume.

Blood pressure continues to decrease as blood flows from major arteries to progressively smaller arteries and finally to arterioles and capillaries. It may seem that pressure should increase because arterioles and capillaries are much narrower than the large arteries that they originate from, but there are so many arterioles and capillaries that their cumulative lumen diameters are much larger than the parent artery diameter. The resistance to fluid flow within a closed fluid channel decreases as the diameter of the channel increases. The fluid pressure within the channel increases as the resistance to fluid flow increases. Therefore, at the arteriolar/capillary level the resistance to blood flow is much less than in the parent artery and the blood pressure is much lower than in the parent artery.

Glomerular Filtration Rate (GFR)

In the renal corpuscles, the effects of blood pressure on the movement of fluids from the capillary into the lumen of Bowman's capsule are much greater than the movement of fluids out of capillaries elsewhere in the body. The fluid pressure within the lumen of Bowman's capsule is potentially much lower than in the extracellular spaces elsewhere in the body. It is almost exclusively the pressure gradient between the capillary interior and the lumen of Bowman's space that drives fluids from the capillary into the lumen of Bowman's space. The amount of fluid that passes from capillaries into Bowman's capsule is called the glomerular filtration rate (GFR). By far the most important determinant of GFR is the body's arterial blood pressure.

Determinants of Blood Pressure

There are three primary determinants of arterial blood pressure 1) the total volume of blood in the cardiovascular system, 2) the force of contraction of the left ventricle of the heart and 3) the resistance of the arterial vessels to arterial blood flow. The **force of ventricular contraction** can be influenced by the autonomic nervous system by increasing or decreasing the contractive force of cardiac myocytes in the cardiac tissue. Sympathetic stimulation increases the force of ventricular contraction and also increases contraction of smooth muscles within arterial wall. By contracting smooth muscle within arterial walls, pressure increases on the blood within the arteries and increases blood pressure. The degree of contraction of arterial smooth muscle is called **arterial tone**. When arterial tone increases, arterial blood pressure increases.

Determinants of Total Body Water

The remaining major determinant of blood pressure is the **total volume of blood** within the blood vessels. Most of this volume is due to the volume of water within the blood. The volume of water is directly determined by the amount of water that is ingested through the digestive tract and the amount of water that is lost through urine and through **insensible water loss.**

Insensible water loss occurs through sweating, evaporation from the lungs and by chemical reactions in the body. There is an **absolute minimum water loss that cannot be prevented** through these processes.

Water loss through sweat can be almost eliminated by regulation of sweat production by the autonomic nervous system. Water loss through evaporation through the lung, by consumption in chemical reactions and by the limit imposed by the maximum capacity of the kidney to concentrate urine cannot be prevented and must be replaced by oral fluid intake. **Euvolemia** is the state where there is normal a volume of total body water. **Hypovolemia** is the state where there are inadequate volumes of total body water. **Hypervolemia** is the state where there abnormally high volumes of total body water.

If total body water volume falls below a critical level, there is insufficient blood volume in the circulatory system to maintain a minimum survivable blood pressure. This occurs when the heart is contracting as strongly and rapidly as possible, when the blood vessels are at maximum tone and the kidney is concentrating urine at the highest possible level. As we will discuss, the maximum urine concentrating capacity of the kidney is directly dependent on the osmolality of the extracellular fluid in the renal medulla.

Intravascular Volume and Sodium Ion Concentrations

The volume of water that is confined to the intravascular and extracellular spaces is determined primarily by the concentration of sodium ion in the intravascular and extravascular fluids. When sodium ion concentrations fall below optimum levels (hyponatremia), the volume of water within blood vessels decrease and can be inadequate to maintain a minimum blood pressure even when there is a normal or even excessive volume of total body water. The kidney's response to this is to reabsorb the maximum possible amount of sodium ion from fluids that are filtered by the kidney.

While the kidney plays a crucial role in maintaining adequate blood pressure, in large part this is related to the requirement of a minimum blood pressure for adequate kidney function. Since glomerular filtration rate depends on blood pressure, inadequate blood pressure results in inadequate glomerular filtration rate. The rate of production of soluble waste products such as organic acids and urea then exceeds the rate that they can be secreted by the kidney. Urea, ammonia levels

then rise and pH levels fall to fatal levels if an adequate blood pressure is not restored. The kidney has the capacity to directly adjust the blood pressure within glomerular capillaries within a range of 80-180 mmHg through a process called autoregulation.

Another critical role of the kidney is to directly maintain the optimum osmolarity of the blood and indirectly the osmolality of the intravascular fluid space and the osmolarity of the fluid within cells - the intracellular fluid space. This is also accomplished by regulating the excretion of water and sodium from the body.

A third critical function of the kidney is to maintain an optimal blood pH. This requires that the kidney have a mechanism to get rid of hydrogen ions when pH is too low and to retain hydrogen ions when blood ph is too high. This is accomplished by regulating the amount of bicarbonate ion in the bloodstream. Blood pH is also decreased by organic acid waste products produced by the body. The kidney does not regulate the levels of these organic acids, but strives to excrete all of these as well as all other soluble waste products with the exception of small amounts of urea that is concentrated in the renal medulla.

All of these functions require a complex interaction with other organ systems including systems and with systems that can detect the levels of water sodium blood osmolarity and blood pH. This information then needs to be transmitted to the kidney. This is usually in the form of hormones secreted elsewhere in the body or by signals sent via the autonomic nervous system.

The kidney also is involved in maintaining adequate levels of red blood cells in blood vessels and in maintaining the optimum level of calcium ions and phosphate in the body. Again, these require detectors for calcium and red blood cell levels and signals to the kidney relaying this information. In many cases it is the kidney itself that directly or indirectly detect the levels of the physiological parameters that it is responsible for optimizing.

The kidney requires a complex suite of structural and cellular functions that can respond to these signals. In the case of red blood cell levels this is the synthesis and secretion of the hormone erythropoietin. For calcium levels, it includes the synthesis and secretion of calcitriol - the activated form of vitamin D. For other functions, it includes the synthesis and secretion of the hormone renin.

Of course, the kidney must have receptors for hormones that participate in maintaining optimum fluid electrolyte and pH. These include the hormones aldosterone, atrial natriuretic hormone, and antidiuretic hormone (ADH or vasopressin). Finally, the kidney uses specialized cells and specialized local environment regions that can respond in a manner that maintains these optimum levels.

An important feature of the renal collection system - the renal tubules, collecting ducts calyces and renal pelvis is that the lumens of these structures are continuous - they are all connected and continuous with the lumens of the ureters, with the internal cavity of the urinary bladder and with the lumen of the urethra. The distal opening of the urethra - the urethral meatus in the glans of the penis in males and in the vulvar surface in females - is potentially open to the external environment. This means the entire internal space of this system is literally outside of the body. Anything that passes into Bowman's capsule from the body has been excreted from the body. And must be reabsorbed through the renal tubules or the renal collecting ducts in order to return to the interior of the body.

Reabsorption

Filtration and reabsorption are the primary processes utilized by the kidney to perform its numerous functions. By definition - in the kidney - reabsorption is the movement of a substance out of the lumen of a renal or collecting tubule into the extracellular space surrounding the tubule or into a peritubular capillary. When this movement is down a substance's concentration gradient it is usually a passive diffusion process - a process that does not require energy.

In the case of water this commonly is simple diffusion through segments of the renal tubule whose tubular walls are permeable to water. After substances are filtered into Bowman's capsule from glomerular capillaries, they almost always must be reabsorbed through specialized transmembrane transport systems located in the cell membranes of the cells that form the interior wall of renal tubules. These are simple cuboidal epithelial cells called **parafollicular cells**. Parafollicular cells have dense **microvilli** located on their apical borders - the surface of the cells that are exposed to the tubule lumen. This creates a **brush border** similar to the brush border of the small intestine.

As is the case with the intestinal epithelia cells' brush border - the parafollicular cells brush border vastly increases the cells' absorptive surface area. This greatly enhances the ability of parafollicular cells to reabsorb substances from the lumen of renal tubules.

Different segments of the renal tubule - the proximal convoluted tubule, the loop of Henle and the distal convoluted renal tubule - have unique complements of transmembrane transporters and permeabilities to water and other substances. The loop of Henle has several sub-regions that have very different membrane permeabilities (by simple diffusion) to various substances and have very different abilities to passively transport substances by facilitated diffusion or to reabsorb substances by actively transport.

Both **glucose and amino acids** are filtered from capillaries into Bowman's capsule. It is detrimental to the body to lose these crucial molecules through the urine and under normal circumstances the kidney is able to nearly completely reabsorb all of the glucose and amino acid molecules that are filtered into the renal tubules. It is logical for the kidney to reabsorb these substances as rapidly as possible and consequently nearly all of the active transporters for the reabsorption of glucose and amino acids are located in the walls of the **proximal convoluted tubule** (PCT) which is the tubular segment directly adjacent to Bowman's capsule. the transporter for amino acids is a sodium ion cotransporter.

The transporter for glucose - a sodium ion glucose cotransporter - can be saturated when the concentration of glucose in tubular fluid exceeds a critical level corresponding to a plasma glucose level 350 mg/dL. Glucose in tubular fluid cannot be completely reabsorbed and glucose is lost from the body in the urine (glucosuria). The presence of glucose in the urine is an indication that an individual is experiencing excessive blood glucose levels (hyperglycemia) usually due to diabetes mellitus.

Most bicarbonate ion (90%) is indirectly reabsorbed in the PCT, as well as about 65% of sodium and chloride ions and 65% of water. Angiotensin II stimulates the reabsorption of sodium ion and bicarbonate ion from the PCT. The increased reabsorption of sodium ion also indirectly increases the diffuse of water out by decreasing the osmotic pressure of tubular fluid.

Parathyroid hormone (PTH) - which is secreted when blood phosphate ions levels in the body are too high - inhibits the reabsorption of phosphate ion. The distal convoluted tubule is the site of most of the reabsorption of calcium ions. Parathyroid hormone (PTH) increases the reabsorption of calcium ion at this site. The levels of sodium ion in the blood are fine-tuned by variable reabsorption of sodium ions. This is usually about 10% of the total amount of sodium ion that is reabsorbed by the kidney.

Reabsorption in the Loop of Henle

One of the most critical features of the kidney is the creation of a very high osmolality within the extracellular compartment of the renal medulla. The renal medulla is composed mostly of loops of Henle. The tips or papillae of renal pyramids are adjacent to the renal calyces and are the deepest region of the renal medulla. The papillae are composed primarily of the sharp bend or u turn in the loops of Henle. The renal collecting duct importantly also travel from the renal cortex through the adrenal medulla to their termination at the renal calices.

The segment of the loop of Henle that originate at the PCT and descends to the U-turn of the loop in the renal papilla is the descending limb of the loop of Henle. The adjacent limb of the loop is the ascending loop of Henle. The lower segment of the ascending loop, originating from the u turn is called the thin ascending segment. The second segment of the ascending limb is called the thick segment of the

ascending limb. The thick ascending limb terminates at the DCT.

It is the loop of Henle's function to create the hyperosmolar environment of the renal medulla. The osmolarity of the adrenal medulla steadily increases as one [proceeds from the superficial regions nearest to the adrenal cortex to the region of maximal hyperosmolarity at the renal papillae. The loop of Henle accomplishes this by virtue of the manner in which various regions have variable permeability to water and by which various regions have variable permeability to sodium and variable ability to reabsorb sodium ion.

The lower end of ascending limb of the loop - the thin ascending segments - is lined by simple squamous epithelium. The distal portion of the ascending limb - the thick ascending segment - and is lined by simple cuboidal epithelium. Water is reabsorbed in the medulla at the descending loop of Henle. This region is permeable to water consequently water diffuses out of the descending limb into the extracellular medullary space due to the high osmotic pressure of the medullary space. This process increases the osmolarity of the tubule fluid.

The thin segment of the ascending limb is also permeable to water and consequently water continues to be reabsorbed by passive diffusion. The ascending thick segment of the loop is impermeable to water and actively reabsorbs sodium from the tubular fluid. This is the process that creates the high osmolarity of the renal medulla and simultaneously decreases the osmolarity of the tubular fluid. This tubular fluid continues through to the DCT and then to a collecting tubule. The tubular fluid in the DCT is maximally dilute. The osmolarity of this fluid corresponds to the minimum osmolarity of the urine that can be produced by the kidney and therefore corresponds to the maxim limit to the ability of the kidney to excrete excess water.

Reabsorption of Water from Collecting Tubules

Tubular Fluid flows from the DCT in the renal cortex into a collecting tubule at a level within the renal cortex. As the fluid descends through the collecting tubule, it again passes through the adrenal medulla.

HESI A² - Spire Study System

Although collecting tubules are generally impermeable to nearly all substances, they are remarkable for their ability to alter their permeability to water. The walls of collecting tubules - in the absence of **antidiuretic hormone (ADH)** - are completely impermeable to water. When ADH molecules bind to receptors on collecting tubules, specialized water pores called **aquaporins** are inserted into the walls of the tubule.

The number of aquaporins that are inserted into the collecting tubule walls - and correspondingly the permeability of collecting tubules to water - increases as the levels of of ADH that bind to collecting tubules increases. This is a critical mechanism in the kidney's ability to adjust the osmolality of urine - from maximally concentrated to maximally dilute. It is important to note that water is still diffusing down its concentration gradient from the collecting tubule into the surrounding extracellular space. The human body does not possess any transmembrane systems that can actively transport water against its concentration gradient.

The maximum urine concentrating ability of the kidney is about equal to the osmolarity of the renal medulla. Additional water cannot be reabsorbed by passive diffusion from the collecting tubule once the osmolarity of the tubular fluid is equal to the osmolarity of the surrounding extracellular space within the renal medulla.

Integration of Renal Functions

It is remarkable that there are some many factors that influence the kidney's functions as the body attempts to maintain optimal levels of total body water of blood osmolarity of blood pressure by regulating intravascular blood volume and arterial tone and contractility of the heart. There are cells and structures that detect the osmolality of the blood - osmoreceptors in the hypothalamus and kidney and blood pressure - baroreceptors - in blood vessels. that interact with hormone systems consisting of renin produced and secreted by the kidney, aldosterone produced and secreted by the adrenal cortex, angiotensin I and II, and ADH produced and released by the posterior pituitary.

It is helpful in the understanding of how these systems interact to first consider that ADH causes the kidney to maximally reabsorb water. Renin aldosterone and angiotensin II causes the kidney to maximally reabsorb sodium ion. Next, consider that there is a baseline state where all of these systems have optimized levels of blood pressure, of total body water and of blood osmolality. This corresponds to the baseline levels of renin, aldosterone, angiotensin II and ADH that are maintaining these levels.

In this state, the kidneys roles are primarily to excrete waste products and to maintain an optimum blood pH. In this scenario, the kidney will produce the minimum amount of urine required to excrete waste products. Additionally, it will produce a urine with an osmolality that is equal to the blood osmolality. this minimizes the loss of body water and sodium ion and maintains the desired osmolality of the blood. This corresponds to maximal levels of ADH and intermediate levels of other hormones.

When the body is hypervolemic with high osmolality (corresponding to hypernatremia), the kidney will maximize the excretion of both water but will also maximally excrete sodium. In this case, the kidney will produce a maximum volume of urine with a maximum osmolality (most maximally concentrated urine). If the body is hypovolemic and hyponatremic - too little body water and too little sodium - the kidney will produce a minimum volume of urine with a minimum or most dilute osmolality - this conserves body water and sodium.

This state corresponds to a maximum level of ADH and a maximum level of other hormones -renin, aldosterone and angiotensin II. The same logical analysis can be applied to determine how the kidney should respond to any combination of abnormal levels of body water and Blood osmolarity.

The basic details of the ADH and renin-aldosterone-angiotensin hormone systems are as follows.

ADH

Osmoreceptors in the hypothalamus and the pituitary gland directly detect plasma osmolality from adjacent capillaries. When plasma osmolality is undesirably high, the osmoreceptors relay this information to the pituitary. The pituitary response is to release antidiuretic hormone (ADH). the effect of antidiuretic hormone on the kidney is to increase the permeability of the renal tubules and collecting ducts to water. This results in the diffusion of water out of the filtrate solution and into the renal medulla where it can be reabsorbed into the circulation by renal capillaries within the renal medulla. This concentrates urine and reduces the loss of additional water from the body that occurs through the excretory system.

The Renin-Aldosterone-Angiotensin Hormone System
The kidney is able to directly detect the sodium ion concentration of plasma within renal arterioles. A response of the kidney to an undesirably low plasma sodium ion concentration (and also to low blood pressure) is the release of the hormone renin. Renin in the bloodstream leads to the production of angiotensin II. Angiotensin II is the activated form of angiotensin hormone.

Angiotensin II has a direct effect on circulatory vessels causing contraction of smooth muscle cells located in the walls of arteries and veins. This increases the force of the vessel walls on the blood within the vessels resulting in increased blood pressure. Angiotensin II has a direct effect on the proximal tubules to increase Na+ reabsorption. Angiotensin II is a potent vasoconstrictor and also stimulates the release of aldosterone from the adrenal gland. Aldosterone causes the kidney to increase the reabsorption of sodium ion thereby helping to restore plasma ion concentrations to normal levels. Several other mechanisms can lead to the release of aldosterone.

This is only a general summary of the complex interactions between kidney functions blood pressure effects and hormone interaction. Many other hormones influence kidney functions directly and indirectly, including atrial natriuretic peptide - that stimulates sodium ion excretion. As we have also mentioned, the kidney also secretes erythropoietin, which is a hormone that stimulates the production of red blood cells. The kidney is able to detect the levels of oxygen in the bloodstream and releases erythropoietin in response to low oxygen levels in arterial blood. The kidney secretes

calcitriol (activated vitamin D) in response to PTH, which increases the intestinal absorption of calcium from the small intestine.

Gluconeogenesis
It certainly appears that numerous critical functions of the kidney are more than sufficient for any single organ of the body, but the kidneys have another vital function as well. The kidney is capable of gluconeogenesis - the ability to synthesize new glucose molecules from other precursor molecules such as amino acids and fats. The liver is the major source of gluconeogenesis, but the kidney provides the last line of defense in supplying glucose to the body in states of severe hypoglycemia.

Abnormal Conditions of the Kidney
Polycystic kidney disease is an autosomal dominant condition that will eventually affect 1 in 1000 adults. The condition is responsible for 10% of cases of kidney failure in the U.S. Kidney stones or chlelithiasis is the formation of solid materials in the renal collecting system. The condition is common and acute attack when the stones pass through the ureters causes one of the most painful condition that humans can experience.

The nephrotic syndrome is another common condition that is the result of many types of damaging kidney processes. The condition results in the loss of proteins in the urine and can be fatal if it does not respond to treatment. Many autoimmune diseases affect the kidneys, most notably systemic lupus erythematosus (SLE). There are many other types of autoimmune conditions that cause various types of damage to the renal glomeruli (glomerulonephritis). Diabetes is one of the major causes of mortality in the U.S. and worldwide. A high percentage of diabetics succumb to kidney failure caused by diabetes (diabetic nephropathy). Pyelonephritis is an infection - usually bacterial - of the kidney that requires hospitalization and aggressive antibiotic therapy. Abscesses of and around the kidney are also not rare and are life threatening medical emergencies.

The Immune System and the Lymphatic System
The immune system's complexity tends to render discussion of the topic confusing unless we define a few terms for this review. Since nearly anything can trigger

an immune response by the body, we can refer to anything that can trigger an immune response as an **immunogenic agent** or an **immunogenic substance**. These substances or agents can include multicellular organisms, single-celled organisms (bacteria, fungi and protozoans), viruses, and foreign or abnormal chemicals or molecules (toxins and venoms, other foreign proteins or abnormal proteins produced by the body, and other types of molecules).

Cells or molecules that are members of the body's immune system will often be referred to in general as **immune system elements, agents, or substances**.

Generally, the body's immune system does not intentionally attack the body's own normal healthy cells. Intentional attacks are usually directed against abnormal cells of the body- particularly if they are infected with a cellular organism or virus or have mutated into a benign (non-malignant) abnormal mass of cells (tumor) or a malignant form (cancer). We will often refer to these cells as "**abnormal-self**" cells.

Regardless of what causes an immune response, we can refer to all specific immune responses as **immune events**. We can be more specific by using the term **initial immune event** or **initial immune encounter** for the first step in an immune response and **ongoing immune event** for latter phases of an immune response.

Although infection and other ongoing immune events can be generalized or "spread out" throughout the body (usually viral or blood-borne disease), the immune system generally operates at distinct sites or locations. These can be sites of infections by a biological or viral agent, but many other processes can trigger localized immune responses. We will often refer to all of these as **immune event sites**.

The Lymphatic System

The immune system is a complex and widely distributed network of cells, organs and other structures. The lymphatic system is a body-wide circulatory system that includes lymphatic vessels, lymph nodes and lymphoid organs. The lymphatic vascular system is closely associated in both structure and distribution to the blood vessels of the cardiovascular system. The lymphatic system functions include the removal of excess fluids and debris from the extracellular or interstitial compartments of the body (the area surrounding cells not including spaces inside blood vessels). The lymphatic system is also a major component of the immune system.

Capillary-size lymphatic vessels are found throughout the body. They are terminal branches of the lymphatic vascular system. Lymphatic fluid moves from interstitial spaces into the lymphatic capillaries, then to progressively larger vessels and then to lymph nodes. Lymph nodes are nodular structures that are widely distributed throughout the body. Lymphatic fluid is filtered at lymph nodes and continues in vessels leaving the lymph nodes to reach one of the two major lymphatic vessels; either the right lymphatic duct or the thoracic duct. The right lymphatic duct delivers lymph fluid into the right subclavian vein and the thoracic duct delivers lymphatic fluid into the left subclavian vein.

The lymphatic circulation is also responsible for the absorption of fats and fat-soluble vitamins (vitamins A, C, D and E) in the small intestines and subsequently for transport to the bloodstream.

Lymph Nodes

For the HESI, the anatomy of lymph nodes is significant in that the cortex of the lymph node is a site where T-cells accumulate and interact with B-cells and that the medulla of lymph nodes is one of the anatomical regions where the maturation of B-cells occurs.

The Spleen

The spleen is the largest lymphoid organ in the body and one of the largest organs of the body in general. It is located in the left upper quadrant of the abdomen just superior to the stomach and just inferior to the diaphragm. The spleen has structures similar to lymph nodes that contain B- and T-cells. The spleen filters blood that arrives via the splenic artery arteries. The spleen contains macrophages that consume damaged and elderly red blood cells and recycles iron to the liver. The spleen also contains a large volume of white blood cells that serve as a readily accessible reserve for immune activities that may be required by the body.

The Thymus
The thymus is an organ located in the midline of the thoracic cavity immediately posterior to the sternum and anterior to the trachea, directly between the lungs. The thymus is the organ where the maturation of T-cells occurs.

The Appendix and the Tonsils
The appendix, an appendage of the cecum of the large intestine and the tonsils, located in the lateral walls of the pharynx are also lymphoid organs that contain B- and T-cell functional regions.

Bone Marrow
The medulla (central region) of most skeletal bones - and in particular the long bones of the arms and legs and the pelvic bones - contain bone marrow. Both red blood cells and white blood cells (including immature T-and B-cells) are produced in the bone marrow.

Immune Responses
Immune responses describe activities of the immune system. Immune responses may be broadly categorized as **innate** (immune system) responses or **adaptive** (immune system) responses. They may also be broadly categorized as **cell-mediated** responses and **humoral** responses. There are humoral and cell-mediated responses that occur in both the innate and adaptive immune system responses.

Inactivate Immune System Chemicals and Cells
Cells and chemicals of the immune system are often present or prepositioned within the body - usually within the interstitial or extracellular spaces of a potential immune event site or within the circulatory system before an initial immune encounter occurs. These cells and chemicals are often inactive - either inactive chemicals such as **proenzymes** that can be triggered into an active form by immune events, "native" immune cells, or cells that have "reset" to an initial state from activities in a previous immune response. We will often refer to theses as inactivated or unactivated substances or immune cells.

Cells of the immune system that have never participated in an immune event will often be referred to a "naive" cells. In particular this applies to B-cells and T-cells of the adaptive immune system that have never participated in immune events.

Barriers to Infection
The first line of defense in the human immune system is the bodies barriers to entry of foreign substances. This is the outer surface of the integumentary system - the skin and the epithelial lining of the bodies aerodigestive system and the conjunctival tissue of the eyes.

Passive Mechanical Barriers
The outer layers of epidermal keratinocytes of the skin - the stratum corneum - are tightly joined by desmosomes that create a relatively **impermeable physical barrier** to nearly all substances including water and atmospheric gases. Additionally, the flaking of the outermost layers of epidermal keratinocytes tends to prevent the accumulation of foreign substances on the outer skin surface.

Active Mechanical Barriers
Physical defenses that remove or decrease the amount of potentially harmful substances on body surfaces and in body cavities include **flushing** actions of tears on the corneas of the eyes and the **outward transport of substances** from the lungs and trachea by the coordinated rhythmic motions of cilia on the outer or apical surfaces of bronchial epithelial cells. This process begins with the secretion of mucous by specialized cells that are interspersed in the outer or apical layer of epithelial cells in the respiratory tract.

The Mucociliary Conveyor Belt
Mucous is also secreted by mucous cells in the epithelial lining of the digestive tract. Mucous is a thick watery substance that protects underlying epithelial cells from various harmful substances within the lumen of the respiratory and gastrointestinal tract. The mucus traps microorganisms and other foreign particles in the respiratory tract and the rhythmic coordinated motion of the cilia located on the respiratory epithelial cells moves the mucous and any entrapped particles out of the tract where it is coughed or sneezed out or

swallowed. This process is informally termed "the mucociliary conveyor belt".

Chemical Barriers

The highly acidic environment within the stomach, as well as proteolytic (protein cutting) enzymes within the stomach and elsewhere within the remainder of the digestive tract also contribute to the destruction of potentially harmful agents (viruses, microorganisms and toxic chemicals).

Secretory substances from the sweat and oil glands of the skin create a hostile environment for the growth of organisms on the skin surface. Organic acid molecules secreted onto the surface of the skin also creates an unfavorably acidic environment for the growth of microorganisms.

The mucosal lining of the vaginal walls is also sufficiently acidic to suppress the growth of most foreign organisms (the yeast *Candida albicans* is a frequent exception).

Saliva and tears also contain substances with antimicrobial properties including lysozyme and phospholipase A2.

Lysozyme

Lysozyme is a hydrolytic enzyme that attacks specific regions of bacterial cell walls. Polymorphonuclear leukocytes (PMNLs) and macrophages (professional immune cells) and breast milk also contain lysozyme. Lysozyme is considered a humoral component of the innate immune system.

Phospholipase A2

Phospholipase A2 catalyzes the release of arachidonic acid from triglycerides and phospholipids of cell membranes.

Arachidonic Acid

Arachidonic acid is another key molecule in humoral immune biochemical pathways biochemical pathways - Arachidonic acid can directly induce **localized pain and inflammation** to surrounding tissue. and can be converted to two other important general classes of

molecules in the humoral immune - **prostaglandins** and **leukotrienes**.

Microbiological Colonization Barriers

A stable community of a variety of microorganisms within the GI tract also suppresses the ability of harmful microorganisms to survive within the GI tract. Stable beneficial colonization of the skin and the vaginal mucosa by microbiological communities also contribute to the barrier defenses at these regions of the body.

The Active Immune Systems

Traditionally, the elements of the non-barrier or active human immune system is described as consisting of two sub-systems - the innate immune system and the adaptive immune system. The innate immune system evolved in vertebrates (including humans) before the adaptive immune system and is theoretically capable of functioning without or independently of an adaptive immune system.

The Innate Immune System

The innate immune system responds to foreign agents in a general manner - it cannot precisely identity foreign agents based on the specific antigens that the agent presents to the immune system. The innate immune system functions in the same ways to any substance that it encounters and then recognizes as a foreign agent.

The activity of the innate immune system proceeds in a specific series of cellular and biochemical steps that are the same regardless of what stimulus is triggering the innate immune responses. This is somewhat of a simplification of the innate response. There are many variations in the type and degree of innate response that can result from an initial triggering of the system by an immunogenic agent.

The Adaptive Immune System

The adaptive immune response is able to identify a specific infectious agent and over time becomes progressively more selective and effective in eradicating that agent from the body. The adaptive immune system is also able to "remember" a specific infectious agent that triggered an initial or first-encounter adaptive immune response. Upon a subsequent identification of this agent in the body, the adaptive immune response is then able to mount a much more rapid and powerful immune response to that particular agent.

Antibodies and Antigens
The adaptive immune system is capable of identifying specific molecular features (antigens) that are possessed by a foreign agent and can generate specific molecules (antibodies) that bind to these specific antigens.

Antibody-Producing Cells
Antibodies are synthesized by B-cells and plasma cells. B-cells are a key cell type of the adaptive immune system. Plasma cells are derived from B-cells that have transformed after activation by an immunological event. Plasma cells synthesize and secrete specific antibodies into the surrounding regions of the body. These antibodies can diffuse into the local interstitial (extracellular) space surrounding the plasma cell. Many of these antibodies then enter the circulatory system and subsequently are widely distributed throughout the body. Antibodies are the primary humoral components of the adaptive immune system.

Antibody-Antigen Specificity
Antibodies can tightly bind to (attack) a vast number of unique or "specific" small molecules and larger molecules which contain these molecular molecules as subunits of their overall molecular structure. Small specific molecules and small specific regions of larger molecules that can be targeted by a specific antibody are called **antigens** ("anti" for "antibody" and "gen" for "genesis") - Antigens by definition are capable of triggering a direct attack by a specific antibody.

All antibodies that can specifically bind to a particular antigen are classified as complementary antibodies to that particular antigen. Conversely, all antigens that can be specifically bound to a particular antibody are - by definition - complementary to that particular antibody.

The Hypervariable Antibody Region
Antibodies are the defining immunological protein complexes of the adaptive immune system. they are small "Y"-shaped molecules composed of protein subunits called light-chains and heavy-chains. One heavy-chain protein forms either side of the "Y" and one light-chain protein is bound - one apiece - to the outer sides of the "V" region located at the top of the "Y" structure. The ends of the "V" portion of the antibody is a **hypervariable region**.

Antibody Gene Rearrangement
There are tens-to-hundreds of thousands of different amino-acid sequences that can form these hypervariable regions. This hypervariable region is the binding site for a particular antigen and is very similar to an active site on an enzyme for the enzyme's substrate molecule.

During B-cell maturation, every maturing B-cell will randomly rearrange segments of DNA in genes that code for the amino acid sequence of the proteins that form the hypervariable region of an antibody.

Since this process is random, the result is that there are tens to hundreds of thousands of different antibodies that a population of B-cells can produce. Each individual B-cell produces only one type of antibody. All B-cells have B-cell receptors displayed on the outer surface of their cell membranes. The distal segment of the B-cell receptor is the specific antibody that the B-cell is capable of synthesizing and releasing into the external surroundings of the B-cell. Any plasma cell derived from a particular B-cell will secrete the antibody corresponding to the antibody segment of the progenitor B-cell.

Hypervariable Cell Membrane Receptors
Although only plasma cells synthesize and secrete full-formed antibodies that then distribute throughout the body, many types of cells can also synthesize partial antibodies. These partial antibodies include the hypervariable "V" region of an antibody.

These hypervariable antibody fragments are then coupled with other proteins to form a specific antigen-receptor complex that is transported and anchored to the outer surface of the cell's membrane. Complementary antigens can then bind to the hypervariable antibody fragment of the receptor and activate the cell to begin additional immune functions. These functions depend on the type of cell that is activated and on other factors that are present during an initial or ongoing immune event.

T-Cell and Mast-Cell Membrane Receptors
T-cells are the other major cell type of the adaptive immune system. Hypervariable antibody-receptor subunits are components of all T-cell receptors and T-cell receptors are present on the membranes of all types of T-cells.

Another notable immune cell that that has cell-membrane receptors with hypervariable antibody sites for antigen binding is the mast cell. **Mast cells** are technically members of the innate immune system but obviously they participate in immune functions that involve adaptive immune responses.

Cells that display receptors that include hypervariable antigen components also rearrange segments of their genes that code for the hypervariable region proteins. Consequently, these cells can synthesize the same vast array of possible different hypervariable antigen regions that B-cells (and plasma cells) are capable of synthesizing for their antibodies.

Antibody-Antigen Affinity
It should be noted that although a particular antibody may be able to bind a specific antigen, there may be other antibodies with hypervariable regions that are even more effective at binding to this antigen. Similarly, an antibody may be able to bind with more than one specific antigen - in particular with antigens that have very similar molecular structures. The effectiveness of a given antibody in binding a particular antigen is referred to as the affinity of the antibody for the antigen.

Notice that once a cell has rearranged it hypervariable gene segments, the cell will produce one and only one specific type of hypervariable antibody segment. All the hypervariable regions of a cell receptor on a single cell and all of the antibodies produced by a single B-cell or plasma cell have the exact same molecular structure. If these individual cells undergo mitotic division, many of the daughter cells will also synthesize the exact same hypervariable regions as the progenitor (parent) cell.

PAMPs and CAMPs
Pathogen-associated molecular patterns (PAMPs) and cytosolic-associated molecular patterns (CAMPs) refer to a class of molecular structures that are shared by a wide range of immunogenic agents. These molecular structural patterns are typically present on the exterior surfaces of immunogenic agents, but they may also be elements of substances contained within these agents.

PAMPs and CAMPs are analogous to antigens. They can be recognized by cellular and humoral elements of the immune system without any participation of antibodies. Some complement proteins can bind to these molecular patterns and many immune cells have receptors that are designed to bind to theses molecular patterns. Antibodies may also recognize PAMPs and CAMPs as antigens (or recognize one or more molecular subregions of PAMPs and CAMPs as more than one antigen).

Humoral Immune Responses
Humoral immune responses are those that are mediated by molecules that are present in body fluids or the extracellular spaces of the body. These molecules may be either pre-formed or synthesized and secreted by other cells in response to an immune event. Humoral responses can occur in both the innate and adaptive immune system.

The Humoral Immune Molecules
Humoral immune substances - which are single molecules or complexes of two or more molecules are technically anything produced by the body that is utilized in immune responses and is NOT a cell. This can be confusing because humoral immune responses can and usually do involve the participation of immune and other cells of the body. Also, the term humoral is usually referring to extracellular molecules. There are many immune molecules that act intracellularly against immunogenic agents.

There are also innate humoral responses and adaptive humoral responses. One general category of humoral (non-cellular) agents are the static or independent immunological molecules that can function alone to restrict infectious processes. These include lysozyme, the organic acids secreted onto the surface of the skin and hydrochloric acid of the stomach.

The primary roles of humoral molecules in the immune system can be generalized in three broad categories. One category is direct or indirect killing or deactivation of immunogenic agents. Another class is signaling functions that affect the behavior of other cells - usually immune cells, but others as well - notably epithelial cells and fibroblasts. A third class is inflammatory or anaphylactic functions.

Humoral molecules with these functions generate several effects that are characteristic for inflammation of tissues at an immune event site. One is the dilation of local blood vessels to increase blood flow to the local immune event site.

A second effect is to cause increased permeability (leakiness) of small blood vessels at a local immune event site. These effects together increase the blood flow and movement of fluids and other substances from local blood vessels into the local immune event site.

The signs of these processes are increased redness (rubor), warmth (calor) and tissue swelling (dolor) of the local immune event site. Another effect of inflammatory humoral molecules is pain(dolor) resulting from the molecules ability to increase the sensitivity of local pain fibers.

The physiological effects of the processes that generate these 4 cardinal signs of inflammation result in the fifth cardinal sign of inflammation - loss of function. Inflamed regions of the body usually lose some or all of their normal functions. The normal range of motion of an inflamed body region is often reduced or lost - this is primarily a protective feature that reduces the chance that the local infectious processes will be spread further by mechanical forces at the site of infection.

Loss of other cellular functions, such as in organs like the kidney, liver and heart are unavoidable consequences of the inflammatory and other immune activities. This is a form of collateral damage to the body caused by immune responses and this type of

damage can cause severe injury to the body. The damage can be permanent and even fatal.

Defensins and Porins
In addition to lysozyme, other humoral molecules are capable of directly killing or deactivating harmful immunogenic agents. Defensins are small molecules that disrupt phospholipid membranes of microorganisms and enveloped viruses - potentially killing these foreign agents. Defensins may be present in body fluids or they may be secreted by immune and other cells of the body.

Porins are molecules - usually secreted by various immune cells - that can create small holes in both foreign and abnormal human cell membranes. These holes in turn allow other humoral molecules to enter and kill the targeted cells.

Complement Cascade Proteins
Another class of humoral molecules that are capable of independent and direct killing or deactivation of immunogenic agents are various members of the complement cascade proteins. Some of the activated forms of complement proteins can create membrane attack complexes (MACs) that create large openings in phospholipid membranes of immunogenic agents (bacteria in particular).

Antibodies are humoral molecules of the adaptive immune system that can directly kill or deactivate immunogenic agents (extracellular viruses and toxic compounds in particular).

Autoimmune and Hyperimmune Responses
Although the human immune responses are designed to deactivate dangerous foreign chemical agents such as venoms and other toxic substances and to combat infectious agents such as viruses, bacteria, and eukaryotic organisms - single cell fungi and protist (such as amoeba) and multicellular parasites.

Often immune responses are inappropriate and harmful - including fatal - human immune response. Autoimmune responses (immune reactions that attack the body's own healthy cells and extracellular components) and hyperimmune responses (excessively intense or disproportional responses to non-self substances) are responsible for a large fraction of all human diseases.

Most commonly this damage caused by the immune system to the body occurs through the generation of the inflammatory response. The inflammatory response produces swelling of tissues and a variety of toxic chemicals and cell activity that cause damage to normal cells and non-cellular structures in the body.

This damage can be rapidly destructive and potentially fatal when the inflammatory response is particularly severe. Anaphylactic shock is a frequently fatal even that is a direct consequence of a severe and rapid inflammatory response.

Inappropriate and prolonged generalized inflammatory states are proven or strongly suspected to be a primary cause of many common and severe human diseases including asthma, psoriasis, inflammatory bowel disease (Crohn's and ulcerative colitis) and type 1 diabetes, rheumatoid arthritis, systemic lupus erythematosus (SLE) progressive neurodegenerative diseases such as multiple sclerosis, amyotrophic lateral sclerosis (AML or Lou Gehrig's disease) Parkinson disease, severe kidney disease (glomerulonephritis) and very likely atherosclerosis, which is the primary cause of cardiovascular heart disease and stroke. Localized regions of chronic inflammation have also been proven to cause malignant changes to cells resulting in cancer at the site of the inflammation.

Self vs Non-Self
One principal of the human immune system is that the human body strives to identify and eliminate anything from within the body that is "non-self". Non-self includes any cells or other substances that are not produced by the body. These other substances do not include essential macro- and micro-nutrients, water and oxygen obtained from the environment through the respiratory and digestive systems.

The Major Histocompatibility Complex (MHC)
The body identifies cells as "self" primarily based on the MHC proteins (class I and II) that are displayed on the outer surface of the bodies cell's membranes. Cells without the precise specific set of MHC molecules that are present on the cell membranes of a particular individual are readily identified by the individual's immune system as "non-self".

MHC class I and II cell membrane proteins are also referred to as the human leukocyte antigens (HLA). All nucleated cells in the human body display MHC class I markers. MHC class II markers are displayed primarily by dedicated immune system cells - macrophages and dendritic cells in particular.

This initial identification step of "non-self" by an initial immune system event triggers a series of immune functions that attempt to disable or kill these cells and then eliminate the resulting cellular remnants from the body.

MHC Incompatibility
The probability that a **random** person will have the same MHC molecules as another person is much less than 1 in 50,000 (**siblings** have a 25% chance of having identical MHC molecules). The same events can lead to rejection of MHC mismatched tissue transplants - such as skin grafts and rejection of immune cells in bone marrow transplants.

Tissue and Organ Transplant Rejection
When it is only the variation in MHC proteins that identifies a cell as non-self, the cell is almost always a cell of the body. This is a "self" cell that usually is infected, injured or otherwise "abnormal self". An important example where these cells are normal human cells but literally "not self" occurs with organ transplants. The donor-organ cells are normal, healthy human cells, but they are cells belonging to another individual. The recipient's immune system will reject these transplanted cells if they (the donor cells) do not have the same MHC molecules as the recipient's cells.

Graft vs Host Disease
The topic of graft vs host disease illustrates the differing roles of MHC class I markers compared to MHC class II markers. As we mentioned, class II markers are displayed almost exclusively by certain dedicated immune cells and MHC class I markers are displayed by nearly all human cells that have a nucleus. In graft vs

host disease, transplanted material (usually an organ) from a donor to a recipient may include donor immune cells.

These cells can be targets of the recipient's immune system due to the presence of non-donor MHC class I markers and other cell membrane markers on the donor immune cells. In graft vs host disease, the donor immune cells evade destruction by the recipient immune system and also are able to engage in their own immune attack upon the recipients nucleated cells by identifying the recipient's MHC class II markers (or other membrane markers) as "non-self". In effect, cells of the donor's immune system attack the recipient. These graft vs host immune responses can be fatal to the recipient if not controlled by immunosuppressive medications or radiation treatments.

"Non-self "can also include substances other than foreign cells. Virtually none of the potential infectious agents have MHC class molecules, but it is generally not the absence of these MHC molecules that triggers an immune response against the agent. These agents can be single and multicellular organisms, viruses and foreign molecules such as toxins, venoms and other potentially harmful chemicals. Even non-biological objects such as slivers of metals or wood can trigger immune responses called "foreign body reactions".

There are, in fact, very few substances that can be introduced into the body that will not result in some form of immune or rejection reaction. These non-self agents can, as we have discussed, also be the body's own cells.

ABO Blood Types
Mature red blood cells are non-nucleated and do not display MHC cell markers. The immune system rejects donor red blood cells from transfusions when there is a mismatch in another class of cell markers that are present on RBC membranes - the ABO markers (also called ABO antigens). Persons may have blood types where their RBCs have an A antigen only (type A), a B Antigen only (type B) or both an A and a B antigen (type AB) The "O' antigen is not an antigen at all - it is a lack of both A and B antigens (type O). an individual's immune system will attack transfused

RBCs that display ABO antigens that are not present on the individual's own RBCs.

ABO Incompatibility
One can see that individuals with type O blood have neither A nor B antigens on their RBCs. They will therefore reject transfused blood from any other blood type (A, B or AB) since these blood types have RBCs with foreign or non-self antigens, either the A or B antigen or both the A and B antigens (type AB). Type O individuals can therefore only be transfused with type O blood.

Notice that type O blood can be transfused to the other blood types. By similar reasoning, type B individuals can be transfused with type O or type B blood, but not with type A or type AB blood. Type A cannot be transfused with type B or type AB blood. Type AB individuals may be transfused with any of the ABO types.

Rh Factor - Universal Blood Donors and Recipients
Another important self vs non-self RBC antigen is the Rh factor. Individuals may be either Rh positive - their RBCs display the Rh antigen, or they may be Rh negative - their RBCs do not display the Rh antigen. Persons with Rh positive blood may receive transfusions of Rh negative blood but persons with Rh negative blood will reject Rh positive transfused blood. Therefore, type O-negative blood - which has no A, B or Rh antigens on their RBCs - are universal donors. Type O negative blood can be transfused to any other blood type individuals. By similar reasoning, type AB-positive individuals may receive transfusions from any other blood-type individuals. Blood type AB-positive is therefore a universal recipient.

Rh Factor Incompatibility in Pregnancy
Rh incompatibility is important in another important context. pregnant women who are Rh- negative may have a developing child in the womb who is Rh-positive. During pregnancy and during delivery, some of the child's blood enters the mother's circulatory system. The immune system will recognize the foreign (non-self) Rh antigen and attack these fetal RBCs. A firstborn Rh-positive child is often spared from any

significant attack by the mother's immune system against the child's Rh-positive blood.

The mother's adaptive immune system will, however, retain a memory of this encounter with the Rh antigen and any Rh-positive children during subsequent pregnancies of can be aggressively attacked within the mother's womb by the mother's own immune system. This can lead to miscarriage or severe intrauterine damage to the child. This is the reason that Rh-negative women are treated with **RhoGam** - an antibody that will suppress the mother's immune system from attacking Rh-Positive blood in the developing child.

"Abnormal-Self" Cells

Cells of the body that are infected with pathogenic agents - viruses, unicellular organisms such as fungi and bacteria and multicellular parasites can change the composition of molecules on the outer surface of their cell membranes and thereby identify themselves to the immune system as "abnormal-self" cells. In some cases, infected cells can present fragments of the infectious biological agent on their membrane surfaces along with their Class I MHC molecules. In other cases, the change is a simple decrease in the number of cell markers on the cell's membrane. In this case it is a simple deficiency in numbers of normal or "self" markers that signals the immune system that a cell is abnormal.

Apoptosis - Cell "Suicide"

Sometimes when they are infected, injured or are otherwise abnormal, an individual's cells actually commit suicide in a process termed apoptosis, Apoptosis can be triggered by the cell itself or it can be induced by various interactions with the immune system. when cells become malignant or cancerous, they often display non-self markers on their cell membranes or release substances that are identified as non-self by the immune system. This typically results in immune responses by the body that attempt to eradicate the cancerous cells. Usually this is successful, but clearly not always since cancer is among the most common causes of death in humans.

Dedicated or Professional Cell Types

Cells whose exclusive or primary functions are of a certain type are frequently referred to as "professional" or "dedicated" cells of that type. For instance, the primary cells of the immune system are professional or **dedicated immune-system cells**.

A dedicated or **professional phagocyte** has a primary role as a cell that phagocytizes cells or other substances; a professional or **dedicated antigen-presenting cell** has a primary function of presenting antigen. Many other cell types may participate in immune events, or be capable of phagocytosis or antigen presentation - but this is not their primary role - Epithelial cells, for instance, are capable of phagocytosis and nearly all nucleated cells are capable of antigen presentation - but this is not normally a primary function of these cells.

Often a cell may have more than one professional function. Macrophages, for example, are dedicated phagocytes and they are also often dedicated antigen presenting cells. Dedicated cells may often have other roles within and outside of the immune system.

Professional Immune System Cells

Immune Cell Lineages

Most Mature cells of the body differentiate from precursor or progenitor cells through one or more cycles of mitotic division. Most cells of the body differentiate from a totipotent stem cell. Totipotent stem cells give rise to pluripotent stem cells which in turn give rise to nearly all other mature cells of the human body. The sequence of progenitor cell through immature cell types to a mature cell is referred to as the **cell lineage** of the mature cell. The two major subcategories of professional immune system cells based on cell lineage are the lymphocytic lineage cell types or lymphocytes and the myeloid lineage cell types.

Leukemias and lymphomas usually occur when there is a defect in the maturation pathway of a mature immune cell. This is called maturation arrest. The cells at a less mature stage are unable to differentiate into the next stage of cell maturation. The body detects the lack of the mature form of the cell and instructs the progenitor cells to continue to replicate. This process leads to an often-fatal accumulation of the immature cell types and lack of any of the mature immune cell type.

Lymphocytes (Lymphocytic-Lineage Cells)

All lymphocytes are professional immune cells. There are three major subtypes of lymphocytes, which are all derived from a common lymphocytic progenitor cell type. All three have a common lymphoid progenitor (stem) cell that is usually located in the bone marrow.

B-Cells and Plasma Cells

B-cells are professional immune cells. B-Cells are lymphocytes. When an inactive B-cell is activated, it often undergoes several rounds of mitotic division to form a clonal population of identical B-cells. These B-cells can then differentiate (transform) into plasma cells. Plasma cells synthesize and secrete antibodies. B-cells and plasma cells - by most definitions - participate in humoral adaptive immune system events.

This is because B-cell and Plasma cell activity ultimately results in the production and release of antibodies and antibodies are not cells. Therefore, antibodies are considered to be humoral agents of the immune system. Of course, plasma cells are required to produce antibodies, so this can be a point of confusion regarding the difference between cell-mediated and humoral immune agents and events. Also, B-cells frequently participate in direct-contact interactions with other professional immune cells - In our discussion summary we will provide our best explanation for how one may - for the HESI - classify immune activities as cell-mediated or humoral and as innate or adaptive.

T-Cells

T-cells, like B-cells, are lymphocytes. There are several important subtypes of T-cells. These are T-helper cells, cytotoxic T-cells, memory T-cells, suppressor (or "regulatory") T-cells and natural killer T-cells (these are not the same as natural killer cells). We will not discuss the roles of suppressor T-cells and another type of T-cell - the gamma delta T-cell - these are almost certainly outside of the scope of the HESI examination.

Natural Killer (NK) Cells

NK cells are the third major class of lymphocyte (the others being B-cells and T-cells). NK cells are able to attack virally infected and cancerous cells of the body ("abnormal-self" cells). NK cells can attack these cells without interacting with other cells or other substances of the adaptive immune system. For this reason, NK cells are considered to be members of the innate immune system. NK cells nevertheless often do interact with the adaptive immune system. Again, do not confuse NK cells with natural-killer T-cells. N-K T-cells cannot attack immunogenic agents without assistance from other elements of the adaptive or innate immune system.

Myeloid Lineage Professional Immune Cells

All myeloid lineage cells are descended from a common myeloid progenitor cell (usually located in the bone marrow). The subcategories of myeloid cell types are erythrocytes (red blood cells or "RBCs") platelets (cell fragments of megakaryocytes) and the myeloid immune cell types. Of the immune cell types, there are two subclasses - granulocytes and monocytes.

Granulocytes

Granulocytes are myeloid-lineage cells. There are four general types of granulocytes, neutrophils or **polymorphonuclear leukocytes** ("leuko" means "white", these are usually referred to by their initials as PMNLs or "polys") eosinophils, basophils and mast cells. These cells contain cytoplasmic granules specific for each cell type that are prominently visible under the microscope with various cellular-staining techniques. All of the granulocytes are capable of chemotaxis to immune event sites via amoeboid locomotion and all are capable of phagocytosis to varying degrees.

Neutrophils (PMNLs)

Neutrophils are usually referred to as PMNLs but many authorities classify all granulocytes as PMNLs, so we will refer to them as neutrophils to avoid confusion. Neutrophils are usually the most abundant type of professional immune myeloid cell type. The majority of the body's population of neutrophils is usually located within the bloodstream. Neutrophils are capable of phagocytosis and can migrate rapidly from within a blood vessel to an immune event via diapedesis and amoeboid locomotion. When neutrophils encounter immune associated molecules diffusing from the event site these molecules activate the neutrophils and provide a chemotactic diffusion gradient for the neutrophils to follow directly to the event site.

Defensins
Neutrophil granulocytes (and all epithelial cells) contain small (18-45 amino acid) polypeptide substances called defensins that contribute to the killing of many types of viruses, bacteria and fungi. Defensins function primarily by creating punctures in cell membranes of bacteria and fungi cells and in the membranes of enveloped proteins (derived from host cells when viruses bud off from viral- infected cells).

Eosinophils
Eosinophils are granulocytes that have some ability to phagocytize substances but less so than neutrophils. Eosinophils have chemical components in their specific granules (eosinophilic granules) that are unique within the body and can be highly toxic to various immunogenic organisms - **multicellular parasites** in particular. Eosinophils are also professional antigen-presenting cells and play vital roles in regulation of other immune processes.

Basophils
Basophils are the least abundant of the granulocytes. Basophil immune functions are associated with their ability (when activated) to release histamine and other substances that generate inflammatory effects at an immune event site. Basophils are most commonly involved in immune activities associated with parasitic infections and in allergic reactions.

Mast Cells
Mast cells are granulocytes that are principally located in tissues that are in close proximity to the external environments. They are abundant in the upper layers of the dermis, in the mucosal layers of the respiratory bronchial tree, the GI system the nasopharyngeal cavity and the conjunctivae (outer layers) of the eyes. Mast cells release a vast array of chemicals when activated and can be activated by number of different triggering mechanisms of both the innate and adaptive immune system.

Mast-Cell Degranulation
The release of mast cell components in response to immune events is referred to as degranulation. The most well-known of the substances that mast cells release during degranulation is histamine. **Histamine** is a potent humoral immune agent that cause dilation of blood vessels (resulting in localized swelling, warmth and redness) and also sensitizes (irritates) local pain fibers, resulting in itchiness and pain.

Mast Cells and Allergies
Mast cell degranulation can be triggered by activated components of the complement system proteins and by binding to PAMPs, CAMPs, specific antigens and antibodies. Mast cell degranulation is the key event in many types of allergic reactions including hay fever and the potentially fatal anaphylactic reactions seen in hyperimmune responses to insect stings (bee venom in particular) food allergies (peanuts, strawberries, etc.), and other types of allergens.

Recall that mast cells have membrane receptors that can bind specific antigens with a hypervariable-antibody segment that is part of the histamine cell membrane receptor. This fact explains how individuals can develop allergies to any of a vast array of very specific environmental substances. Since histamine receptor hypervariable antibody regions can have affinities to almost any small molecular structure, individuals may possess large numbers of mast cells that have an affinity to virtually any antigen-possessing substance in the environment.

Monocytes
monocytes are the largest of the granulocyte class of professional immune cells. They are unique among the granulocytes in that one of their primary function is to differentiate into either macrophages or dendritic cells, which are also professional immune cells. After maturing from a progenitor stem cell in the bone marrow, monocytes enter the bloodstream and subsequently accumulate in the spleen or migrate into tissues located throughout the body where they differentiate into macrophages or dendritic cell. macrophages and dendritic cells tend to remain at a given location until they are activated by an immune

event.

Monocytes are capable of recognition and phagocytosis of immunogenic agents via several mechanisms, including recognition of CAMPs on the immunogenic agent, recognition of complement protein fragments attached to an immunogenic agent or recognition of antibodies attached to an immunogenic agent. Monocytes can phagocytose and subsequently kill or deactivate immunogenic agents through fusion of the phagosome with a lysosome.

Fragments of a phagocytized immunogenic agent can then be coupled to a MHC class II molecule and transported to a monocytes outer membrane surface for antigen presentation to other elements of the immune system. Monocytes can also kill or deactivate immunogenic agents through a process defined as **antibody-dependent cell-mediated cytotoxicity.**

Macrophages
Macrophages, as we just mentioned, are descended from monocytes. Macrophages reside in locations throughout the body, where they patrol for substances that require removal from the body (a custodial function).

Macrophages that patrol specific locations in the body often are given other names; in the liver sinusoids, they are called **Kupffer cells**; in the lungs - **alveolar macrophages**. In the central nervous system, they are called **microglia** (microglia may be a separate form of differentiated monocyte in contrast to other resident macrophages).

Macrophages also patrol for immunogenic substances and are capable of presenting antigens from ingested immunogenic agents in the same fashion described for monocytes.

Dendritic Cells
Dendritic cell are phagocytic cells that are residents of tissues throughout the body, particularly at sites that are likely portals of entry for foreign immunogenic substances. Dendritic cells possess **Toll-like receptors** on their cell membranes which are able to bind to pathogen-associated molecular patterns (**PAMPs**) that

are present on or in a wide variety of foreign microorganisms. After recognizing and then phagocytizing a foreign immunogenic substance, dendritic cells are usually able to digest the substance and present the digested fragments as antigens coupled to their MHC class II molecules on their outer cell membrane surfaces.

Dendritic cells are also capable of migrating to lymph nodes and other lymphatic tissues where they can present these antigen-MHC class II membrane complexes to B-cells and T-cells. B- and T-cells are activated by binding of their respective receptors with these antigen-MHC complexes. Natural Killer (NK) cells can also be activated through this process.

There are several types of dendritic cells and most if not all are differentiated daughter cells descended from a monocyte progenitor cell, or a lymphoid progenitor cell. In addition to activating T and B cells and NK cells by binding of antigen-MHC complexes, dendritic cells also induce additional changes in these cells through the release of an interleukin (IL-12). Il-12 is also released by activated macrophages. IL-12 stimulates the release of interferons by T-cells and NK cells. The most notable of these is Interferon gamma (IFγ). Interferon gamma has a wide range of effects on other cells of the immune system, including stimulation of phagocytic activity in macrophages and the production of intracellular chemicals in infected cells that can kill intracellular infectious organisms located inside the infected cells.

Phagocytes
Although we have already discussed several types of cells with a primary phagocytic function in the immune system - most importantly macrophages and dendritic cells - it is helpful to consider all phagocytes as a separate topic.

Phagocytes are a class of cell types that participate in immune responses and also function as custodians by engulfing other undesirable substances that serve no purpose in the body. These include fragments of dead cells and other molecular remnants that are essentially "trash" such as protein or other macromolecular fragments. Phagocytic cells also participate in the formation and remodeling of structures within the body. Bone formation and remodeling by osteoclasts is a notable example.

Phagocytic cells in the human body include dedicated phagocytes. Many types of cells are capable of phagocytosis but dedicated or professional phagocytes of the immune system have cell surface receptors for foreign agents they are designed to detect and engulf. Neutrophils, (PMNLs), monocytes, macrophages, dendritic cells, mast cells and microglia (in the central nervous system) are dedicated phagocytes. Most dedicated phagocytic cells are capable of independent purposeful locomotion via pseudopodial (amoeboid) movements. This allows these cells to move from a distant site in the body to a site where an immune response is occurring. This process is called chemotaxis. Chemical attractant molecules are generated by an ongoing immune response. These chemoattractant molecules then diffuse outward from the site of the immune response. As the attractants diffuse their concentration decreases as the distance from the initial diffusion site increases. This establishes a concentration gradient that phagocytic cells can follow to the site of the immune response.

In addition to their movement through intercellular (interstitial) spaces of the body towards an immunological event site, phagocytic (and other cells capable of chemotaxis) are frequently initially located inside of a blood vessel. In order to exit the vessel, the cells must squeeze between the cells that comprise the walls of the vessel. This squeeze-through process is termed diapedesis. diapedesis is usually triggered by the same chemicals that create the chemotactic concentration gradient leading to the immune event site.

Phagocyte Activation
Phagocytosis is initiated when a phagocytic cell is activated. Activation of a phagocytic cell may occur when the cell encounters and then binds to particular pattern of chemicals on an infectious cell (PAMPs or other distinctive membrane molecules) or particular assemblies of complement proteins that have attached themselves to an infectious cell's outer membrane. Often the phagocyte is activated or induced to proceed further in its phagocytic processes when it binds to one or more antibodies that have attached to their target antigens on a cell or other foreign substance.

Activation of a phagocytic cell can also occur before the cell is in close proximity to a target cell or substance. This usually occurs when signaling chemical diffuse from an immune event site and encounter the phagocytic cell. This activation at a distance usually is by signal chemicals that have established a concentration gradient from the immune event site and provides a chemotactic path to the site for the phagocytic cell. These chemicals may be products of the infectious agent or products produced by the body during an immune event.

These substances include activated protein fragments of the complement cascade, other chemicals produced in the non-cellular inflammatory reactions at an immune event site or by cells that are infected or injured or by other cells of the immune system that are present at an immune event site.

In addition to triggering an engulfment sequence for a target substance by the phagocyte, the activation process also frequently triggers other processes in the phagocyte, including cell division to increase the number of phagocytes, release of chemicals that can directly injure or kill infectious organisms and/or increase the efficiency of the phagocytosis of the target organism.

Activation of phagocytic cells can also cause the cell to release signaling molecules that are chemoattractants for other immune cells or that induce changes in other immune cells or interact with non-cellular chemicals in the complement and inflammation reactions occurring at the immune event site.

Once a target substance (infectious cell, viral particle or harmful chemical) target substance has been phagocytized by a cell.

Most commonly this involves the fusion of the phagocytic vesicle (the target substance enclosed within a segment of the phagocytic cell membrane) with a lysosome - a cell vesicle that contains various chemicals that can digest or deactivate the phagocytized substance. The result is a phagolysosome that encloses the target substance and the contents of the lysosome within a new vesicle that is the combined membrane of the phagosome and the lysosome. Aft Once a cell has phagocytized and digested a target substance it may subsequently transport an intact antigen or digested fragments of the antigen of the target substance to the cell's outer surface membrane. This process is termed antigen presentation. Many cells of the body can present antigen, but certain cells of the immune system are dedicated or professional antigen-presenting cells. Among the most notable of these professional antigen-presenting cells are macrophages and dendritic cells.

A particularly important type of dendritic cells is the Langerhans cell. Langerhans cells are located in the dermal layer of the skin. Other dendritic cells are located in other regions of the body close to the boundary with the external environment - such as the linings of the lungs and the GI tract.

One key feature of dendritic cells (Langerhans cells in particular) - is that they maintain their positions within tissues until they encounter and phagocytize a target substance. This activates the dendritic cell to migrate to a lymph node or other lymphoid organ.

When the dendritic cell arrives at the lymphoid organ it encounters B-cells and T-cells. Through subsequent bindings of T-cell or B-cell membrane receptors with the presented antigen and other cell membrane molecules on the dendritic cell, these B- and T-cells are activated to perform further immune actions directed against the antigen-possessing agent.

When a potentially harmful non-viral agent (bacteria, fungi and multicellular pathogens or parasites) succeeds in breaching the outer barrier defenses (skin or mucous membranes) the first active immune response usually occurs by the recognition of a pattern of molecular components that are found on the surface of or contained within the cell or cells of many of these organisms. These patterns of molecular components are referred to as pathogen-associated molecular patterns (PAMPs). PAMPs are recognized by cells of the immune system that possess pattern recognition receptors (PRRs) on their outer cell membrane surfaces.

There are several varieties of PRRs that a human cell may possess. A series of cellular responses is triggered in a PRR-possessing cell when it encounters a PAMP and subsequently forms a ligand-bond between its PRR and the PAMP. There are two general types of responses, signaling responses and endocytic responses.

Signaling responses are triggered by Toll-like receptors. toll-like receptors or found primarily on immune sentinel or surveillance cells such as dendritic cells and macrophages, but also on natural-killer cells B-cells, T-cells and non-immune system cells such as fibroblasts, epithelial cells and endothelial cells.

Endocytotic PRR binding to a PAMP triggers the phagocytosis and intracellular destruction of the substance or biological agent that possesses the receptor PAMP by the cell whose PPR is ligand bonded to the PAMP.

Ligand bonding of PAMPs to toll-like receptors initiates an intracellular series of biochemical reactions. The result of these reactions depends on the type of toll-receptor cell that binds to a PAMP. Effects can include stimulation of cell division, synthesis and release of cell-signaling molecules such as interleukins and cytokines. In some cases, toll-like receptor binding to a PAMP triggers apoptosis or "suicide" of the toll-like receptor cell. PAMPS can also bind with proteins that are members of the complement protein system.

The Complement System
The complement system is an important subsystem of the immune system. The system comprises at least 30 different individual complex proteins and other molecular factors that can be activated by a wide variety of foreign substances and by interactions with cells and antibodies and infectious microorganisms - bacteria in particular.

Most of the complement proteins are synthesized by the liver Complement proteins that are not participating in active immune reactions within at sites of immune response are most abundant within the bloodstream. Circulating proteins in the bloodstream Within the bloodstream, the complement proteins are in inactive or proenzyme forms. The complement system is activated when one of these proteins (C3) is cleaved into two fragments - C3a and C3b. This first cleavage step occurs when various initial events occur during invasion by a foreign agent.

In most cases an earlier component or components of the complement reaction cascade sequence has attached itself to the outer cell membrane surface of an infectious organism. These components begin to assemble a C3 convertase complex. The first component attaches to the cell membrane at a site that has a particular affinity for the complement component. This site may be a PAMP or another distinctive molecular feature of or located on the cell membrane. A convertase complex can also be initiated by binding of antibodies of the humoral immune response. When two antibodies to an antigen located on the cell membrane of an infectious organism bind alongside each other on the cell membrane. The convertase complex is progressively assembled at an anchor point on two adjacent antibodies.

Regardless of what triggered the formation of the complex, when a C3 protein encounters a convertase complex the complex cleaves the C3 protein into two fragments - C3a and C3b. This leads to an immediate series of subsequent cascade reactions that progressively activate other proteins in the complement cascade. The product of each step of the cascade creates activated fragments of a complement protein in the inactive form into one or more active protein fragments. These fragments in turn activate the next complement protein in the cascade reaction. The result is that only one or a few molecules that begin the C3a convertase complex assembly can rapidly trigger the formation of a huge number of activated complement proteins.

There are three major consequences of activation of the complement cascade. The first is direct killing of an infectious cell as an innate immune response or as a consequence of adaptive immune responses.

The Complement Membrane Attack Complex (MAC)
When activated C5-C9 proteins assemble alongside activated C3b fragments that remain attached to C3 convertase complexes on the membrane of an infectious cell, these fragments form a membrane attack complex (MAC) that creates a large opening in the infectious cell membrane. This opening is large enough to allow the infectious cell cytoplasm to escape from the cell interior. As additional MACs form, the cell is killed as its cytoplasm is lost through the openings created in the cell membrane by the MACs.

By this process the complement system functions as an element of the innate immune system and is capable of killing infectious organisms either independent of other elements of the immune system or in concert with other immune system activities. Notice that when MAC formation begins with C3 convertase formation on adjacent antibodies on an infectious cell surface that the complement system is in effect triggered by activities of the humoral response of the adaptive immune system (since the humoral response is the production of antibodies that attack specific foreign antigens).

Opsonization
Complement proteins directly enhance the effectiveness of phagocytosis of infectious cells by other cells of immune system. Activated complement protein fragments attached to the surface of an infectious cell's outer membrane promote the recognition and engulfment of infectious cells by phagocytic cells of the immune system.

Inflammation
Activated complement proteins also promote the inflammatory processes associated with innate immune responses. Either directly or indirectly these proteins participate in the processes resulting in the four cardinal signs of inflammation - swelling, redness, warmth and pain. Permeability of local blood vessels resulting in increased fluid leakage from the vessels into the intravascular spaces and localized swelling at an infection site. Blood vessels at the site also dilate, resulting in increased blood flow. This causes the increased temperature and redness associated with localized infection. These four components of the local inflammation immune response produce the fifth sign of inflammation - incapacitation or impairment of

function of the cells, tissues and/or organs at the infection site.

Mast Cell Degranulation

Activated complement proteins may cause these inflammatory effects directly, but often their effect is indirect by stimulating mast cell degranulation. The granules of mast cells contain histamine, a protein that directly stimulates increased blood flow in and permeability of local blood vessels. Histamine is also irritating to local pain fibers and this causes the itching associated with the inflammatory response as well as triggering the sneezing and watery eyes in "hay-fever" allergic reactions.

The pain associated with inflammatory reactions is caused by increased pain receptor firing due to increased pressure at the site of inflammation and by several other chemicals including prostaglandins and leukotrienes produced by the body as part of the inflammatory process -, these chemicals also irritate local pain fibers resulting in additional pain sensation at a site of inflammation. They also are involved in causing fever - (an increase in the body's core temperature) that tends to inhibit viral replication in infected cells.

Chemotaxis

Activated complement proteins also functions as chemoattractants for other cells of the immune system such as macrophages and PMLS. These proteins can initiate diapedesis - the movement of cells out of the blood vessels into the local extracellular space. Once the immune cells have moved out of local blood vessels they migrate to an infection site by following the concentration gradient of complement proteins that have diffused from an infection site. Complement proteins also indirectly produce other chemoattractant gradients via interactions with various steps in immune responses.

There are numerous other interactions between complement proteins and the immune system that enhance both the innate and adaptive immune response. Among these are effects that trigger replication and differentiation in immune system cells. This widespread ability of the complement system to enhances or 'complement" many aspects of both the innate and adaptive immune system activities is the source of its designation as the 'complement" system.

Antigen Presentation

This activation of a B-cell or T-cell by an interaction with an antigen presented by a dendritic cell is an example of a common theme in the immune system where a cell of the body presents a foreign antigen or other membrane marker to an immune system cell.

Injured or infected non-immune cells of the body - may display a "kill me" membrane marker this binds to an immune cell membrane receptor. This triggers subsequent immune events that lead to the death of the cell. As we mentioned earlier, cellular and chemical elements of the immune system may bind directly to a PAMP or similar feature of a foreign substance - the complement cascade reactions can initiate immune responses in this manner. Injured, infected or otherwise stressed cells of the body can initiate immune responses by displaying "kill me" membrane markers and can also initiate immune responses by releasing chemoattractant and inflammatory signal chemicals.

Immune System Response Pathways

In general, an immune system response is a series of actions by the immune system that is capable of detecting potentially harmful foreign substance when it enters the body and then disabling the substances ability to potentially cause injury to the body. These responses are often categorized as either innate or adaptive immune system responses but innate and adaptive immune responses often overlap during infectious events.

Innate Immune Response Pathways

Perhaps the best definition of a purely innate immune response is one that does not involve the participation of any antibodies or any T-cells at any stage of the immune response.

There are two general categories of such purely innate immune responses. The first is the extracellular response. This is a response to an infectious cell (or cells if the agent is a multicellular organism) that is encountered within the body, but not within a cell of the body. The most well-studied of these extracellular infectious events is the innate immune response to infection by bacteria. The second general category of a purely innate immune response is the intracellular response. This is the response to the infection of a living cell of the body by an infectious agent. Usually, this is a viral infection, but there are other organisms that can cause an ongoing infectious process by infecting and reproducing inside human cells.

The diagrams below illustrate the series of events that occur in purely innate immune response to an extracellular bacterial infection and to a viral infection of a living human cell.

Activation of the Innate Immune System - PAMP Binding to Sentinel Cell PRRs

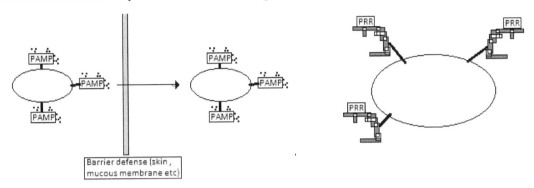

One pathway for activation of the innate immune system occurs when a foreign cellular organism such as a bacterium that possesses pathogen-associated molecular pattern (PAMP) sites breaches the outer barrier defenses of the body. As the infectious organism enters the body it encounters a sentinel cell that possesses pattern recognition receptors that can bind to the particular PAMP sites on the infectious organism. Sentinel cells (or immune surveillance cells) are usually tissue macrophages (resident macrophages) or dendritic cells.

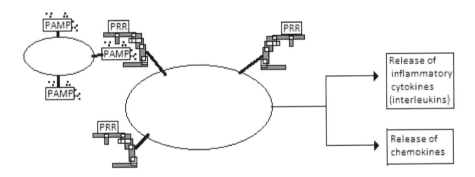

PAMP-PRR binding triggers activation of the sentinel cell. One of the primary consequences of sentinel cell activation is the release of inflammatory cytokines and the release of chemokines.

The scale of the diagram is greatly exaggerated. The size of PAMPs and PRRs are much smaller relative to the size of the infectious cell and the sentinel cell. They are enlarged to illustrate the interaction between PAMPs and PRRs. Sentinel cells - such as resident macrophages and dendritic cells - are usually much larger than unicellular infectious cells - particularly when the infectious organisms are bacterial cells.

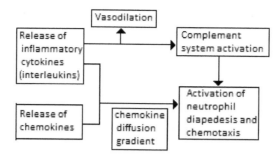

One of the primary purpose of the release of chemokines and inflammatory cytokines by activated sentinel cells is to rapidly attract large numbers of neutrophils to the infection site. Inflammatory cytokine cause vasodilation and activation of the complement system.

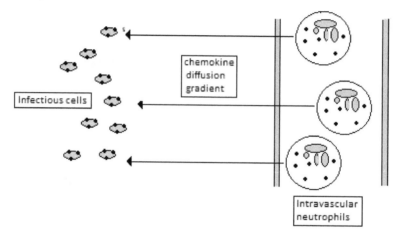

The first step in the migration of neutrophils to the site of infection requires the neutrophils within a nearby blood vessel to squeeze through the endothelial cells that form the walls of the vessel - This process is called diapedesis. Several cytokines released by sentinel cells result in the expression of intercellular adhesion molecules (ICAMs) by the endothelial cells and integrin molecules on the neutrophil cell membrane.

Interactions between the ICAMs and integrin molecules allow the neutrophils to first attach to and then pass between endothelial cells of the vessel wall. Once neutrophils exit the vessel they move toward the infection site by following the chemotactic concentration gradient generated by sentinel cell release of cytokines and also by fragments of complement proteins resulting from activation of the complement system (also triggered by cytokines released by sentinel cells or through other activation pathways).

Complement System Activation in the Innate Immune Response
One of the effects of the triggering of the innate immune response by sentinel cell binding to PRR receptors to PAMPs on an infectious cell leads to the release of inflammatory cytokines by the sentinel cell. One of the effects of the released inflammatory cytokines is the activation of the complement system. There are over 20 types of complement proteins. These proteins can be released by numerous types of cells including sentinel cell, but there is also a significant amount of complement proteins in nearly all extracellular body fluids. There are multiple pathways that lead to activation of the complement system in addition to activation by inflammatory cytokines released by sentinel cells.

At least two of the activation pathways for the complement system can be triggered directly by infectious cells themselves. This is a second pathway for the initiation of the innate immune response against infectious cells (the other being the PAMP-PRR receptor binding of sentinel cells).

All complement system activation pathways converge on the conversion of complement protein C3 to complement protein C3a and C3b fragments. The results of this C3 conversion is summarized in the diagram below.

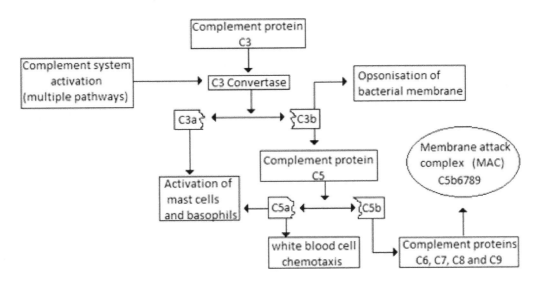

Notice that there are four critical functions that activation of the complement system accomplishes. One is the production of the complement protein fragment C5a which creates a chemotactic diffusion gradient that attracts most types of white blood cells to the activation site (which is also the site of an infectious event). Additionally, C5a and C3a are potent activators of mast cells and basophils.

A third function is the opsonization of infectious cells - this is principally accomplished by the binding of C3b fragments to the cell membranes of infectious cells. These C3b fragments are recognized by neutrophils, macrophages and other phagocytic cells and their presence on the cell membrane of infectious cells greatly enhances the ability of theses of these immune system cells to phagocytize the infectious cells.

Finally, activation of the complement system results in the formation of membrane attack complexes (created from C5b fragments and C6-C9 complement proteins. These complexes insert through infectious cell membranes, creating large transmembrane pores that allow cell contents to escape, resulting in the death of the infectious cell.

Another important feature of activation of the complement system is the activation of local basophils and mast cells by complement protein fragments (C3a and C5a). The recruitment of white blood cells to the infection site is enhanced by this release of histamine.

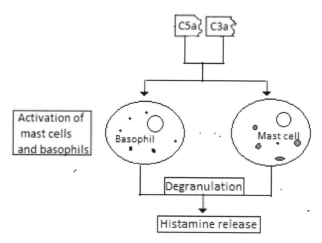

The activation process for basophils and mast cells includes degranulation - the release of histamine molecules into the local environment. The effects of histamine in this innate immune response are diagrammed below.

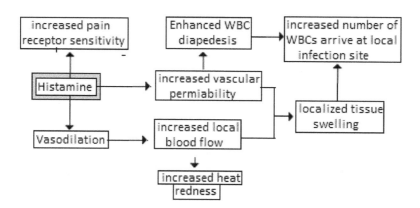

Histamine effects include the irritation of local pain fibers causing pain and loss of function of tissues at the infection site. Histamine causes endothelial cells that form the walls of local blood vessels to shrink - increasing the ability of white blood cells to move out of the vessel (diapedesis) and then to migrate to the infection site. Histamine also causes smooth muscle cells in local vessel walls to relax. This relaxation increases blood flow in the local vessels.

The shrinkage of endothelial cells combined with the increased blood flow in local vessels allow fluids in the vessel to move into the local interstitial space. This causes swelling of the local tissue at the infection site. Swelling of the local tissues increases the ability of white blood cells to move from the local vessels to the infection site. Increased blood flow also causes increased warmth and redness at the infection site.

The final phase of this type of innate immune response is the accumulation of large numbers of white blood cells at the infection site. At the infection site, infectious bacterial cells are already being destroyed by membrane attack complexes generated by the complement system. Complement proteins (C3b) have also begun to coat the bacterial membranes which increases the susceptibility of the bacterial cells to phagocytosis by neutrophils, macrophages and other phagocytic cells.

The first white blood cells to arrive at the site - neutrophils - continue killing infectious bacterial cells by releasing bactericidal chemicals into the infectious region and by phagocytizing bacteria - particularly those coated by complement proteins. Neutrophils arrive within minutes to hours after the innate immune response is triggered. If the infection continues for greater than 24 hours, monocytes and macrophages arrive to participate in the killing of bacteria.

Macrophages that phagocytize the infectious bacteria will be able to digest the bacterial cells and then present fragments of the bacteria (as foreign antigens) along with MHC class II molecules to T-cells and B-cells of the adaptive immune system. This is one pathway for a triggering of an adaptive immune response to the infection event.

The Innate Immune System Response to Intracellular Infection

The second major pathway for a purely innate immune system response occurs when normal human cells are infected with a virus or other intracellular pathogen (bacteria or another intracellular parasite). This type of invasion of the body by infectious agents often avoids the innate immune response we have described for extracellular infectious agents.

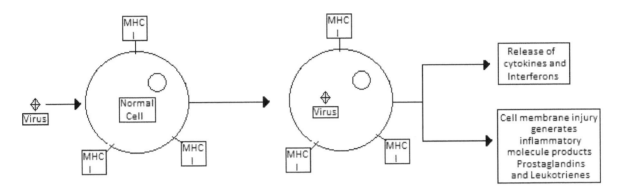

When a normal human cell is infected with a virus (or other intracellular infectious agent), The cell releases a number of cytokines that can attract and activate other cell types of both the innate and adaptive immune system. Interferons are a class of these released cytokines that have several important effects. One is the suppression of viral replication, another is the activation of natural killer cells.

Viral infection results in damage to the infected cell's cell membrane. Products of injured cell membranes cause similar effects as the inflammatory cytokines generated in an extracellular innate immune response. These inflammatory effects increase the ability of other types of immune cells to migrate to the site of viral infection.

If the body has not been previously infected by a particular virus, there is no rapidly available source of antibodies that can be generated to attack the viral particles. The adaptive immune response must be generated through a series of steps beginning with the display of viral antigens along with MHC class II molecules on the membrane of the infected cell.

Natural Killer Cells in the Innate Immune Response

A more rapid response to the viral infection is an innate immune response by natural killer (NK) cells. Natural killer cells are lymphocytes that do not require interaction with antibodies to attack virally infected cells. Natural killer cells that are in the vicinity of virally infected cells will tend to be activated by interferons produced by the virally infected cells.

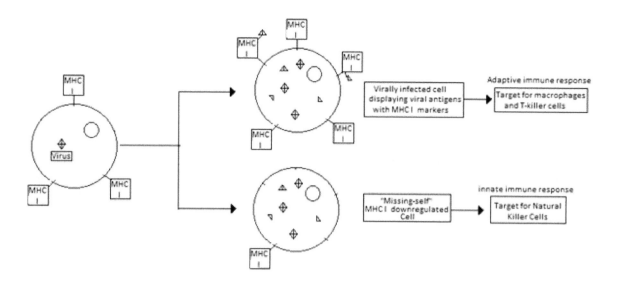

Once activated, the NK cell identifies the infected cells - one hypothesized detection method occurs when the virally infected cells decrease the number of MHC class I displayed on their cell membranes. This downregulation of MHC I membrane markers is actually caused by the infectious agent in the cell. This is a strategy of the infecting virus or other intracellular pathogen uses to avoid the immune system - without MHC Class I markers, antigens of the infecting agent cannot be displayed to trigger an innate immune response.

This decrease in MHC I markers can also in itself be evidence that cells are infected (or otherwise abnormal - such as cancer cells). Natural killer cells are able to identify cells with reduced MHC I markers. The combination of interferons and other activating cytokines in the local environment released by the infected cells and the decreased numbers of MHC I markers on the infected cell's membrane cause nearby natural killer cells to attack the infected cell.

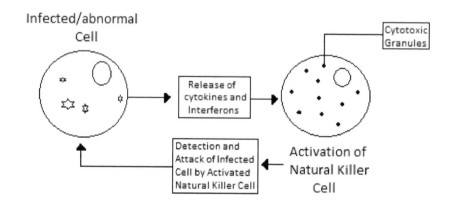

Natural-Killer Cell Cytotoxicity - Perforins and Granzymes
Upon activation by interferons and other cytokines in the local environment Natural killer detect virally infected (or otherwise abnormal) cells in their vicinity. When this natural killer/infected/abnormal cell encounter occurs, the natural killer cell releases the contents of cytotoxic granules within the NK cell into the local environment.

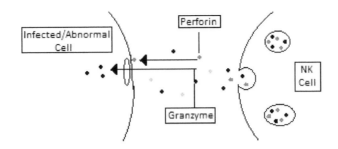

The contents of these cytotoxic granules include two primary types of molecules. One of these is perforin molecules, which attach to the membrane of nearby infected/abnormal cells and create small holes or pores in the infected cell's membrane. The second type of molecule released from NK cytotoxic granules are granzymes. Granzymes diffuse through the pores created by perforins in the infected cell's membrane and subsequently cause a fatal series of events within the cell known as apoptosis.

Adaptive Immune Response Pathways

The adaptive immune system responses require the participation of antibodies and /or T-cells. Antibodies are produced when the immune system detects a foreign infectious agent and subsequently identifies specific small molecular segments possessed by the infectious agent. Furthermore, these molecular segments are not otherwise found in the body and are therefore foreign molecular segments. These small molecular segments are classified as foreign antigens.

If the immune system has never previously encountered a particular foreign antigen (a novel foreign antigen), there are several immune system response pathways that result in the production of antibodies that are precisely designed to bind to the novel foreign antigen.

There are countless numbers of different antigens that can be identified by the immune system. The immune system is able to produce specific antibodies that can efficiently bind to nearly any specific foreign antigen. Since nearly every infectious agent possess antigens that are unique or highly specific to that agent, the antibodies produced against the infectious antigens are highly specific for the agent.

The ability of the immune system to recognize any one of the huge number of possible foreign antigens that can be present on an infectious agent and then produce antibodies that are able to specifically bind any one of these foreign antigens is explained in part by the general molecular structure of antibodies.

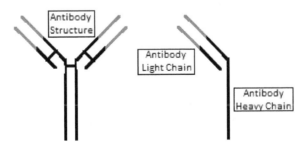

In the diagram above, the general "Y"-shaped structure of an antibody is shown on the left. Antibodies are composed of two types of protein subunits - heavy chains and light chains. These are identified in the illustration on the right. Notice that two identical heavy chain proteins form the core of an antibody and that a single light chain is attached to the upper-lateral segment of each heavy chain.

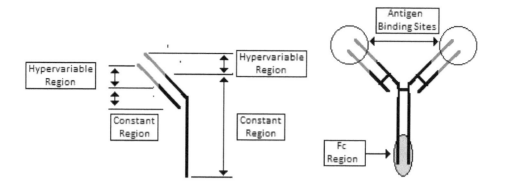

The most distal segments of the heavy and light chain of an antibody are hypervariable regions - regions that can vary enormously in their precise amino acid sequence and local molecular structure (secondary and tertiary protein structure). The precise molecular structure of an antibodies hypervariable region determines which specific antigen the antibody is capable of binding. The molecular structures of the two antigen binding sites are identical.

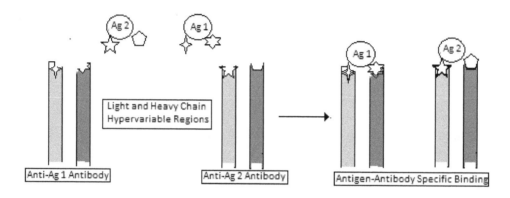

The enormous variability of antibody hypervariable regions allows for the production of antibodies that can bind to almost any possible foreign antigen molecular structure. Although there are countless possible molecular structures for the hypervariable regions of an antibody, any single antibody producing cell (a plasma cell) produces antibodies with one and only one precise hypervariable region structure.

Antibodies also form the antigen-binding segment of T-cell receptors and B-cell receptors. If a B-cell is activated and subsequently differentiates (after several rounds of mitotic division) into plasma cells, all of the daughter plasma cells will only produce antibodies with the exact hypervariable region structure as the hypervariable region of the progenitor B-cell's B-cell receptor.

The "Fc" Antibody Segment
The Fc region of an antibody is located at the "stem" of an antibody. The Fc region consists of two distal constant segments of the two heavy chains. Many immune cell types have membrane receptors for the Fc region of antibodies. The binding of Fc-antibody regions to these receptors can activate and or enhance the immune functions of the immune cells. One class of antibodies - the complement fixation antibodies - have a region that can bind and activate complement proteins.

Antigen Activation of B-Cells
The production of antibodies directed at a new foreign antigen requires that one of the antigen particles binds to a B-cell with a B-cell receptor that is complementary to the antigen.

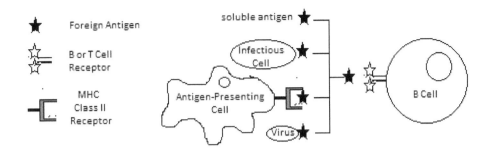

The diagram above illustrates the forms in which a new foreign antigen may be presented a "novel" B-cell (a B-cell that has never been previously activated). Although T-Cells cannot bind a foreign antigen unless the antigen is presented as an MHC I or II antigen complex, B-Cells can bind a foreign antigen in an unbound or free (native) form as well as in the MHC-antigen complex form. In all cases, the antigen travels from the infection site to local lymphatic vessels and then to the lymph node attached to the lymphatic vessel.

Once the antigen reaches the connecting lymph node, it progresses into the medulla (middle region) of the lymph node where it encounters the population of B-cells that occupy this medullary region. The antigen may arrive in the form of a small dissolved (soluble) molecule or as part of an intact virus or infectious cell.

Antigen/B-Cell Matching
There are thousands of novel B-cells in any single lymph node and there are many local lymph nodes that a may be accessible from an infection site. Each of these novel B-cells has a B-cell receptor that has a unique hypervariable antigen-binding region. It is a near certainty that within a lymph node a new foreign antigen will encounter at least one or a few novel B-cells that possess a B-Cell receptor that can efficiently bind the antigen.

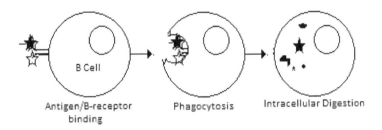

Soluble antigens and antigens transferred from antigen-presenting cells are easily phagocytized by the B-cell. The B-cell is also able to phagocytize the antigen along with the entire attached virus or the entire attached infectious cell if it arrives in either of these forms (attached to a virus or infectious cell). In these cases, the virus or cell is digested and the antigen obtained as a fragment of the digestion process.

Very often the antigen is carried to the B-cell by a migrating antigen-presenting cell that has phagocytized an infectious agent that possesses the antigen. In this case, the antigen is presented to the B-cell along with a MHC class II membrane marker. The antigen is transferred from the antigen-presenting cell MHC marker to the B-Cell receptor. The antigen presenting cell is not phagocytized by the B-cell.

B-Cell Antigen Presentation

Once the antigen is available as a fragment within the B-cell, the fragment is attached to a MHC class II marker and the antigen-MHC complex is transported to and then displayed on the outer surface of the B-cell membrane.

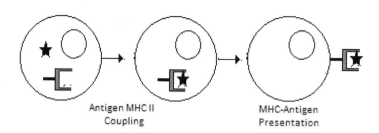

Antigen MHC II Coupling   MHC-Antigen Presentation

Once a naive B-cell has been activated and subsequently presented the activating foreign antigen with a MHC Class II marker on its outer cell membrane, the MHC-antigen complex can be recognized by a T-cell that possesses a T-cell receptor that is also complementary to the presented antigen on the B-cell. The segment of the T-cell receptors (and B-cell receptors) That bind foreign antigens are essentially antibodies that are anchored to the cell membrane.

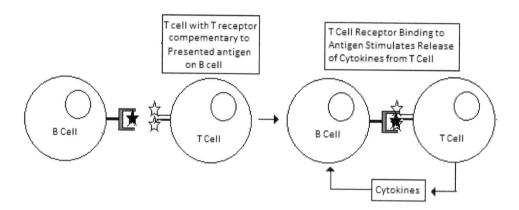

B-Cell/T-Cell Matching

The population of naive T-cells in the body have individual T-cells that may have any one of a vast array of possible antigen binding site structures. T-cells constantly patrol through lymph nodes and intermingle with B-cells within the lymph nodes. Some of these T-cells will have a particular T-cell receptor that can bind to the B-cell's presented antigen. When one of these patrolling T-cells encounters the B-cell, The T-cell binds the B-cell MHC-antigen complex with its T-cell receptor.

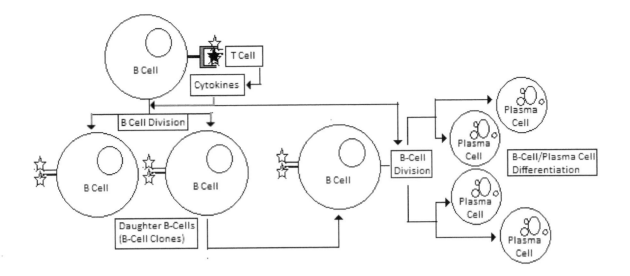

T-Cell Promotion of B-Cell Maturation

This B-cell/T-cell binding event results in the release of several types of cytokines by the T-cell. One of the major effects of these cytokines is to cause the B-cell to undergo numerous rounds of mitotic cell division. This results in the production of a population of daughter B-cells that are identical to the original B-cell (a clonal B-cell population). All of the daughter B-cells will have B-cell receptors that are identical to the original B-cell.

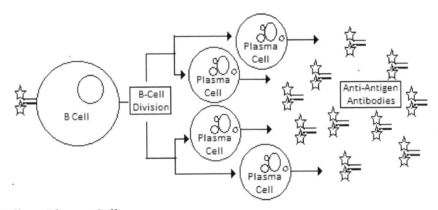

Differentiation of B-Cells to Plasma Cells

A second major effect of the cytokines released by the T-cell is to induce a large fraction of the clonal B-cells to transform (differentiate) into plasma cells. Plasma cell are the cells that synthesize and release antibodies that are able to subsequently diffuse throughout the body. Any single plasma cell only secretes antibodies that have that have identical antigen binding sites.

These binding sites are identical to the binding site of the B-cell receptors located on the B-cell from which the plasma cells are derived. Therefore, the antibodies will bind to the same antigen that binds to the progenitor B-cell's B-cell receptor.

The overall result of the activation of a single B-cell by a single foreign antigen is the production of a clonal population of plasma cells that release of a vast number of antibodies specifically targeted against the foreign antigen. These antibodies will be distributed throughout the body and will bind to the targeted foreign antigen wherever the antigen is located almost anywhere in the body.

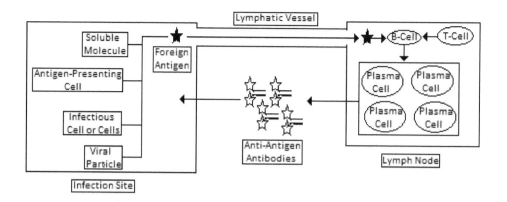

Antigen Presentation by Professional Phagocytes

If a foreign antigen has not been previously encountered by the immune system, the innate immune system can present the foreign antigen to the adaptive immune system by a sequence of events shown in the diagrams below.

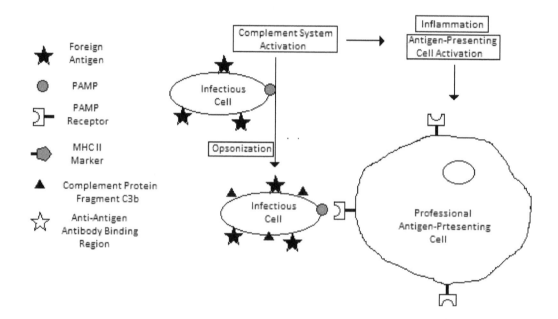

PAMP Activation of the Complement System

In the case where the foreign antigen is present in an extracellular infectious cell (such as a bacterial cell) PAMPs possessed by the infectious cell can directly trigger activation of the complement system. One of the effects of complement system activation in this manner is the creation of large numbers of complement protein fragments (primarily C3b fragments). These fragments can attach to the infectious agent's cell membrane (opsonization).

Pathogen Opsonization and PAMP-PRR Binding

Opsonization increases the ability of professional antigen-presenting cells (usually a macrophage) to phagocytize the infectious cell (pathogen). The infectious cell is recognized by the antigen-presenting cell by the PAMPs located on the cell. Pathogen recognition receptors (PPRs) such as Toll-like receptors on the antigen presenting cell bind to the PAMPs on the infectious cell and the infectious cell is subsequently engulfed and internalized by the antigen presenting cell (phagocytized).

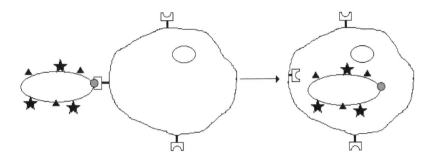

Phagocytosis and Digestion of Pathogens

The phagocytized infectious cell is initially confined within a membrane bound vesicle called a phagosome. The phagosome is subsequently fused with other membrane bound vesicles called lysosomes. The fusion of a phagosome and lysosomes creates a new membrane-bound vesicle known as a phagolysosome. Lysosomes contain proteolytic (protein cutting) and other digestive molecules that are able to digest the infectious agent within the phagolysosome. This digestion process creates small fragments of the infectious agent including fragments that can be presented as foreign antigens.

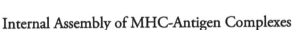

Internal Assembly of MHC-Antigen Complexes

Internal (cytosolic) MHC II markers are attached to theses foreign antigens to form an antigen-MHC complex. These complexes are then transported to the cell membrane and displayed on the outer surface of the cell membrane. In this form, the antigen can be presented to B-cell in lymph nodes. This presentation to B-cells initiates the processes where the adaptive immune system generates circulating antibodies directed against the foreign antigen. This antibody response is classified as the humoral adaptive immune system response.

Activation of the Cell-Mediated Immune Response

The cell-mediated response of the adaptive immune system can be initiated by the presentation of the foreign antigen by the antigen presenting cell. In this case the antigen is presented to a T-cell rather than to a B-cell. Often this occurs within lymph nodes, but it can also occur at or near the site of infection.

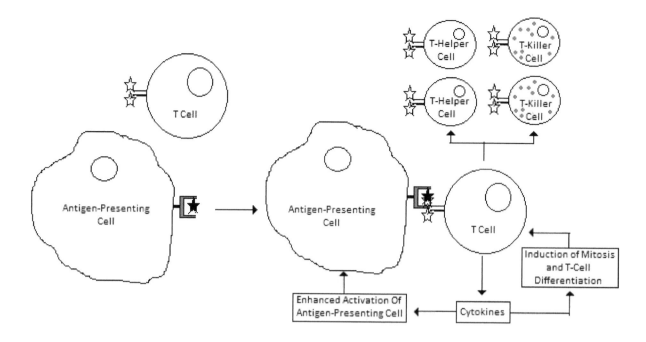

T-Cell Receptor Binding to the MHC-Antigen Complex

Since the antigen presented is a new antigen, No T-cell in the immune system has ever previously encountered the foreign antigen. Therefore, the T-cell that participates in antigen presentation is a novel T-cell. Since T-cell receptors (and B-cell receptors) have unique antigen binding site structures, the only T-cells that can be presented with the antigen are T-cells that have a unique antigen binding site on their T-cell receptors that can bind to the antigen. Only a few of the novel T-cells that encounter the antigen-presenting cell will have a complementary T-receptor to bind the antigen.

Cytokine Effects of T-Cell Activation

When a novel T-cell is able to bind to the complementary antigen, The T-cell is activated and releases several types of cytokines. These cytokines have an effect on the adjacent antigen-presenting cell (by definition, a paracrine effect) and also on the T-cell itself (by definition, an autocrine effect). The cytokine effects on the antigen -presenting cell include an enhancement of the cell to phagocytize, and digest other infectious cells.

More importantly are the effects of the cytokines on the novel T-cell. These effects trigger the novel T-cell to undergo several rounds of mitosis and to cause the daughter T-cells to differentiate into helper T-cells and killer (cytotoxic) T-cells. All of the daughter T-helper and T-killer cells will have T-cell receptors that are identical to the original novel T-cell, so all will be able to bind to the foreign antigen. This process rapidly generates a large number of T-cells that can participate in increasingly powerful immune responses against the infectious agent that possesses the foreign antigen.

Antibody Neutralization of Viral Particles

Antibodies that are generated against antigens possessed by a virus that is infecting the body can bind to viral particles that are present in extracellular locations. As the diagram below illustrates, the antibodies targeted against the viral antigen can coat viral particles and render the particles incapable of infecting other cells of the body (neutralization). These viral -antibody complexes can then be phagocytized by other immune cells and subsequently internally digested. Macrophages with membrane receptors for the Fc region of antibodies are particularly efficient at this type of clearance of virus-antibody complexes.

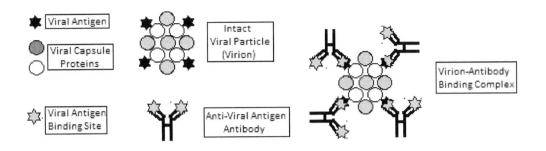

Antibody neutralization of viral particles is a specific example of the general category of antibody neutralization of harmful immunogenic agents. It is an essentially physical effect of the coating of these immunogenic agents by antibodies that disables the agent's capacity to cause injury to the body. One important category of such immunogenic agents is toxins and venoms - harmful molecules that are generated by infectious organisms (cholera toxin and botulinum toxin are examples), injected by noxious animals (wasps, bees, spiders, snakes etc.) and poisons produced by plants, fungi and other organisms that are absorbed through the skin or ingested.

Complement-Fixation Antibodies

After a foreign antigen possessed by an infectious cell has been recognized by the adaptive immune system, plasma cells release antibodies targeted against the antigen. When these antibodies encounter a cell that displays the antigen, the antibodies bind the antigen at the antibody hypervariable region. There are usually numerous locations on the cell that display the antigen. Consequently, the cell becomes coated (opsonized) by anti-antigen antibodies.

The class of antibodies that are directed against antigens associated with cellular infectious agents are predominantly complement-fixation antibodies (in contrast to neutralizing antibodies, which are targeted against viral particles and immunogenic molecules such as toxins).

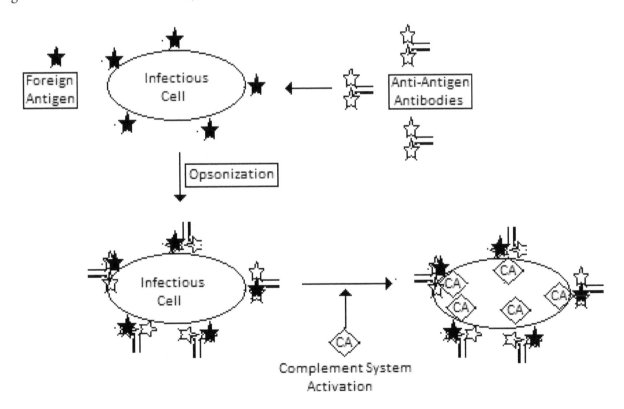

Fc-Region Antibody Receptor Cells

Once an infectious cell is opsonized by antibodies it becomes highly susceptible to attack by both innate and additional adaptive immune responses. Numerous types of immune cells have FC region antibody receptors on their cell membranes. When one of these cells encounters the antibody opsonized cell, the immune cell binds to the Fc region of an attached antibody via the immune cell's Fc receptor.

If the cell is a professional phagocy such as a macrophage, the Fc-receptor/antibody binding activates the immune cell to phagocitize the opsonized cell. If the immune cell displays additional types of antigens after digesting the cell, T-cells and B-cells can generate additional antibodies directed against any and all of the different antigens associated with the phagocytized cell. This can greatly increase the effectiveness of the immune response against any other infectious cells that possess these antigens.

Neutrophils have Fc receptors and can phagocytize antibody-opsonized cells, but they also have another cell-killing mechanism - the release of highly toxic granules that can directly kill attached opsonized cells. Neutrophils are not noted to present antigen to any significant extent. Natural Killer cells possess Fc receptors and can kill attached opsonized cell via the same mechanism that they kill infected cells of the body (perforin granzymes release and induction of cell death). The immune sequence of an immune cell binding to an antibody attached to a target antigen on infectious cell, followed by the killing of the infectious cell is defined as **antibody-dependent cell-mediated cytotoxicity.**

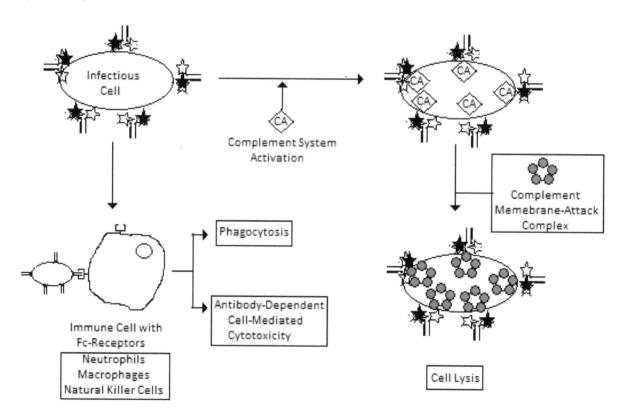

Complement Activation

As their name implies, complement-fixing antibodies attached to their complementary antigens on an infectious cell can efficiently activate the complement system. The anaphylactic, immune-cell activating and chemotactic effects of various complement proteins enhance the accumulation and activity of immune cells to the infection site. The formation of complement-protein membrane-attack complexes on the membrane of the infectious cell is also enhanced and contributes substantial independent cell-killing activity.

T-Killer Cell Cytotoxicity

It is important to note that T-cells can not bind antigens without simultaneously binding to a MHC class I or class II membrane markers. Additionally, T-cells do not have Fc antibody region receptors. For these two reasons T-killer cells have little or no capacity to attack extracellular immunogenic agents such as bacteria, viruses or multicellular parasites (since they do not possess MHC membrane markers). The primary targets of T-killer cells are cells of the body that are infected by viruses or other intracellular pathogens. The diagrams below illustrate the sequence of events that lead to the killing of infected cells of the body by T-killer cells.

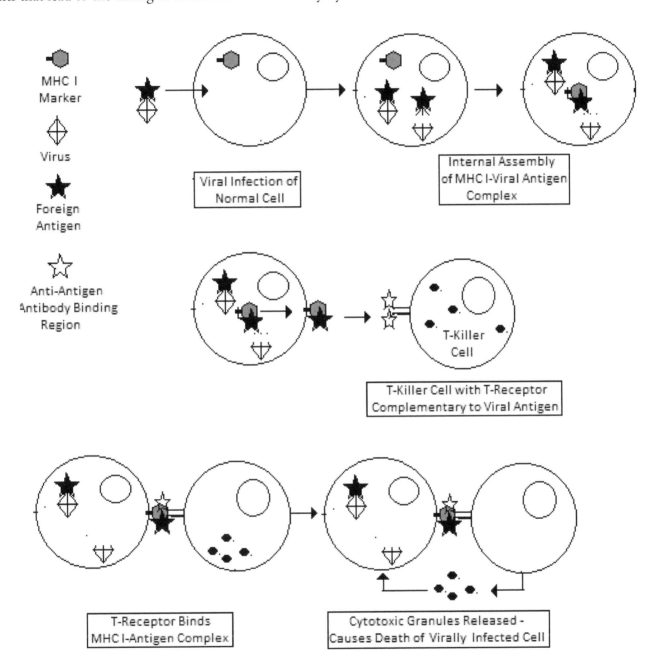

Notice that the T-killer immune response does not involve antibodies. It seems logical to define this type of immune response as non-antibody-dependent cell-mediated cytotoxicity. Such is not the case, however. This type of immune response is classified as **cell-mediated cytotoxicity**.

Adaptive Immunity

Perhaps the most important feature of the adaptive immune system is its capacity to retain a "memory" of nearly any foreign antigen that it has previously encountered. When novel B-cells and T-cells are activated by a first-time encounter with a foreign antigen, the immune sequences that follow includes the production of memory B and T-cells. These cells can respond immediately to a subsequent infection by agents that possess the antigen.

Of comparable importance is that the immune system continues to produce antibodies against the foreign antigen. These antibodies circulate throughout the body at low levels often for the lifetime of the previously exposed individual. These circulating antibodies frequently provide such a rapid response to reinfection by agents with the antigen that there that no apparent signs or symptoms of the reinfection occur. This is the definition of naturally acquired immunity to a particular infectious agent. This naturally occurring acquired immunity would be very beneficial to any species for this reason. In humans, it has an additional enormously important benefit. It is the basis for the ability of modern medicine to create and provide vaccines against many of the deadliest pathogens that historically have plagued human beings.

The Reproductive System

The male and female human reproductive systems are responsible for the generation of human offspring. The first stage of this process begins with the production of male and female gametes. Recall that gametes are the haploid (N) cells that result from meiotic cell division. In males, the gamete is a sperm cell and in females the gamete is a mature ovum.

The second stage of this process is fertilization, where male gametes are transported to the female reproductive system and a sperm cell fuses with an ovum to produce a diploid (2N) cell - a zygote. The zygote is a hybrid cell that contains one set of chromosomes 1 through 21 (the human autosomal chromosomes) and one sex chromosome (chromosome 22) either an X or a Y chromosome from the sperm cell and one set of chromosomes 1 through 21 and one X sex chromosome (chromosome 22) from the ovum. The resultant zygote has a full set of 21 pairs of autosomes and two sex chromosomes - either an X or a Y chromosome or two X chromosomes. Zygotes with an X and a Y chromosome develop into male human offspring and those with two X chromosomes develop into female offspring.

The zygote then begins the process of cell division and cell differentiation that eventually leads to the production of a mature human fetus that is capable of independent survival outside of the female reproductive system. At this stage, the fetus is born from the mother to the outside world through the process of labor and delivery.

The synthesis and secretion of the sex hormones - testosterone in the male and estrogen in the female also occurs in the gonads of the reproductive system.

The Male Reproductive System

The male reproductive system consists of the external male genitalia - the penis, the scrotum and the testis, and the internal male genitalia - The distal segment of the urethra, the seminal vesicles, and the prostate gland, bulbourethral glands and the Cowper's gland. The penis consists of a central canal - the urethra - which also serves as the passageway for the delivery of urine from the bladder to the exterior of the body, and the distensible surrounding erectile tissue - the **corpus cavernosum**. The distal end of the penis forms the head or **glans** of the penis which contains the external opening of the urethra - the **meatus** and surrounding tissue called the foreskin.

The scrotum is an external anatomical pouch or sack consisting of skin and smooth muscle. The scrotum is divided into two chambers. Each chamber contains a single **testis** along with the associated structures of the testis - the **epididymis** and the **ductus deferens**. The scrotum allows the testis to experience a slightly lower temperature environment than internal body temperature. This is necessary to allow the proper functioning of spermatogenesis (sperm production) that occurs within the testis.

The testes are ovoid-shaped organs that are responsible for the first stages of the production of sperm cells. The testes are enclosed by a tough outer membrane - the **tunica albuginea**. The interior of the testis consists of a collection of thin coiled tubules called the **seminiferous tubules**. The cells lining the interior of the seminiferous tubules include specialized epithelial cells called **Sertoli cells** and **germ cells** that are capable of undergoing cell division and differentiation to produce sperm cells (spermatozoa).

The seminiferous tubules connect proximally to the **rete testis** - a short stalk of common connecting tubules where developing sperm cells are concentrated before they proceed to **efferent ducts** and into the epididymis. The epididymis is a highly convoluted tubule that forms a mass at the superior surface of the testis. Developing sperm cells are retained within the epididymis for 2-3 months. During this time, the developing sperm cell reach maturity.

The distal end of the epididymis is continuous with the **vas deferens**. The vas deferens are short -length segments of tubules that connect the epididymis to the **ejaculatory ducts** located in the interior of the pelvic cavity. The ejaculatory ducts connect to the **urethra** and also have connections with ducts of the **prostate gland, the bulbourethral glands and Cowper's glands**. These glands provide contributions to the seminal fluid that serves as the fluid medium that nourishes and supports the transportation of sperm cells during ejaculation.

Testosterone Production

A primary function of the male gonads - the testis - is the production of the male sex hormone testosterone. Testosterone is a steroid hormone whose synthesis and secretion is regulated by the **hypothalamus** through the release of gonadotrophin releasing hormone (**GnRh**) which regulates the synthesis and release of luteinizing hormone (**LH**) and follicle-stimulating hormone (**FSH**) by the **anterior pituitary**.

Both FSH and LH stimulate the testes to synthesize and release testosterone. **Luteinizing hormone directly stimulates the production of testosterone**. Testosterone production occurs in **Leydig cells**. Leydig cells interstitial cells (located in loose connective tissue) that are located alongside the seminiferous tubules of the testis. Testosterone produced by the Leydig cells stimulates the sexual maturation of prepubescent males and during puberty stimulate the development of **male secondary sexual characteristics**. Secondary male sexual characteristics include the development of pubic and facial hair, an increase in muscle and bone mass, a deepening of the voice and the maturation of the gonads and external male genitalia. After puberty, **testosterone plays critical roles in the maturation of sperm cells.**

Spermatogenesis

The production of mature sperm cells begins with male diploid germ cells called **spermatogonia**. Spermatogonia cells are located on the basement membrane of seminiferous tubules. Spermatogonia are surrounded by specialized epithelial cells called **Sertoli cells**. As sperm cell development proceeds from spermatogonia, the developing sperm cells move upward through the Sertoli cells. During this process, the Sertoli cells provide critical functions that support the development of the sperm cells. **The functions of sertoli cells are under the direct influence of the hormone FSH.**

Spermatogonia mitotically divide to form daughter cells called **primary spermatocytes**. These primary spermatocytes undergo meiotic division to produce **haploid gamete cells called spermatids**. Under the influence of testosterone, spermatids begin to mature into spermatozoa. As this maturation process continues, the developing spermatozoa move upward through their surrounding Sertoli cells and are released into the lumen of the seminiferous tubules. The spermatozoa are then transported by peristaltic action to the lumens of the tubules of the epididymis where they undergo final maturation and attain the ability of independent locomotion via a flagellum or tail located on each spermatozoa.

The Female Reproductive System

The female reproductive system consists of the external and internal female genitalia. The functions of the female reproductive system are the production of female gametes the support of the fertilization of the fusion of female and male gametes to create a human zygote, and the physical support, protection and nourishment of the development of the zygote to a mature human fetus and the subsequent delivery of the fetus to the outside world. The gonads of the female reproductive system are also responsible for the synthesis and release of the female sex hormone estrogen.

The External Female Genitalia

The external female genitalia as a group are called the **vulva**. The vulva consists of the **mons pubis** which is a mound of fatty tissue overlying the pubic bone that forms the anterior segment of the vulva. The mons pubis consists of the **labia majora.** The labia majora are outer folds or lips that are divided into right and left labia by the **pudendal cleft.** The two folds of the labia majora are lateral to the underlying labia minora, clitoris, vaginal introitus (external opening), urethral meatus, the greater and lesser vestibular glands (Bartholin's glands and Skene's glands) and the vulvar vestibule.

The **labia minora** are similar in structure to the labia majora and are laterally located adjacent to and inferomedial to the labia majora and adjacent and lateral to the central regions of the vulva. The central vulvar regions include the midline superiorly located **clitoris** and the centrally located **vulvar vestibule.** The **urethral meatus** and the **vaginal introitus or orifice** is located in the midline of the vulvar vestibule. The urethral meatus is located immediately superior to the vaginal orifice. The **greater vestibular glands** or **Bartholin's glands** and the **lesser vestibular glands** or **Skene's glands** are located lateral to the vaginal orifice. The Bartholin's glands secrete mucous which provides lubrication of the vagina and the surrounding vestibular regions.

The Female Internal Reproductive System

The female internal reproductive system consists of four major components, the vagina, uterus, fallopian tubes and the ovaries. In contrast to the male reproductive system, the female urethra does not communicate with any female reproductive structures and has no role in the female reproductive system.

The Vagina

The vagina is an anatomical tube consisting of muscular and fibrous tissue. The lumen of the vagina begins at the vaginal orifice and extends internally to the pelvic cavity where it terminates at the cervix of the uterus. The cervix is the inferior portion of the uterus and protrudes into the lumen of the vagina. The walls of the vagina encircle the cervix and the interior lining of the vaginal lumen is continuous with the external surfaces of the cervix.

The Uterus

The functions of the uterus are to serve as a site for the **implantation of a developing embryo** and to provide a continuous supportive, nurturing and protective environment for the continued development of the embryo into a viable human fetus. When the fetus is sufficiently developed to survive outside of the uterus, the uterus undergoes a series of muscular contractions that expel the fetus from the internal uterine cavity through the cervical canal and into the lumen of the vagina.

The uterus is a pear-shaped muscular organ located in the pelvic cavity in a position immediately adjacent and dorsal to the urinary bladder and immediately adjacent and ventral to the rectum. The four major anatomical regions of the uterus are the **cervix** or neck of the uterus, the internal os, the **corpus or body** of the uterus and the **fundus** or superior region of the uterus. The cervix or neck of the uterus is the conically shaped inferior segment of the uterus that extends into the vagina forming the cap to the internal end of the vagina. In the central region of the cervix is a passageway that is continuous with the lumen of the vagina and extends into the central cavity of the uterus.

The walls of the uterus consist of three layers. The innermost layer, which includes the internal surface of the central uterine cavity, is the **endometrium.** The endometrium includes an innermost epithelial layer which in turn consists of a **basal layer** and an overlying **functional layer.** The functional layer includes the surface layer cells that are exposed as the lining of the central uterine cavity. The functional layer consists of epithelial cells, mucous glands and blood vessels that are responsive to a number of hormones.

The functional layer undergoes an approximately once-per-month cycle of growth, degeneration and regeneration (menstrual cycle) that occurs in response to the variations in the levels of hormones that regulate the menstrual cycle. The middle layer of the uterus is called the **myometrium**. The myometrium is composed of several thick layers of smooth muscle tissue. The outermost encapsulating layer of the uterus - the **parametrium** - consists of a continuation of the peritoneum, the epithelial surface layer of the abdominal cavity. The Uterus is structurally supported in its position within the pelvic cavity by the three pairs of suspensory ligaments the **uterosacral, cardinal and round ligaments.**

The Fallopian Tubes

The fallopian tubes are a pair of structures that extend from superior-lateral positions on the uterus, one on the left and one on the right - medial to a position directly opposite of the respective left or the right ovary. The fallopian tubes contain a central lumen that is lined with ciliated epithelium. One end of the lumen is continuous with the central cavity of the uterus and the other end is open to the pelvic cavity and faces the respective ovary. There is a short gap between the ovary and the lateral opening of the lumen of the fallopian tube. During ovulation -when a mature follicle within the ovary ruptures and releases a mature ovum (female gamete) - the ovum is drawn into the fallopian tube by local peritoneal fluid currents generated by the motion of cilia within the fallopian tube. Once inside the tube, the ovum is carried by the same ciliary motions into the central cavity of the uterus. Fertilization of the ovum by a sperm cell (which sometimes occurs within the fallopian tubes) triggers a set of reactions that allow the developing embryo to implant within the wall of the endometrium of the uterus.

The Ovaries

The ovaries are the female gonads. Ovaries are 3-to-4 cm in size and ovoid shaped. There are two ovaries in females, one located in the pelvic cavity on either the left or right side just medial to distal end of the respective left or right fallopian tube. The ovaries are connected to the uterus by a ligament - the **ovarian ligament** and to the peritoneal wall of the pelvis by another ligament - the **suspensory ligament.**

In addition to their role as the primary **estrogen producing glands** the ovaries also are the organs that contain all of a female's germ cells that will eventually mature and be released by the ovaries during ovulatory cycles. All of these progenitor germ cells are present at birth in a human female's ovaries.

The general structure of an ovary includes an outer region called the **cortex** and an inner region called the **medulla**. The medulla of the ovary contains loose connective tissue that surrounds the blood vessels that provide the blood supply for the ovary.

The Ovarian Cortex

The ovarian cortex is composed of dense connective tissue including fibroblast cells that can change functionally in response to various hormone levels. The cortex also has an outer layer of cuboidal epithelial cells called the germinal layer. As female germ cells mature into functional gametes (eggs) they acquire an organized collection of cells called **granulosa cells**. The granulosa cell mass and the embedded germ cell together are called an **ovarian follicle**. The ovarian follicles at all stages of development are located in the ovarian cortex.

Oogenesis

The process of producing human female gametes is called oogenesis. The process begins during fetal development with female **primordial germ cells**. These cells appear in the fetal ovaries. Primordial germ cells then differentiate into **oogonia**. Oogonia are diploid germ cells that undergo further mitotic divisions and differentiation into **primary oocytes**. Primary oocytes then enter meiotic division and progress to the prophase 1 stage of meiosis.

Primary Follicles and Maturation Arrest

Prior to the onset of puberty, all primary oocytes remain in the **prophase 1 stage of meiosis**. This is called maturation arrest. These primary oocytes acquire a collection of granulosa cells and together they comprise a primary ovarian follicle. No primary oocytes within a female's ovaries will proceed to subsequent phases of meiosis until the female reaches puberty. At puberty, the cyclic processes of ovarian follicular development and the menstrual cycle of the uterine endometrial tissue begins. The onset of this process at puberty is called **menarche**.

Hormonal Regulation During the Menstrual Cycle

With the onset of puberty, the **hypothalamus** begins to release **GnRH** in a controlled fashion that varies throughout the menstrual cycle. For the first half of the cycle GnRh is released in increasing amounts. This triggers the **anterior pituitary** to release **FSH** and **LH** also in increasing amounts. FSH stimulates the ovaries to begin the next stage of oogenesis. Some of the primary follicles randomly begin to mature into **secondary follicles**.

During this process, the primary oocytes of the developing secondary follicle emerge from maturation arrest and proceed from the prophase 1 stage of meiosis and complete the first round of meiosis. This results in the production of a haploid (N) daughter cell called a **secondary oocyte**. The other daughter cell of this first round of mitosis degenerates into a structure called a **polar body**.

Ovulation and the FSH and LH Peaks

As this process is occurring the ovaries are also producing increasing amounts of estrogen. This increasing estrogen level reaches a critical level at about day 15 of the menstrual cycle. The critical estrogen level feeds back to the hypothalamus and the pituitary resulting in a rapid spike in FSH and LH levels. In response, one of the developing secondary follicles randomly becomes dominant and further matures. The LH spike stimulates this dominant secondary follicle to rupture at the surface of the ovary. This event is called ovulation. The secondary oocyte of the ruptured follicle escapes and is drawn into the lumen of the fallopian tube.

Progesterone and the Corpus Luteum

At this time, the secondary follicle undergoes a **second round of meiosis** resulting in daughter cell that is a mature female gamete called an **ovum**. The ovum is now capable of being fertilized by a sperm cell. The second daughter cell of the meiotic division degenerates into a polar body. The remaining cells of the ruptured secondary follicle reorganize into a structure called the **corpus luteum** which remains in the cortex of the ovary. The corpus luteum begins to produce the steroid

hormone **progesterone** which stimulates the endometrium of the uterus to continue to thicken in anticipation of the potential implantation of a fertilized ovum. If implantation occurs the corpus luteum will persist and continue to produce progesterone to maintain the endometrium. If implantation does not occur, the corpus luteum degenerates, progesterone levels fall and the blood vessels of the endometrium degenerate. The endometrial tissue then sloughs off and is expelled from the uterus during menstruation.

Abnormalities of the Reproductive System

During gestation developing human fetus undergoes differentiation of the reproductive system. This differentiation results in female genitalia under the influence of the hormone estrogen. If high levels of testosterone are present during genitalia development, the genitalia develop into male genitalia. When a female fetus is exposed to abnormally high levels of testosterone or when a male fetus experiences abnormally low levels of testosterone the result is **ambiguous external genitalia** - highly underdeveloped male genitalia in genetic males and external genitalia resembling a male in genetic females. The genetic males do not have internal female reproductive organs - ovaries and uterus, and the females do not have male gonads, prostate glands or other functional internal male reproductive structures. Most commonly ambiguous genitalia result from genetic conditions associated with dysfunctional enzymes in the biochemical synthetic pathway of steroid hormone precursors in the adrenal cortex. Most frequently this is a **21-hydroxylase enzyme deficiency** resulting in **congenital adrenal hyperplasia**.

In males, **failure of the testes to descend** from the abdominal cavity into the scrotum requires surgical correction to preserve fertility and to reduce the risk of testicular cancer which is very high in undescended testicles. **Prostate cancer** is a very common cancer in males, particularly after the age of 50.

Females often suffer from abnormalities of ovarian function - usually related to endocrine disorders. These conditions often cause irregular menstrual cycles, heavy menstrual bleeding and low fertility rates. **Polycystic ovarian disease** is a common abnormality of this type and often includes symptoms of excessive testosterone levels - a deepening of the voice and hirsutism - male pattern hair distribution. Benign smooth muscle tumors of the myometrium of the uterus are also common. These tumors are called **fibroids** and can become quite large. Occasionally the tumors cause excessive menstrual bleeding and can interfere with fertility. In these cases, surgical removal may correct the conditions.

Endometriosis and Ectopic Pregnancy

Another common abnormality in females is **endometriosis**. This condition occurs when **endometrial cells** within the uterus escape - presumably through the fallopian tubes - and implant on tissue surfaces throughout the abdomen. This tissue responds to hormones in the same manner as endometrial tissue in the uterus during menstrual cycles. During the proliferative phase of the menstrual cycle the endometrial tissue implanted outside of the uterus - called ectopic tissue - can enlarge and invade local abdominal tissue and cause severe pain.

In a similar fashion, a fertilized ovum may also escape into the abdominal cavity and can implant and begin to develop just as a fertilized ovum develops in a normal implantation site within the uterine cavity. This condition is called an ectopic pregnancy. Ectopic pregnancies are very dangerous and can cause death due to internal hemorrhaging if not detected and treated in a timely manner.

Infectious Diseases

Viral, bacterial, fungal and parasitic infections of the external genitalia internal reproductive systems are extremely common and run the gamut in levels of severity from the uncomfortable and unsightly to fatal without proper treatments. Some of these conditions are the result of hormonal abnormalities or poor hygiene but most are the result of sexual transmission. The most serious of the sexually transmitted diseases progress to generalized infections of the body.

Mild to Moderately Severe Sexually-Transmitted Diseases

Vaginal yeast infections caused by the fungal species **Candida albicans** occur commonly in most females and causes itching and superficial tissue damage but is otherwise harmless and easily treated with topical antifungal medications. The **pubic or crab louse** - *Pthirus pubis*, also pubic louse) is an insect that lives on human pubic hair. Infestation causes intense itching but is otherwise not harmful and is treated with topical antiparasitic medications. **Bacterial Urinary tract infections (UTIs)** are very common in healthy females and originate from bacterial in the anogenital regions that migrate through the urethra to the urinary bladder. UTIs cause severe discomfort and require oral antibiotic treatment. Vaginal yeast infections and UTIs are not considered to be sexually transmissible diseases.

Granuloma inguinale is a sexually transmitted bacterial disease caused by *Klebsiella granulomatis* that causes of disfiguring external genital ulcerations. **Genital warts** are a relatively benign sexually transmitted condition caused by certain strains of the **human papilloma virus (HPV)**. Genital warts are cosmetically unsightly but do not cause significant illness. Sexually transmitted Infection of the cervix by other strains of the human papilloma virus are associated with high incidences of **cervical cancer**. The majority of infections by these dangerous strains of HPV can be prevented by immunization with the vaccine **Gardasil**.

Trichomoniasis is a sexually transmitted infectious disease caused by the parasite *Trichomonas vaginalis*. There are no symptoms in 70% of cases. When symptoms do occur they include genital itching, and burning with urination. The condition is treated with oral antibiotics. Complications of trichomonas infections include an increased risk of **infection and transmission of the HIV** virus and increased risk of **premature birth and low infant weight**.

Chlamydia is a very common sexually transmitted disease caused by the bacteria *Chlamydia trachomatis*. The disease of goes unnoticed or may have symptoms of itching. It is treated with antibiotics. Untreated and or repeated infection greatly **increases the risk of pelvic inflammatory (PID)** disease in women. Pelvic inflammatory disease affects the uterus fallopian tubes and ovaries. The consequence of the disease is scarring of the reproductive organs which often results in **infertility** and increased risk for **ectopic pregnancy**.

Genital herpes is a sexually transmitted viral disease caused by the **herpes simplex type 2 virus**. The infection persists for life and causes periodic outbreaks of painful genital ulcers. Active herpes infection in mothers can infect infants during delivery. This can cause eye infections resulting in **blindness.**

Severe Sexually Transmitted Diseases

The most severe sexually transmitted infections are the bacterial and spirochete infections **gonorrhea** and **syphilis**, the viral diseases **hepatitis B and C** and most severe - **acquired immunodeficiency disease (AIDS)** caused by the **human immunodeficiency virus (HIV).**

Gonorrhea is caused by the bacteria *Neisseria gonorrhoeae*. If untreated the disease often results in both male and female infertility and can also cause arthritis, meningitis and damage the valves of the heart. Gonorrhea infections also greatly increase the risk of pelvic inflammatory disease. Syphilis is caused by the spirochete *Treponema pallidum*. If untreated, syphilis infections can progress to secondary and tertiary forms of the disease. The tertiary form - **neurosyphilis,** causes dementia and eventually death. Both gonorrhea and syphilis are treated with antibiotics.

The hepatitis B and C viruses cause severe liver disease including rapid **liver failure** and long-term liver failure. Both diseases greatly increase the risk for **liver cancer** - hepatitis C in particular. Hepatitis C can now be cured if treated early through the use of newly approved antiviral drug therapy. HIV infection is **universally fatal** if untreated but can be managed through lifelong treatment consisting of multi-antiviral drug therapy.

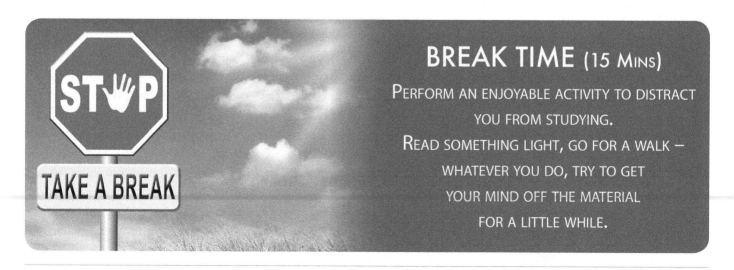

STOP — TAKE A BREAK

BREAK TIME (15 Mins)
PERFORM AN ENJOYABLE ACTIVITY TO DISTRACT YOU FROM STUDYING.
READ SOMETHING LIGHT, GO FOR A WALK — WHATEVER YOU DO, TRY TO GET YOUR MIND OFF THE MATERIAL FOR A LITTLE WHILE.

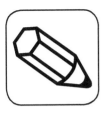

VOCABULARY

YOU COMPLETED A CROSSWORD PUZZLE FOR THE VOCABULARY CHAPTER IN MODULE 3. LET'S TRY ANOTHER ONE. BELOW IS A CROSSWORD PUZZLE TO HELP YOU LEARN SOME ADDITIONAL WORDS AND EXPAND YOUR VOCABULARY.

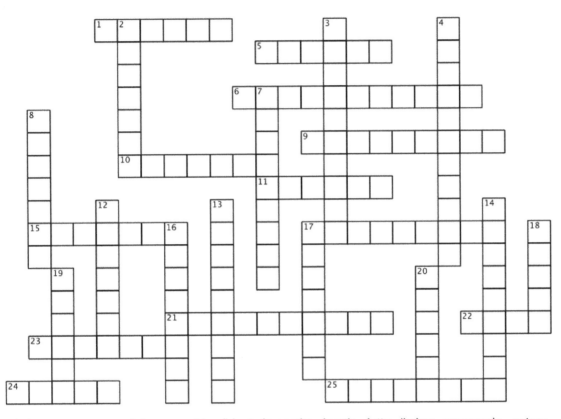

accost boggy canvass defy eccentric fidget hypocrite inertia jetty limber menagerie notary obliterate prestige reluctant spontaneous turmoil vestibule abdicate belligerent corrugated dilemma profane sublime thrift vagrant

Across

1. aggressively approach and speak to someone
5. flexible or supple
6. hostile and aggressive
9. unwilling or hesitant
10. moral or spiritual
11. a person authorized to perform legal formalities, usually relating to contracts or other documents
15. the mechanics principle where an object will remain in motion or at rest unless acted on by another force
17. a space adjacent to a main room or area
21. when a material is molded into a network of ridges and grooves
22. resist or refuse to obey
23. a difficult choice
24. a small pier at which boats can dock
25. deep respect and admiration

Down

2. to survey someone about his/her opinion
3. completely destroy
4. suddenly or instantly
7. somewhat strange or uncoventional
8. a great disturbance or uncertainty
12. irreverent or disrespectful
13. someone who claims to have certain principles or beliefs, but does not act in the same manner
14. a strange collection of items
16. to renounce or fail to carry out
17. a person without a settled home
18. very wet and muddy
19. a characteristic of being wise with money
20. wiggle or squirm about

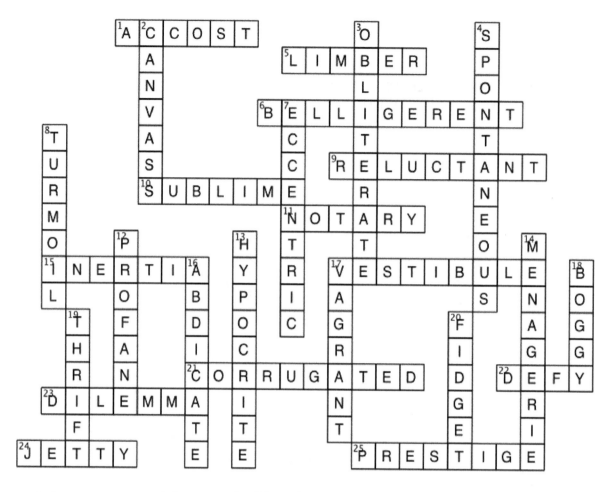

accost boggy canvass defy eccentric fidget hypocrite inertia jetty limber menagerie notary obliterate prestige reluctant spontaneous turmoil vestibule abdicate belligerent corrugated dilemma profane sublime thrift vagrant

Across

1. aggressively approach and speak to someone [ACCOST]
5. flexible or supple [LIMBER]
6. hostile and aggressive [BELLIGERENT]
9. unwilling or hesitant [RELUCTANT]
10. moral or spiritual [SUBLIME]
11. a person authorized to perform legal formalities, usually relating to contracts or other documents [NOTARY]
15. the mechanics principle where an object will remain in motion or at rest unless acted on by another force [INERTIA]
17. a space adjacent to a main room or area [VESTIBULE]
21. when a material is molded into a network of ridges and grooves [CORRUGATED]
22. resist or refuse to obey [DEFY]

Down

2. to survey someone about his/her opinion [CANVASS]
3. completely destroy [OBLITERATE]
4. suddenly or instantly [SPONTANEOUS]
7. somewhat strange or uncoventional [ECCENTRIC]
8. a great disturbance or uncertainty [TURMOIL]
12. irreverent or disrespectful [PROFANE]
13. someone who claims to have certain principles or beliefs, but does not act in the same manner [HYPOCRITE]
14. a strange collection of items [MENAGERIE]
16. to renounce or fail to carry out [ABDICATE]
17. a person without a settled home [VAGRANT]
18. very wet and muddy [BOGGY]
19. a characteristic of being wise with money [THRIFT]

CRITICAL READING

VOCABULARY-IN-CONTEXT

Vocabulary-in-Context questions ask you for the definition of a word as it is used within the context of the passage. The format of these questions is similar to that of Word Knowledge questions. You will be given a word and asked to select the closest meaning from a list of four choices. The difference, though, is that where Word Knowledge questions test straightforward vocabulary, the words chosen for Vocabulary-in-context questions are often words that can have more than one meaning. You will need to use context clues from the passage in order to figure out which meaning is correct.

It's also important to note that many questions on the exam will not always ask you to simply determine the meaning of a vocabulary word. Many times, instead of asking you for a synonym or definition of a vocabulary word, the question will ask you what the vocabulary word "most nearly means". For these types of questions, you'll need to use context clues and your

existing vocabulary knowledge to determine which answer choice has a meaning that is closest to that of the vocabulary word.

To answer these questions, reread the sentence from the passage that the word is taken from. Come up with a prediction—your own definition or synonym of what the word means as used in that sentence. Then, look at the answer choices and choose the one that best matches your prediction. If you do not see your prediction among the answer choices, read each of the answer choices as part of the sentence, replacing the original word, and choose the one that makes the most sense.

Let's look at some examples.

Some of the questions you'll encounter will ask you to fill in the blank in a sentence. For the questions below, select the word that fits best in the sentence.

1. The bolt was _____. It took a lot of effort to loosen the fastener.

A. Rusted
B. Shiny
C. Loose
D. Strong

Answer: A.

Using the context clues in the sentence, you can assume that the missing word is somehow related to the phrase "loosen the fastener". Something about the bolt made it difficult to remove. You can immediately eliminate "shiny" since it is not related to the action of removing a fastener. Likewise, "loose" is not correct because if the bolt were loose, it wouldn't be difficult to remove it. "Strong" could possibly fit if there wasn't a better answer choice, but it's not typically used to describe how difficult a fastener is to remove. The word that best fits in the sentence is "rusted" because rust directly increases the difficulty of removing a fastener.

2. As the commanding officer's eyes widened and his face turned red, he proceeded to _____ the lance corporal.

    A. Tease
    B. Scold
    C. Compliment
    D. Correct

Answer: B.

Using the context clues in the sentence, you can assume that the missing word is somehow linked to widened eyes and a red face, which are associated with anger. You can immediately eliminate "tease" and "compliment" since those words connote lightheartedness and sincerity, not exactly similar to the demeanor described in the sentence. "Correct" could possibly fit if there wasn't a better answer choice, but it's not necessarily associated with widened eyes and a red face. The word that best fits in the sentence is "scold" because scolding connotes anger or irritation, which correlate with widened eyes and a red face.

Sure, those were fairly easy, but those are just one type of vocabulary-in-context questions you'll probably encounter on the exam. For the questions below,

select the word that MOST NEARLY means the same as the underlined word.

1. The chairman of the board abandoned his position after a damaging scandal.

A. Squandered
B. Resigned
C. Ignored
D. Neglected

Answer: B.

All the answer choices connote negative characteristics of the position of chairman of the board, but only "resigned" most closely matches the underlined word. "Squandered" suggests a wasted opportunity. "Ignored" means deliberately taking no notice of. "Neglected" signifies a failure to pay attention to. "Resigned" indicates voluntarily leaving a job, which MOST nearly means the same as "abandoned", leaving permanently.

2. Sarah considered herself a parsimonious shopper. She loved finding great shopping deals.
A. Cheap
B. Frugal
C. Economical
D. Thrifty

Answer: A.

All the answer choices reflect the general meaning of "parsimonious", being careful with money, but only one choice has a negative association. "Frugal", "economical" and "thrifty" are all adjectives with a positive connotation, but "cheap" is usually used as a negative description.

Those were a bit more difficult, but let's try a few more. For the questions below, select the word that LEAST LIKELY means the same as the underlined word.

1. The evidence of the murder was destroyed before the trial.

A. Devastated

B. Obliterated
C. Ruined
D. Incinerated

Answer: D.
While all the answer choices can be used in place of "destroyed", "incinerated" suggests a specific type of damage: destruction by fire. Technically, "incinerated" is a logical answer, but the question isn't asking which choice is not logical. It's asking which choice LEAST likely means the underlined word. This was a tough one, but you should expect to see some questions like this on the exam.

2. While trying to negotiate a peace treaty, one side was being entirely <u>hostile</u> to the other.

A. Belligerent
B. Threatening
C. Averse
D. Combative

Answer: C.

While all the choices are mostly synonyms of "hostile", only one choice excludes a violent implication in its definition. "Averse" means strongly opposed to, but "belligerent", "threatening" and "combative" all suggest harm or death, as does "hostile".

Sometimes, you will need to read a passage before answering the questions. Let's look at some examples of those questions.

"American elections consist of citizens voting for their government representatives. Today, this includes members of the U.S. Senate, but this was not always the case. When the United States Constitution was first written, the people did not get to elect their senators directly. Instead, the senators were appointed by state legislators (who are elected

directly by the people in their respective states). This changed in 1913, however, with the 17th Amendment to the Constitution. This amendment allows for the direct election of U.S. Senators by the citizenry. While this election process can make the senators more accountable to their constituents, since the citizens will decide whether a senator will keep his or her job at the next election, it diminishes the voice that state legislatures have in the federal government."

1. The word <u>constituents</u> in the passage most nearly means:

A. Elements
B. Employees
C. Senators
D. Voters

Answer: D.

By reading the choices back into the sentence, you can see that the best synonym for "constituents" is "voters". It is the voters who decide whether or not to reelect the senators. The word "constituents" on its own can have several meanings, including voters, elements, members, components and parts. In the context of this passage, however, "voters" is the best definition.

2. The word <u>amendment</u> in the passage most nearly means:

A. Rule
B. Principle
C. Alteration
D. Truth

Answer: C.

By reading the choices back into the sentence, you can see that the best synonym for "amendment" is "alteration". The passage states how the Constitution originally provided for senator selection. However, the passage explains the difference in process after the 17th amendment. Because "alteration" means "change", it is the best choice.

ARITHMETIC REASONING

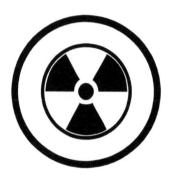

SCIENTIFIC NOTATION

Scientific notation was originally developed as a simplified way for scientists to express extremely large or small numbers. In mathematics, scientific notation is used to easily compare large and small numbers. Let's take a look at how to translate a real number to its scientific notation equivalent.

Converting standard numbers to scientific notation is performed without calculation, although counting place values is still essential. For example:

The number 2,345,000 is equal to 2.345 * 1,000,000. By writing the value of 1,000,000 as 106 (10 multiplied by itself 6 times), the formulation of the scientific notation equivalent of the original number is completed: 2.345 * 106.

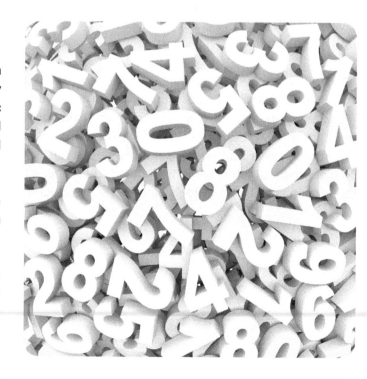

Similarly, small decimal numbers can be written using scientific notation as well. For example:

The number 0.00736 is equal to 7.36 * 0.001. By writing the value of 0.001 as 10^{-3} (1 divided by 10, three times), the formulation of the scientific notation equivalent of the original number is completed: $7.36 * 10^{-3}$.

Instead dividing (or multiplying) by 10, the translation to scientific notation can also be simplified by counting the number of places that the decimal point is transferred in the conversion process. In the first example above, when the scientific notation was written, it began with writing 2.345. This number was formulated by moving the decimal point six places to the left in the original number. Therefore, the exponent of 10 was 6 (10^6).

Similarly, in the second example, the decimal part of the scientific notation number, 7.36, was written by moving the decimal point three places to the right. Therefore, the exponent of 10 was -3 (10^{-3}).

Using this method, no calculation is required. The included benefit is that the "significance" of numbers is easily determined. Answering the question of the number of significant figures for the two examples is a simple matter when using scientific notation. The number of digits in the decimal part of the scientific notation is always the number of significant figures. 2,345,000 has four significant figures. 0.00736 has three. The zeros in these numbers are often referred to as "place holders" when converting to scientific notation.

Notice that the exponent is NOT determined by counting zeros, but by counting the number of decimal places that are moved when formulating the scientific notation. The decimal part in scientific notation always has only one digit to the left of the decimal point.

MATHEMATICS KNOWLEDGE

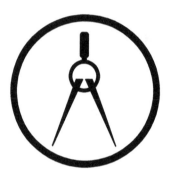

GEOMETRY

To tackle geometry questions on a mathematical reasoning test, there are a few formulas and rules that you need to know. This section takes you through those basic rules. It covers intersecting lines, triangles, squares and rectangles, and circles.

BASIC VOCABULARY

Vocabulary that is important to know for geometry questions includes the following:

LINE – A line is a set of all points between two endpoints. Lines have no area or width, only length.

ANGLE – An angle is the corner formed by two intersecting line segments, and it is measured in

degrees. Degrees measurements show the magnitude of the "sweep" of the angle. In the figure below, angle x is shown as the measure between the two line segments.

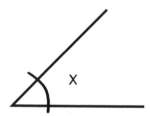

360° describes the angle measurement all the way around a full circle. Half of that, 180°, is the angle measurement across a straight line. Two lines at right angles to each other, called perpendicular lines, have an angle measurement of 90°.

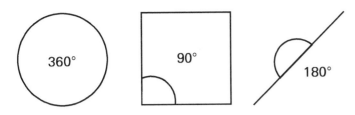

AREA – The area is the measure of space inside a two-dimensional figure. It has units of length * length, or length². For example, rooms are described as being a number of square feet. Counties are described as being so many square miles. Each basic shape has a special formula for determining area.

PERIMETER – The perimeter is the measure of the length around the outside of a figure.

VOLUME – For three-dimensional figures, the volume is the measure of space inside the figure. Volume has three dimensions: length * width * height. Because of this, it has units of length³ (cubic length). For example, you may have heard "cubic feet" used to describe the volume of something like a storage unit. This formula applies only to square and rectangular three-dimensional shapes. Other figures have their own formulas for determining volume.

INTERSECTING LINES

There are two important properties to know about pairs of intersecting lines:
1. They form angles that add up to 180° along the sides of each line.

2. They create two pairs of equal angles.

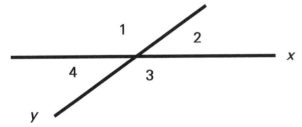

For example, in the diagram above, line x intersects line y, forming the four angles 1, 2, 3 and 4. Any two angles along one side of a line will add up to 180°:

Angle 1 + Angle 2 = 180°
Angle 2 + Angle 3 = 180°
Angle 3 + Angle 4 = 180°
Angle 4 + Angle 1 = 180°

All four of the angles added together would equal 360°:

Angle 1 + Angle 2 + Angle 3 + Angle 4 = 360°

The two angles DIAGONAL from each other must be equal. For the figure above, we know that:

Angle 1 = Angle 3
Angle 2 = Angle 4

This property is very useful: if you are given any one of the angles, you can immediately solve for the other three. If you are told that Angle 1 = 120°, then you know that Angle 2 = 180° - 120° = 60°. Since Angle 3 = Angle 1 and Angle 4 = Angle 2, you now know all four angles.

PARALLEL/PERPENDICULAR LINES

Parallel lines are lines that lie on the same 2-D plane (i.e., the page) and never intersect each other. The thing to remember about parallel lines is that if a line intersects two parallel lines, it will form a bunch of corresponding angles (like the ones discussed above). Also, you can never assume that two lines are parallel just from a diagram. You need to be told or given enough information that you can deduce it. Parallel lines have the same slope.

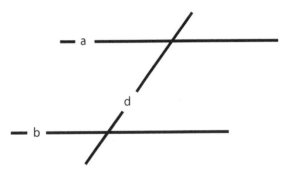

Lines a and b are parallel and are intersected by line d.

In the diagram above, all four of the acute angles (the ones smaller than 90°) are equal to each other. All four of the obtuse angles (the ones greater than 90°) are equal to each other. Why? Because a line intersecting parallel lines forms equivalent angles. This is simply an expanded case of the intersecting lines concept discussed earlier.

SQUARES AND RECTANGLES

By definition, a square has four sides of equal length and four angles of 90°. A rectangle has two pairs of sides of equal length and four angles of 90°. This means that the sum of all four angles in a square or rectangle is 360°.

In the diagram above, the shape on the left is a square. So, if you are given the length of side *a*, you automatically know the length of every side. You already know the measure of every angle, because they are all 90° - the measure of right (perpendicular) angles.

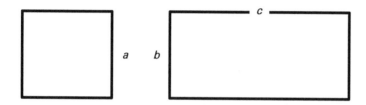

The shape on the right is a rectangle. So, if you are given the length of side *b*, you know the length of the opposite side. However, you do not know the length of the longer two sides unless they are given.

The perimeter of a square is the sum of all four line segments. Since the line segments are equal, the equation is as follows:

Perimeter of a square = 4 ∗ (side length)

The perimeter of the square above is 4*a*.

The perimeter of the rectangle is also the sum of its sides. However, since there are two pairs of equal length sides in a rectangle, the equation is as follows:

Perimeter of a rectangle =
2 ∗ (long side length) + 2 ∗ (short side length)

The perimeter of the rectangle above is 2*b* + 2*c*.

The area of a square is its length times its width. Since length and width are the same for a square, the area is the length of one of its sides squared (that's where the term "squared" comes from) and the equation is as follows:

Area = a^2

For a rectangle, length times width is not equal to one side squared (it's not a square, so the sides are not all the same length). The equation for the area of a rectangle is as follows:

Area = $b * c$

TRIANGLES

A triangle is a polygon (closed shape) made of three line segments. While the four angles in a square and rectangle always add up to 360°, the three angles in a triangle always add up to 180°. However, these angles are not always the same measure, as they are for squares and rectangles.

Below are the different types of triangles:

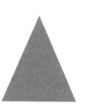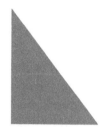

EQUILATERAL
SIDES OF SAME LENGTH

ISOSCELES
TWO SIDES OF SAME LENGTH
TWO ANGLES OF SAME

RIGHT
ONE ANGLE OF 90°

The area of a triangle will always equal one half of the product of its base and its height. You can choose any side to be the base (the one at the bottom of the triangle is probably best), and the height of a triangle is the perpendicular line from the base to the opposite angle. The height is NOT the length of a side, unless the triangle is a right triangle. For example:

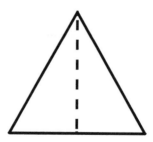

In this triangle, the bottom leg is the base, and the dotted line is the height.

A = 1/2 (base ∗ height)

Another important formula to know when working with triangles is the Pythagorean Theorem. This tells you how to relate the lengths of the sides of right triangles – the ones that include 90° angles.

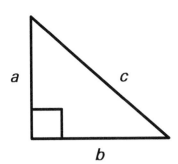 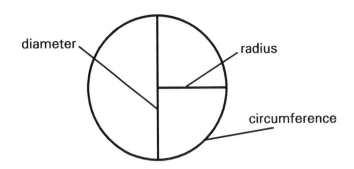

In the diagram above, you have right triangle ABC. You know it's a right triangle because it has a 90° angle – not because it *looks* like one. Never assume the measure of an angle without being given that information. Side c is called the hypotenuse, which is the longest side of a right triangle. Sides a, b and c are related to each other according to the Pythagorean Theorem:

$$c^2 = a^2 + b^2$$

Regardless of how the sides of the right triangle are labeled, the length of the longest side squared is equal to the sum of the lengths of the two shorter sides, each squared. There will likely be a few problems that will require you to use this relationship to solve.

Here are some important details to remember about triangles:

- A triangle has three sides and three angles.
- The angles of a triangle will always add up to 180°.
- A triangle is a "right triangle" if one of the angles is 90°.
- If a triangle is equilateral, all angles are 60°, and all sides are the same length.
- The area of a triangle is one half times the base times the height.
- For right triangles, you can relate the lengths of the sides using the Pythagorean Theorem.

CIRCLES

A circle is a figure without sides. Instead, it has a circumference with a set of points equidistant from the center of the circle.

Here are some important details to remember about circles:

- The measurement around the outside of a circle is called the circumference.
- The line segment going from the center of the circle to the circumference is called the radius.
- The line segment that goes across the entire circle, passing through the center, is the diameter.
- The number of degrees in the central angle of a circle is 360°.

The circumference of a circle can be found using the following formula:

$$C = 2\pi r$$

In this formula, r is the radius (or the distance from the center of the circle to an outside point on the circle). If you are given the diameter, then you can find the circumference using this formula:

$$C = \pi d$$

The radius is twice the length of the diameter:

$$D = 2r$$

The area of a circle can be found using this formula:

$$A = \pi r^2$$

So, the area is equal to the radius squared times the constant (pronounced pi). Sometimes, answer choices are given with as a part of the value, , for example. When you see this, work out the problem without substituting the value of (approximately 3.14). You can, in fact, estimate that is 3.14 or 22/7 in your calculations, but you'll end up with a decimal or fraction for your answer.

PRACTICE TEST 1

So, you think you're ready for Practice Test 1? Or maybe you just started, and you need to take the Pre-test.

Either way, it's time to test what you know. Turn to the next page to begin.

MATHEMATICS

1 – The number of students enrolled at Two Rivers Community College increased from 3,450 in 2010 to 3,864 in 2015. What was the percent increase?

    A. 9%

    B. 17%

    C. 12%

    D. 6%

2 – Find the median in this series of numbers: 80, 78, 73, 69, 100.

    A. 69

    B. 73

    C. 78

    D. 80

3 – Solve this equation: $\sqrt{11 * 44} =$

    A. 36

    B. 24

    C. 18

    D. 22

4 – Amy drives her car until the gas gauge is down to 1/8 full, then she fills the tank to capacity by adding 14 gallons. What is the capacity of the gas tank?

    A. 16 gallons

    B. 18 gallons

    C. 20 gallons

    D. 22 gallons

5 – Which of these numbers is largest?

    A. −345

    B. 42

    C. −17

    D. 3^4

6 – Which of the following is a prime number?

    A. 81

    B. 49

    C. 59

    D. 77

7 – The area of a triangle equals one-half the base times the height. Which of the following is the correct way to calculate the area of a triangle that has a base of 6 and a height of 9?

    A. $(6 + 9)/2$

    B. $\frac{1}{2}(6 + 9)$

    C. $2(6 * 9)$

    D. $\dfrac{(6)(9)}{2}$

8 – Calculate the value of this expression: $2 + 6 * 3 * (3 * 4)^2 + 1$

    A. 2,595

    B. 5,185

    C. 3,456

    D. 6,464

9 – If $x \geq 9$, which of the following is a possible value of x?

    A. 2^3

    B. 9

    C. –34

    D. 8.5

10 – Solve this equation: $-9 * -9 =$

    A. 18

    B. 0

    C. 81

    D. –81

11 – Solve this equation: $x = a^2 * a^3$

    A. $x = a$

    B. $x = a^5$

    C. $x = 1$

    D. $x = 0$

12 – Jean buys a textbook, a flash drive, a printer cartridge, and a ream of paper. The flash drive costs three times as much as the ream of paper. The textbook costs three times as much as the flash drive. The printer cartridge costs twice as much as the textbook. The ream of paper costs $10. How much does Jean spend altogether?

    A. $250

    B. $480

    C. $310

    D. $180

13 – Which of the following is the smallest possible integer value of x in this equation: $x > 3^2 - 4$

    A. 3

    B. 5

    C. 6

    D. 7

14 – In the graduating class at Emerson High School, 52% of the students are girls and 48% are boys. There are 350 students in the class. Among the girls, 98 plan to go to college. How many girls do not plan to go to college?

    A. 84

    B. 48

    C. 66

    D. 72

15 – A cell phone on sale at 30% off costs $210. What was the original price of the phone?
   A. $240
   B. $273
   C. $300
   D. $320

16 – Seven added to four-fifths of a number equals fifteen. What is the number?
   A. 10
   B. 15
   C. 20
   D. 25

17 – If the sum of two numbers is 360, and their ratio is 7:3, what is the smaller number?
   A. 72
   B. 105
   C. 98
   D. 108

18 – Alicia must have a score of 75% to pass a test of 80 questions. What is the greatest number of questions she can miss and still pass the test?
   A. 20
   B. 25
   C. 60
   D. 15

19 – Carmen has a box that is 18 inches long, 12 inches wide, and 14 inches high. What is the volume of the box?
   A. 44 cubic inches
   B. 3,024 cubic inches
   C. 216 cubic inches
   D. 168 cubic inches

20 – The lines in the diagram below are

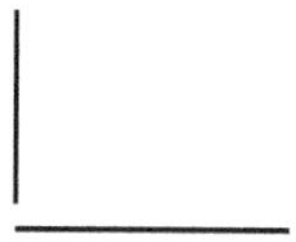

   A. Parallel
   B. Perpendicular
   C. Acute
   D. Obtuse

21 – Find the area.

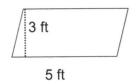

3 ft

5 ft

    A. 16 square feet

    B. 7.5 square feet

    C. 15 square feet

    D. 30 square feet

22 – Which of these numbers is largest?

    A. 5/8

    B. 3/5

    C. 2/3

    D. 0.72

23 – It took Charles four days to write a history paper. He wrote 5 pages on the first day, 4 pages on the second day, and 8 pages on the third day. If Charles ended up writing an average of 7 pages per day, how many pages did he write on the fourth day?

    A. 11

    B. 8

    C. 12

    D. 9

24 – What is the approximate area of the portion of the square that is not covered by the circle?

4 ft

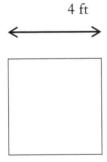

    A. 4.14 square feet

    B. 3.44 square feet

    C. 6.25 square feet

    D. 5.12 square feet

25 – Which of the following is equivalent to the equation: $\dfrac{5}{mp} \div \dfrac{p}{4}$

A. $\dfrac{5p}{4mp}$

B. $\dfrac{20}{mp^2}$

C. $\dfrac{20mp}{4p}$

D. $\dfrac{4mp}{5p}$

---

26 – Danvers is 8 miles due south of Carson and 6 miles due west of Baines. If a driver could drive in a straight line from Carson to Baines, how long would the trip be?

A. 8 miles

B. 10 miles

C. 12 miles

D. 14 miles

---

27 – Lourdes rolls a pair of 6-sided dice. What is the probability that the result will equal 10?

A. 1/36

B. 2/36

C. 3/36

D. 4/36

---

28 – Four friends plan to share equally the cost of a retirement gift. If one person drops out of the arrangement, the cost per person for the remaining three would increase by $12. What is the cost of the gift?

A. $144

B. $136

C. $180

D. $152

---

29 – What is the factorial of 5?

A. 25

B. 5 and 1

C. 120

D. 125

---

30 – Which digit is in the thousandths place in this number: 1,234.567

A. 1

B. 2

C. 6

D. 7

31 – What is the mode in this set of numbers: 4, 5, 4, 8, 10, 4, 6, 7

    A. 6

    B. 4

    C. 8

    D. 7

32 – Which of the following numbers is a perfect square?

    A. 5

    B. 15

    C. 49

    D. 50

33 – Amanda makes $14 an hour as a bank teller, and Oscar makes $24 an hour as an auto mechanic. Both work eight hours a day, five days a week. Which of these equations can be used to calculate how much they make together in a five-day week?

    A. $(14 + 24) * 8 * 5$

    B. $\dfrac{14 + 24}{(8)(5)}$

    C. $(14 + 24)\,(8 + 5)$

    D. $14 + 24 * 8 * 5$

34 – The population of Mariposa County in 2015 was 90% of its population in 2010. The population in 2010 was 145,000. What was the population in 2010?

    A. 160,000

    B. 142,000

    C. 120,500

    D. 130,500

35 – What is the sum of 1/3 and 3/8?

    A. 3/24

    B. 4/11

    C. 17/24

    D. 15/16

36 – In four years, Tom will be twice as old as Serena was three years ago. Tom is three years younger than Serena. How old are Tom and Serena now?

    A. Serena is 28, Tom is 25

    B. Serena is 7, Tom is 4

    C. Serena is 18, Tom is 15

    D. Serena is 21, Tom is 18

37 – A rectangle's length is three times its width. The area of the rectangle is 48 square feet. How long are the sides?

    A. Length = 12, width = 4

    B. Length = 15, width = 5

    C. Length = 18, width = 6

    D. Length = 24, width = 8

38 – Which of the following is the prime factorization of 24?

    A. $24 = 8 * 3$

    B. $24 = 2 * 2 * 2 * 3$

    C. $24 = 6 * 4$

    D. $24 = 12 * 2$

39 – x is a positive integer. Dividing x by a positive number less than 1 will yield:

    A. A number greater than x

    B. A number less than x

    C. A negative number

    D. An irrational number

40 – Solve this equation: $x = 8 - (-3)$

    A. $x = 5$

    B. $x = -5$

    C. $x = 11$

    D. $x = -11$

41 – Which of the following statements is true?

    A. The square of a number is always less than the number.

    B. The square of a number may be either positive or negative.

    C. The square of a number is always a positive number.

    D. The square of a number is always greater than the number.

42 – Marisol's score on a standardized test was ranked in the 78th percentile. If 660 students took the test, approximately how many students scored lower than Marisol?

    A. 582

    B. 515

    C. 612

    D. 486

43 – Sam worked 40 hours at d dollars per hour and received a bonus of $50. His total earnings were $530. What was his hourly wage?

    A. $18

    B. $16

    C. $14

    D. $12

44 – Solve for *r* in this equation: $p = 2r + 3$

    A. r = 2p – 3

    B. r = p + 6

    C. $r = \dfrac{p+3}{2}$

    D. $r = \dfrac{p-3}{2}$

45 – What is the least common multiple of 8 and 10?

    A. 80

    B. 40

    C. 18

    D. 72

46 – Solve this equation: x = –12 ÷ –3

    A. $x = -4$

    B. $x = -15$

    C. $x = 9$

    D. $x = 4$

47 – Convert the improper fraction 17/6 to a mixed number.

    A. $2\dfrac{5}{6}$

    B. $3\dfrac{1}{6}$

    C. 6/17

    D. $3\dfrac{5}{6}$

48 – What value of *q* is a solution to this equation: $130 = q(-13)$

    A. 10

    B. –10

    C. 1

    D. 10^2

49 – Find the value of $a^2 + 6b$ when a = 3 and b = 0.5.

    A. 12

    B. 6

    C. 9

    D. 15

50 – If the radius of the circle in this diagram is 4 inches, what is the perimeter of the square?

    A. 24 inches
    B. 32 inches
    C. 64 inches
    D. 96 inches

SCIENCE

1- Bronchial epithelial cell membranes possess which of the following?
    A. microvilli
    B. cillia
    C. flagella
    D. dendrites

2- Emulsification of fats requires _____ and occurs in the _____.
Which of the following correctly completes the statement above?
    A. amylase; stomach;
    B. bile; stomach
    C. amylase; small intestine
    D. bile; small intestine

3- In immune functions involving T-helper cells, the T-helper cell most likely engages in which of the following?
    A. phagocytosis
    B. cell lysis
    C. circulating antibody production
    D. intercellular membrane binding

4- In a normal human, once blood is pumped out of the heart , which of the following statements is always true?
    A. It passes through capillaries before returning to the internal chambers of the heart
    B. It has been fully oxygenated.
    C. It immediately enters the aorta
    D. It travels to the lungs before returning to the heart

5- Oxygen enters the circulatory system during
    A. inspiration only
    B. inspiration and the interval between inspiration and expiration only
    C. the interval between inspiration and expiration and during expiration only
    D. continuously throughout the entire respiratory cycle

6- The integrative functions of the nervous system requires which of the following?

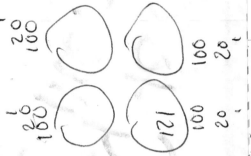

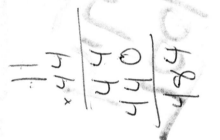

the following biologically active proteins?

en

capacity of the human innate immune system?

lls

e to cytokines

lescribes the relative anatomical positional relationship between
mal human adult?

esophagus.

the vertebral column.

the abdominal aorta.

ral to the pancreas.

nich of the following locations?

    A. the liver

    B. the kidney

    C. the pancreas

    D. red blood cells

11- In humans, which of the organs listed below does NOT receive supplies of both oxygenated and deoxygenated blood?

    A. the lungs

    B. the heart

    C. the liver

    D. the large intestine

12- In humans, which of the skeletal muscles listed below are more often than not under involuntary rather than voluntary control?

    A. the masseters

    B. the diaphragm

    C. the biceps

    D. the tongue

13- In humans, the majority (>50%) of water obtained through oral intake is absorbed into the body through which of the following?

  A. the oral mucosa and the esophagus
  B. the esophagus and the stomach
  C. the small intestines
  D. the large intestines

14- Which of the following cell types secrete perforins?

  A. liver parenchymal cells
  B. natural killer (NK) cells
  C. T-helper cells
  D. vascular endothelial cells

15- In humans, which of the following is true regarding dietary intake of proteins?

  A. It does not occur in individuals who are strict vegetarians
  B. It must include a variety of proteins that consist of all 20 amino acids required for for protein synthesis in the body
  C. inadequate intake during childhood development can lead to the disease kwashiorkor.
  D. breakdown begins when protein reaches the ileum of the small intestine.

16- Among the choices below, which pair of taxonomic categories of organisms are in separate domains?

  A. Eubacteria and Archaebacteria
  B. Fungi and Plantae
  C. Animalia and Protista
  D. Fungi and Protista

17- An absolute requirement for continual adaptation of a species to occur through natural selection is described in which of the following statements?

  A. Mutations in the somatic cells of the fertile members of the species must be able to occur.
  B. Mutations in the germ line cells of the fertile members of the species must be able to occur.
  C. Sister chromatids must be capable of exchanging DNA segments before the completion of meiosis I
  D. Sister chromatids must be capable of exchanging DNA segments before the completion of meiosis II

18- For all biological nucleic acids, a nucleotide is composed of which of the following three components?

  A. a carboxylic acid, a nitrogenous base and a pentose sugar
  B. an amino acid , a hexose sugar and a nitrogenous base
  C. a phosphate group, a pentose sugar and a nitrogenous base
  D. a phosphate group, a hexose sugar and an amino acid

19- Which of the following is a true statement regarding fundamental differences between eukaryotic and prokaryotic cells?

    A. Some, but not all, prokaryotic cells have cell walls, but no eukaryotic cells have cell walls.

    B. Some, but not all, prokaryotic cells have ribosomes, but all eukaryotic cells have ribosomes.

    C. Some, but not all, eukaryotic cells have nucleoids, but all prokaryotic cells have nucleoids

    D. Some, but not all, eukaryotic cells have chloroplasts, but no prokaryotic cells have chloroplasts.

20- Which of the following cellular organelles do not possess an outer encapsulating organellar membrane?

    A. mitochondria

    B. ribosomes

    C. chloroplasts

    D. nuclei

21- which of the following is true regarding the relationship between a complete segment of mRNA and the gene from which the mRNA segment was transcribed?

    A. The mRNA segment base sequence is identical to the DNA gene base sequence

    B. The mRNA segment base sequence is identical to the complementary DNA strand segment of the gene base sequence

    C. The mRNA segment base sequence is identical to the complementary DNA strand segment of the gene base sequence except that adenine is substituted for thymine in the mRNA base sequence

    D. The mRNA segment base sequence is identical to the complementary DNA strand segment of the gene base sequence except that uracil is substituted for thymine in the mRNA base sequence

22- The gastrulation stage of human fetal development is characterized by which of the following?

    A. Individual tissue layers begin to form

    B. The four fundamental cell types begin to differentiate

    C. The first multipotent stem cells begin to appear

    D. The first individual organs begin to function.

23- The interphase stage of a normal somatic cell cycle consists of which three sub-phases?

    A. prophase, G1 and G2

    B. G1, G2, and cytokinesis

    C. G1, S and G2

    D. G1, S and prophase

24- During the metaphase I stage of meiosis, which of the following events occurs at the metaphase plate?

    A. Homologous tetrad pairs align

    B. individual tetrads align

    C. individual chromatids align

    D. homologous chromatid pairs align

25- During photosynthesis, what is the total number of oxygen molecules produced for each molecule of glucose ($C_6H_{12}O_6$) that is synthesized?

    A. 2

    B. 6

    C. 12

    D. 24

26- In human cells, which of the following statements correctly states a true principle of the processing of genetic information?

    A. A single, unique sequence of genes codes for a single unique protein

    B. A single, unique three-base codon will code for only one single, unique type of amino acid.

    C. A single unique protein can only be coded for by a single, unique sequence of codons

    D. A single unique protein can only be coded for by a single, unique sequence of of DNA bases.

27- By a strict genetic definition, perfectly identical twins must have _____ .

Select the answer choice that completes the statement above.

    A. identical phenotypes only

    B. identical genotypes only

    C. both identical genotypes and phenotypes

    D. either identical genotypes or identical phenotypes

28- In the reaction H_2CO_3 ---> HCO_3^- + H^+, if H_2CO_3 if HCO_3^- is a strong base which of the following is true?

    A. H_2CO_3 is a strong acid

    B. H_2CO_3 is a weak acid

    C. H_2CO_3 is a weak base

    D. H_2CO_3 is a strong base

29- The largest fraction of energy that the earth receives from the sun is in the form of which of the following?

    A. kinetic energy of electrons

    B. kinetic energy of neutrons

    C. electromagnetic energy

    D. chemical energy

30- Which of the following has the greatest gravitational potential energy?

    A. a 5 kg mass, at rest, 10 m above the surface of the earth

    B. a 5 kg mass, free-falling, with a current velocity of 10 m/s, 5 m above the surface of the Earth

    C. a 2 kg mass, at rest on the floor of an open vertical shaft, 30 m below the surface of the earth

    D. a 50 kg mass at the instant that it is propelled directly upward with a velocity of 10 m/s

31- An organized functional collection of adipose cells is considered to be which of the following

    A. epithelial tissue

    B. connective tissue

    C. a syncytium

    D. a gland

32- In chemical reactions where a catalyst participates, the catalyst------of the reaction by ------of the reaction

    A. increases the efficiency of the reaction; increasing the activation energy

    B. increases the efficiency of the reaction; decreasing the activation energy

    C. increases the rate of the reaction; increasing the activation energy

    D. increases the rate of the reaction; decreasing the activation energy

33- Which of the following is the correct electron configuration for a neutral neon atom in its lowest electron energy state?

    A. 1s2 2s2 2p6

    B. 1s2 2s2 3s2 3p4

    C. 2s2 2p2 3s2 3p2 3d2

    D. 6s2 2p2

34- In biological chemical systems, an increase in the activity of an enzyme indicates that which of the following has occurred?

    A. The enzyme has increased its optimum functional pH range

    B. The enzyme has increased its optimum functional temperature range

    C. The enzyme has increased its effect on the rate of a chemical reaction

    D. The enzyme has increased the total number of reactions that it is capable of catalyzing.

35- Which of the following lists three substances in DECREASING order of pH value, beginning with the substance with the highest pH on the left?

    A. sulphuric acid, vinegar, water

    B. ammonia, blood, orange juice

    C. water, ammonia, sulphuric acid

    D. vinegar, water, orange juice

36- If an alkane with 6 carbon atoms is converted to an alkyne with 6 carbon atoms, what is the change in the number of hydrogen atoms contained in the alkane compared to the alkyne?

    A. The alkane contains 4 less hydrogen atoms than does the alkyne.

    B. The alkane contains 2 less hydrogen atoms than does the alkyne.

    C. The alkane contains 2 more hydrogen atoms than does the alkyne.

    D. The alkane contains 4 more hydrogen atoms than does the alkyne.

37- which of the following is the site a site of steroid hormone production?

    A. the pancreas

    B. the adrenal gland

    C. the thyroid

    D. the thymus

38- In the unbalanced oxidation-reduction reaction $CH_4 + O_2 \rightarrow CO_2 + H_2O$, which answer choice below shows the correct, balanced half-reaction for oxygen?

    A. $O_2 \rightarrow 2O^- + 2e^-$

    B. $2O_2 + 8e^- \rightarrow 4O^{-2}$

    C. $4H^+ + 2O \rightarrow 2H_2O^+$

    D. $CH_4 + O_2 \rightarrow 1/2CO_2 + 1/2H_2O$

39- A sample of liquid bromine (Br_2) is in an open contained at a pressure of 1 atm and temperature of 20C. As heat is applied to the sample at a constant rate, which of the following will occur beginning at the moment when the bromine sample reaches its boiling point?

    A. The liquid bromine density will increase at a constant rate.

    B. The temperature of the liquid bromine will remain constant.

    C. The volume of liquid bromine that is converted to bromine gas will increase at a constantly increasing rate.

    D. The liquid bromine density will decrease at a constant rate.

40- Water molecules in the liquid state will have____ intermolecular bonding compared to the intermolecular bonding of water molecules in the solid state.

Which of the following correctly completes the statement above?

    A. the same type of

    B. stronger

    C. a different type of

    D. no

41- Which of the taxonomic classification category pairs listed below begin with the broader category followed by the more specific category?

    A. order; phylum

    B. family; class

    C. class; order

    D. genus; family

42- In a single chromosome____

Which of the answer choices correctly completes the statement above?

    A. every DNA strand contains genes

    B. there are always two copies of every gene

    C. every functional gene can be transcribed into a mRNA molecule

    D. there are at least 2 alleles for every gene

43- Which of the sequences listed in the answer choices show the correct RNA transcript of the DNA sequence listed below?

DNA: AGC TAC CCG

RNA: ___ ___ ___

    A. TCG ATG GGC

    B. UCG AUG GGC

    C. TCG UTG GGC

    D. CTA GCA AAT

44- Ribosome construction occurs in which of the following locations inside of a cell?

  A. rough endoplasmic reticulum
  B. peroxisomes
  C. lysosomes
  D. nucleoli

45- In terms of processing of genetic information, ribosomes are to proteins as _____ is/are to DNA Which of the following completes the analogy shown above?

  A. amino acids
  B. codons
  C. RNA polymerase
  D. DNA polymerase

46- In double-stranded DNA, one strand is called the "sense" strand and the other is called the "anti-sense" strand. Which of the following occurs during replication of double-stranded DNA?

  A. The sense strand is completely replicated before replication of the antisense strand begins.
  B. The antisense strand is completely replicated before replication of the sense strand begins.
  C. Either the sense or the antisense is replicated before replication of the complementary strand begins.
  D. Replication of both strands occurs simultaneously.

47- During mitosis, spindle fibers connect which of the following structures?

  A. centromeres and chromosomes
  B. centrosomes and chromosomes
  C. sister chromatids
  D. homologous chromosomes

48- Which of the following correctly describes a role of chlorophyll in living organisms?

  A. transport of oxygen molecules
  B. absorption of sunlight
  C. oxidation of carbon dioxide
  D. production of ATP

49- What are the two general structural categories of nitrogenous bases in nucleic acids?

  A. purines and pyrimidines
  B. thymines and uracils
  C. nucleotides and nucleosides
  D. pyrimidines and hydroxy-ureas

50- Among the choices below, which is the most accurate approximation of the error rate during the replication of DNA that occurs BEFORE any corrective error activities occur.

  A. 1 base error per 1000 genes
  B. 1 base error per 1x10 to the 6 genes
  C. 1 base error per 1x10 to the 6 bases
  D. 1 base error per 1x10 to the 12 bases

ENGLISH & READING

1. Which of the following choices best completes this sentence?
    When asked if the sleeping pill had _____ him at all, the man replied that it had had no _____; nonetheless, he realized that he _____not attempt to drive his car that evening.
    - A. affected; effect; ought
    - B. affected; effect; aught
    - C. effected; affect; ought
    - D. effected; affect; aught

2. Which sentence makes best use of grammatical conventions for clarity and concision?
    - A. Hiking along the trail, the birds chirped loudly and interrupted our attempt at a peaceful nature walk.
    - B. The birds chirped loudly, attempting to hike along the nature trail we were interrupted.
    - C. Hiking along the trail, we were assailed by the chirping of birds, which made our nature walk hardly the peaceful exercise we had wanted.
    - D. Along the nature trail, our walk was interrupted by loudly chirping birds in our attempt at a nature trail.

3. Which word from the following sentence is an adjective?
    A really serious modern-day challenge is finding a way to consume real food in a world of overly processed food products.
    - A. really
    - B. challenge
    - C. consume
    - D. processed

4. To improve sentence fluency, how could you state the information below in a single sentence?
    My daughter was in a dance recital. I attended it with my husband. She received an award. We were very proud.
    - A. My daughter, who was in a dance recital, received an award, which made my husband and I, who were in attendance, very proud.
    - B. My husband and I attended my daughter's dance recital and were very proud when she received an award.
    - C. Attending our daughter's dance recital, my husband and I were very proud to see her receive an award.
    - D. Dancing in a recital, my daughter received an award which my husband and I, who were there, very proud.

5. Which sentence is punctuated correctly?
    - A. Since the concert ended very late I fell asleep in the backseat during the car ride home.
    - B. Since the concert ended very late: I fell asleep in the backseat during the car ride home.
    - C. Since the concert ended very late; I fell asleep in the backseat during the car ride home.
    - D. Since the concert ended very late, I fell asleep in the backseat during the car ride home.

6. Which of the choices below best completes the following sentence?
    Negotiations with the enemy are never fun, but during times of war _____ a necessary evil.
    - A. its
    - B. it's
    - C. their
    - D. they're

7. Which of the verbs below best completes the following sentence?
The a cappela group _____ looking forward to performing for the entire student body at the graduation ceremony.
   A. is
   B. are
   C. was
   D. be

8. What kind of sentence is this?
I can't believe her luck!
   A. Declarative
   B. Imperative
   C. Exclamatory
   D. Interrogative

9. Identify the error in this sentence:
Irregardless of the expense, it is absolutely imperative that all drivers have liability insurance to cover any personal injury that may be suffered during a motor vehicle accident.
   A. Irregardless
   B. Imperative
   C. Liability
   D. Suffered

10. Which of the following sentences is grammatically correct?
   A. Between you and me, I brang back less books from my dorm room than I needed to study for my exams.
   B. Between you and I, I brought back less books from my dorm room then I needed to study for my exams.
   C. Between you and me, I brought back fewer books from my dorm room than I needed to study for my exam.
   D. Between you and me, I brought back fewer books from my dorm room then I needed to study for my exams.

11. Choose from the answers to complete this sentence with the proper verb and antecedent agreement:
Neither of _____ _____ able to finish our supper.
   A. we; were
   B. we; was
   C. us; were
   D. us; was

12. Which word in the following sentence is a noun?
The library books are overdue.
   A. The
   B. library
   C. books
   D. overdue

13. Which of the following is a simple sentence?
   A. Mary and Samantha ran and skipped and hopped their way home from school every day.
   B. Mary liked to hop but Samantha preferred to skip.
   C. Mary loved coloring yet disliked when coloring was assigned for math homework.
   D. Samantha thought Mary was her best friend but she was mistaken.

14. Which of the following is NOT a simple sentence?
    A. Matthew and Thomas had been best friends since grade school.
    B. Matthew was tall and shy, and Thomas was short and talkative.
    C. Matthew liked to get Thomas to pass notes to the little red-haired girl in the back row of math class.
    D. Matthew and Thomas would tease Mary and Samantha on their way home from school every day.

15. Which of the following sentences is punctuated correctly?
    A. "Theres a bus coming so hurry up and cross the street!" yelled Bob to the old woman.
    B. "There's a bus coming, so hurry up and cross the street", yelled Bob, to the old woman.
    C. "Theres a bus coming, so hurry up and cross the street,"! yelled Bob to the old woman.
    D. "There's a bus coming, so hurry up and cross the street!" yelled Bob to the old_woman.

16. Which of the following sentences is punctuated correctly?
    A. It's a long to-do list she left for us today: make beds, wash breakfast dishes, go grocery shopping, do laundry, cook dinner, and read the twins a bedtime story.
    B. Its a long to-do list she left for us today; make beds; wash breakfast dishes; go grocery shopping; do laundry; cook dinner; and read the twins a bedtime story.
    C. It's a long to-do list she left for us today: make beds; wash breakfast dishes; go grocery shopping; do laundry; cook dinner; and read the twins a bedtime story.
    D. Its a long to-do list she left for us today: make beds, wash breakfast dishes, go grocery shopping, do laundry, cook dinner, and read the twins a bedtime story.

17. Which of the following sentences is written in the first person?
    A. My room was a mess so my mom made me clean it before I was allowed to leave the house.
    B. Her room was a mess so she had to clean it before she left for the concert.
    C. You had better clean up your room before your mom comes home!
    D. Sandy is a slob and never cleans up her own room until her mom makes her.

18. Which sentence follows the rules for capitalization?
    A. My second grade Teacher's name was Mrs. Carmicheal.
    B. The Pope gave a very emotional address to the crowd after Easter Sunday mass.
    C. The president of France is meeting with President Obama later this week.
    D. My family spent our summer vacations at grandpa Joe's cabin in the Finger Lakes region.

19. The girl returning home after her curfew found the _____ up the stairs to her bedroom maddening as it seemed every step she took on the old staircase yielded a loud _____.
    Which of the following completes the sentence above?
    A. clime; creak
    B. clime; creek
    C. climb; creek
    D. climb; creak

20. By this time next summer, _____ my college coursework.
    Which of the following correctly completes the sentence above?
    A. I did complete
    B. I completed
    C. I will complete
    D. I will have completed

21. Which of the following choices best completes this sentence?

The teacher nodded her _____ to the classroom _____ who was teaching a portion of the daily lesson for the first time.

    A. assent; aide

    B. assent; aid

    C. ascent; aide

    D. ascent; aid

22. Which of the following sentences is grammatically correct?

    A. No one has offered to let us use there home for the office's end-of-year picnic.

    B. No one have offered to let we use their home for the office's end-of-year picnic.

    C. No one has offered to let ourselves use their home for the office's end-of-year picnic.

    D. No one has offered to let us use their home for the office's end-of-year picnic.

23. Which choice most effectively combines the information in the following sentences?

The tornado struck. It struck without warning. It caused damage.

The damage was extensive.

    A. Without warning, the extensively damaging tornado struck.

    B. Having struck without warning, the damage was extensive with the tornado.

    C. The tornado struck without warning and caused extensive damage.

    D. Extensively damaging, and without warning, struck the tornado.

24. Which word in the sentence below is a verb?

Carrying heavy boxes to the attic caused her to throw out her back.

    A. Carrying

    B. to

    C. caused

    D. out

25. Which choice below most effectively combines the information in the following sentences?

His lecture was boring. I thought it would never end. My eyelids were drooping. My feet were going numb.

    A. His never-ending lecture made my eyelids droop, and my feet were going numb.

    B. My eyelids drooping and my feet going numb, I thought his boring lecture would never end.

    C. His lecture was boring and would not end; it made my eyelids droop and my feet go numb.

    D. Never-ending, his boring lecture caused me to have droopy eyelids and for my feet to go numb.

26. Which choice below correctly completes this sentence?

Comets _____ balls of dust and ice, _____ leftover materials that _____ planets during the formation of _____ solar system.

    A. Comets is balls of dust and ice, comprised of leftover materials that were not becoming planets during the formation of its solar system.

    B. Comets are balls of dust and ice, comprising leftover materials that are not becoming planets during the formation of our solar system.

    C. Comets are balls of dust and ice, comprised of leftover materials that became planets during the formation of their solar system.

    D. Comets are balls of dust and ice, comprised of leftover materials that did not become planets during the formation of our solar system.

Questions 27-35 are based on the following passage about Penny Dreadfuls.

Victorian era Britain experienced social changes that resulted in increased literacy rates. With the rise of capitalism and industrialization, people began to spend more money on entertainment, contributing to the popularization of the novel. Improvements in printing resulted in the production of newspapers, as well as, Englands' more fully recognizing the singular concept of reading as a form of leisure; it was, of itself, a new industry. An increased capacity for travel via the invention of tracks, engines, and the coresponding railway distribution created both a market for cheap popular literature, and the ability for it to be circulated on a large scale.

The first penny serials were published in the 1830s to meet this demand. The serials were priced to be affordable to working-class readers, and were considerably cheaper than the serialized novels of authors such as Charles Dickens, which cost a shilling (twelve pennies) per part. Those who could not afford a penny a week, working class boys often formed clubs sharing the cost, passed the booklets, who were flimsy, from reader to reader. Other enterprising youngsters would collect a number of consecutive parts, then rent the volume out to friends.

The stories themselves were reprints, or sometimes rewrites, of gothic thrillers, as well as new stories about famous criminals. Other serials were thinly-disguised plagiarisms of popular contemporary literature. The penny dreadfuls were influential since they were in the words of one commentator the most alluring and low-priced form of escapist reading available to ordinary youth.

In reality, the serial novels were overdramatic and sensational, but generally harmless. If anything, the penny dreadfuls, although obviously not the most enlightening or inspiring of literary selections, resulted in increasingly literate youth in the Industrial period. The wide circulation of this sensationalist literature, however, contributed to an ever greater fear of crime in mid-Victorian Britain.

27. Which of the following is the correct punctuation for the following sentence from paragraph 1?
   A. NO CHANGE
   B. Improvements in printing resulted in the production of newspapers, as well as England's more fully recognizing the singular concept of reading as a form of leisure; it was, of itself, a new industry.
   C. Improvements in printing resulted in the production of newspapers, as well as Englands more fully recognizing the singular concept of reading as a form of leisure; it was, of itself, a new industry.
   D. Improvements in printing resulted in the production of newspapers as well as, England's more fully recognizing the singular concept of reading as a form of leisure; it was, of itself, a new industry.

28. In the first sentence of paragraph 1, which of the following words should be capitalized?
   A. era
   B. social
   C. literacy
   D. rates

29. In the last sentence of paragraph 1, which of the following words is misspelled?
   A. capacity
   B. via
   C. coresponding
   D. cheap

30. In the first sentence of the paragraph 2, "this demand" refers to which of the following antecedents in paragraph 1?

    A. travel

    B. leisure

    C. industry

    D. market

31. Which of the following sentences is the clearest way to express the ideas in the third sentence of paragraph 2?

    A. A penny a week, working class boys could not afford these books; they often formed sharing clubs that were passing the flimsy booklets around from one reader to another reader.

    B. Clubs were formed to buy the flimsy booklets by working class boys who could not afford a penny a week that would share the cost, passing from reader to reader the flimsy booklets.

    C. Working class boys who could not afford a penny a week often formed clubs that would share the cost, passing the flimsy booklets from reader to reader.

    D. Sharing the cost were working class boys who could not afford a penny a week; they often formed clubs and, reader to reader, passed the flimsy booklets around.

32. Which word in the first sentence of paragraph 3 should be capitalized?

    A. stories

    B. gothic

    C. thrillers

    D. criminals

33. Which of the following versions of the final sentence of paragraph 3 is correctly punctuated?

    A. The penny dreadfuls were influential since they were in the words of one commentator; the most alluring and low-priced form of escapist reading available to ordinary youth.

    B. The penny dreadfuls were influential since they were, in the words of one commentator, "the most alluring and low-priced form of escapist reading available to ordinary youth".

    C. The penny dreadfuls were influential since they were, in the words of one commentator, the most alluring and low-priced form of escapist reading available to ordinary youth.

    D. The penny dreadfuls were influential since they were in the words of one commentator "the most alluring and low-priced form of escapist reading available to ordinary youth."

34. In this first sentence of paragraph, which of the following words is a noun?

    A. serial

    B. novels

    C. sensational

    D. generally

35. In the last sentence of paragraph, which of the following words is an adjective?

    A. circulation

    B. literature

    C. however

    D. greater

36. The author wants to add a sentence to the passage that would list some of the books which were plagiarized into penny dreadfuls. Which paragraph would be the best place to add this information?
    A. Paragraph 1
    B. Paragraph 2
    C. Paragraph 3
    D. Paragraph 4

Questions 37-43 are based on the following passage about Martin Luther King Jr.

Martin Luther King Jr. was an American baptist minister and activist who was a leader in the African-American Civil Rights Movement. He is best known for his role in the advancement of civil rights using non-violent civil disobedience based on his Christian beliefs. In the United States, his racial equality efforts, and his staunchly advocating civil rights is among, undoubtedly, culturally the most important contributions made by King to last century's society.

King became a civil rights activist early in his career. In 1955, he led the Montgomery bus boycott, and in 1957 he helped found the Southern Christian Leadership Conference (SCLC), serving as its first president. With the SCLC, King led an unsuccessful 1962 struggle against segregation in Albany, Georgia, and helped organize the 1963 nonviolent protests in Birmingham, Alabama. King also helped to organize the 1963 March on Washington where he delivered his famous I Have a Dream speech. There, he established his reputation as the greatest orator in American history.

On October 14, 1964, King justly received the Nobel Piece Prize for combating racial inequality through nonviolent resistance. In 1965, he helped to organize the famous Selma to Montgomery marches, and the following year he and SCLC took the movement north to Chicago to work on eliminating the unjust and much-despised segregated housing there. In the final years of his life, King expanded his focus to include opposition towards poverty and the Vietnam War, and he gave a famous speech in 1967 entitled "Beyond Vietnam". This speech alienated many of his liberal allies in government who supported the war, but to his credit King never allowed politics to dictate the path of his noble works.

In 1968, King was planning a national occupation of Washington, D.C., to be called the Poor People's Campaign, when he was assassinated on April 4 in Memphis, Tennessee. His violent death was, not surprisingly, followed by riots in many U.S. cities.

King was posthumously awarded the Presidential Medal of Freedom and the Congressional Gold Metal. Martin Luther King, Jr. Day was established as a holiday in numerous cities and states beginning in 1971, and eventually became a U.S. federal holiday in 1986. Since his tragic death, numerous streets in the U.S. have been renamed in his honor, and a county in Washington State was also renamed for him. The Martin Luther King, Jr. Memorial on the National Mall in Washington, D.C., was dedicated in 2011.

37. In the first sentence of paragraph 1, which of the following words should be capitalized?
    A. baptist
    B. minister
    C. activist
    D. leader

38. Which is the best rewording for clarity and concision of this sentence from paragraph 1?
   A. His efforts to achieve racial equality in the United States, and his staunch public advocacy of civil rights are undoubtedly among the most important cultural contributions made to society in the last century.
   B. His efforts achieving equality in the United States, and to staunchly advocate civil rights are undoubtedly among the most important contributions culturally and societally made in the last century.
   C. Racial equality and civil rights, staunchly advocated by King in the United States, are, without a doubt, last century's greatest contributions, in a cultural way, to society.
   D. Last century, King made cultural contributions to racial equality and civil rights, which are undoubtedly the greatest made in the previous century.

39. Which of the following found in paragraph 2 should be placed inside quotation marks?
   A. Montgomery bus boycott
   B. Southern Christian Leadership Conference
   C. March on Washington
   D. I Have a Dream

40. In the first sentence of paragraph 3, which of the following words is misspelled?
   A. received
   B. Piece
   C. combating
   D. racial

41. In the first sentence of paragraph 5, which of the following words is misspelled?
   A. Posthumously
   B. Presidential
   C. Medal
   D. Metal

42. Which of the following sentences from the passage provides context clues about the author's feelings in regard to King?
   A. He is best known for his role in the advancement of civil rights using non-violent civil disobedience based on his Christian beliefs. (P. 1)
   B. King also helped to organize the 1963 March on Washington where he delivered his famous I Have a Dream speech. (P. 2)
   C. This speech alienated many of his liberal allies in government who supported the war, but to his credit King never allowed politics to dictate the path of his noble works. (P. 3)
   D. King was posthumously awarded the Presidential Medal of Freedom and the Congressional Gold Metal. (P. 5)

43. The author is considering adding a paragraph about King's family to the passage. Should he or she do this?
   A. Yes, because it adds needed personal details to the passage.
   B. Yes, because it would elaborate on information already provided in the passage.
   C. No, because the passage is about King's public life and works, and information about his family would be irrelevant.
   D. No, because information about his family has already been included and an additional paragraph on that topic would be redundant.

44. Which of the following sentences uses correct punctuation for dialogue?
    A. "Hey, can you come here a second"? asked Marie.
    B. She thought about his offer briefly and then responded. "I think I will have to pass".
    C. "I am making pancakes for breakfast. Does anybody want some?" asked mom.
    D. The conductor yelled "All aboard"! and then waited for last minute travelers to board the train.

45. Which of the following is a compound sentence?
    A. She and I drove to the play together.
    B. I woke up early that morning and began to do long-neglected household chores.
    C. The long-separated cousins ran and jumped and sang and played all afternoon.
    D. I trembled when I saw him: his face was white as a ghost.

46. Which of the following is the best order for the sentences below in forming a logical paragraph?
    A. A, B, C, D, E
    B. A, C, E, B, D
    C. A, D, B, D, E
    D. A, C, E, D, B

A. *Walt Disney was a shy, self-deprecating and insecure man in private but adopted a warm and outgoing public persona.*
B. *His film work continues to be shown and adapted; his studio maintains high standards in its production of popular entertainment, and the Disney amusement parks have grown in size and number to attract visitors in several countries.*
C. *However he had high standards and high expectations of those with whom he worked.*
D. *He nevertheless remains an important figure in the history of animation and in the cultural history of the United States, where he is considered a national cultural icon.*
E. *His reputation changed in the years after his death, from a purveyor of homely patriotic values to a representative of American imperialism.*

47. Which of the choices below is the meaning of the word "adopted" in the following sentence?
Walt Disney was a shy, self-deprecating and insecure man in private but adopted a warm and outgoing public persona.
    A. took
    B. began to use
    C. began to have
    D. legally cared for as one's own child

48. Which of the following sentences is written in the second person?
    A. You had better call and RSVP to the party right away before you forget.
    B. She had every intention of calling with a prompt reply to the invitation, but the week got hectic and she forgot.
    C. I am utterly hopeless at remembering things, so I will set up a calendar reminder for myself to call Jan about the party.
    D. "Did you forget to RSVP to the party?!" asked her exasperated roommate.

HESI A² - Spire Study System

49. Which of the following sentences shows proper pronoun-antecedent agreement?
  A. The author published several best-selling novels; some of it was made into films that were not as popular.
  B. Everyone should bring their parents to the town-wide carnival.
  C. Smart companies will do what it takes to hold onto its best employees.
  D. Parents are reminded to pick up their children from school promptly at 2:30.

50. Which of the following sentences shows proper subject-verb agreement?
  A. Danny is one of the only students who have lived up to his responsibilities as a newspaper staff member.
  B. One of my friends are going to be on a TV series starting this fall.
  C. Rice and beans, my favorite meal, reminds me of my native country Puerto Rico.
  D. Most of the milk we bought for the senior citizens' luncheons have gone bad.

ANSWERS PRACTICE TEST 1

MATHEMATICS

1 – C. 12%

To find the percent increase, you first need to know the amount of the increase. Enrollment went from 3,450 in 2010 to 3,864 in 2015. This is an increase of 414. Now, to find the percent of the increase, divide the amount of the increase by the original amount:

$$414 \div 3,450 = 0.12$$

To convert a decimal to a percent, move the decimal point two places to the right:
$$0.12 = 12\%$$

When a question asks for the percent increase or decrease, divide the amount of the increase or decrease by the original amount.

2 – C. 78

To find the median in a series of numbers, arrange the numbers in order from smallest to largest:

$$69, 73, 78, 80, 100$$

The number in the center is the median. If there are an even number of numbers in the series, for example:

$$34, 46, 52, 54, 67, 81$$

then the median will be the average of the two numbers in the center. In this example, the median will be 53 (the average of 52 and 54). Remember: the median is not the same as the average.

3 – D. 22

This question asks you to find the square root of 11 times 44. First, do the multiplication: 11 * 44 = 484. Now multiply each of the possible answers by itself to see which one is the square root of 484.

4 – A. 16 gallons

Amy drives her car until the gas tank is 1/8 full. This means that it is 7/8 empty. She fills it by adding 14 gallons. In other words, 14 gallons is 7/8 of the tank's capacity. Draw a simple diagram to represent the gas tank.

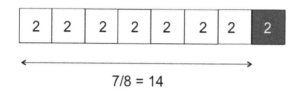

You can see that each eighth of the tank is 2 gallons. So the capacity of the tank is 2 * 8, or 16.

5 – D. 3^4

Positive numbers are larger than negative numbers, so this limits the possible answers to 42 and 3^4. 3^4 equals 81 (3 * 3 * 3 * 3).

6 – C. 59

A prime number is a whole number greater than 1 that can be divided evenly only by itself and 1. In this question, only 59 fits that definition. 81 is not prime because it can be divided evenly by 9; 49 is not prime because it can be divided evenly by 7; and 77 is not prime because it can be divided evenly by 7 and 11.

7 – D. $\dfrac{(6)(9)}{2}$

The area of a triangle is one-half the product of the base and the height. Choices A and B are incorrect because they add the base and the height instead of multiplying them. Choice C is incorrect because it multiplies the product of the base and the height by 2 instead of dividing it by 2.

8 – A. 2,595

The steps in evaluating a mathematical expression must be carried out in a certain order, which is called "the order of operations." These are the steps in order:

Parentheses: The first step is to do any operations in parentheses.
Exponents: Then do any steps that involve exponents.
Multiply and **D**ivide: Multiply and divide from left to right.
Add and **S**ubtract: Add and subtract from left to right.

One way to remember this order is to use this sentence:
Please **E**xcuse **M**y **D**ear **A**unt **S**ally.

To evaluate the expression in this question, follow these steps:

Multiply the numbers in **Parentheses**: 3 * 4 = 12

Apply the **Exponent** 2 to the number in parentheses: $12^2 = 144$

Multiply: 6 * 3 * 144 = 2,592

Add: 2 + 2,592 + 1 = 2,595

---

9 – B. 9

The symbol ≥ means "greater than or equal to." The only answer that is greater than or equal to 9 is 9.

---

10 – C. 81

When two numbers with the same sign (both positive or both negative) are multiplied, the answer is a positive number. When two numbers with different signs (one positive and the other negative) are multiplied, the answer is negative.

---

11 – B. $x = a^5$

When multiplying numbers that have the same base and different exponents, keep the base the same and add the exponents. In this case, $a^2 * a^3$ becomes $a^{(2+3)}$ or a^5.

---

12 – C. $310

The costs of all these items can be expressed in terms of the cost of the ream of paper. Use x to represent the cost of a ream of paper. The flash drive costs three times as much as the ream of paper, so it costs $3x$. The textbook costs three times as much as the flash drive, so it costs $9x$. The printer cartridge costs twice as much as the textbook, so it costs $18x$. So now we have:

$$x + 3x + 9x + 18x = 31x$$

The ream of paper costs $10, so $31x$ (the total cost) is $310.

---

13 – C. 6

Solve the equation:

$$x > 3^2 - 4$$
$$x > 9 - 4$$
$$x > 5$$

We know that x is greater than 5, so the answer could be either 6 or 7. The question asks for the smallest possible value of x, so the correct answer is 6.

---

14 – A. 84

First, find the number of girls in the class. Convert 52% to a decimal by moving the decimal point two places to the left:

$$52\% = .52$$

Now, multiply .52 times the number of students in the class:

$$.52 * 350 = 182$$

Of the 182 girls, 98 plan to go to college, so 84 do not plan to go to college.

$$182 - 98 = 84$$

---

15 –   C. $300

If the phone was on sale at 30% off, the sale price was 70% of the original price. So

$$\$210 = 70\% \text{ of } x$$

where x is the original price of the phone. When you convert 70% to a decimal, you get:

$$\$210 = .70 * x$$

To isolate x on one side of the equation, divide both sides of the equation by .70. You find that $x = \$300$.

---

16 –   A. 10

Use the facts you are given to write an equation:
$$7 + 4/5n = 15$$

First, subtract 7 from both sides of the equation. You get:
$$4/5n = 8$$

Now divide both sides of the equation by 4/5. To divide by a fraction, invert the fraction (4/5 becomes 5/4) and multiply:

$$n = \frac{8}{1} * \frac{5}{4}$$

$$n = \frac{40}{4}$$

$$n = 10$$

---

17 –   D. 108

The ratio of the two numbers is 7:3. This means that the larger number is 7/10 of 360 and the smaller number is 3/10 of 360.

$$\frac{3}{10} * \frac{360}{1} = \frac{1,080}{10} = 108$$

---

18 –   A. 20

Alicia must have a score of 75% on a test with 80 questions. To find how many questions she must answer correctly, first convert 75% to a decimal by moving the decimal point two places to the left: 75% = .75. Now multiply .75 times 80:

$$.75 * 80 = 60.$$

Alicia must answer 60 questions correctly, but the question asks how many questions can she miss. If she must answer 60 correctly, then she can miss 20.

19 –   B. 3,024 cubic inches

The formula for the volume of a rectangular solid is length * width * height. So the volume of this box is:

$$18 * 12 * 14 = 3{,}024 \text{ cubic inches}$$

20 –   B. Perpendicular

Lines that form a right angle are called perpendicular.

21 –   C. 15 square feet

This shape is called a parallelogram. The area of a parallelogram equals the base times the height.

22 –   D. 0.72

The simplest way to answer this question is to convert the fractions to decimals. To convert a fraction to a decimal, divide the numerator (the top number) by the denominator (the bottom number).

$$5/8 = 0.625$$
$$3/5 = 0.6$$
$$2/3 = 0.67$$

The largest number is 0.72.

23 –   A. 11

If Charles wrote an average of 7 pages per day for four days, he wrote a total of 28 pages. He wrote a total of 17 pages on the first three days, so he must have written 11 pages on the fourth day.

24 –   B. 3.44 square feet

Find the area of the square by multiplying the length of a side by itself. The area of the square is 16 square feet. Now find the area of the circle by using this formula:

$$A = \pi r^2$$

The symbol π equals approximately 3.14. The letter r is the radius of the circle. In this case, r is half the width of the square (or 2), so r^2 is 4. Therefore, the area of the circle is

$$A = 3.14 * 4$$
$$A = 12.56$$

To find the area of the square that is not covered by the circle, subtract 12.56 square feet from 16 square feet.

25 –   B. $\dfrac{20}{mp^2}$

To divide by a fraction, invert the second fraction and multiply.

So $\dfrac{5}{mp} \div \dfrac{p}{4}$ becomes $\dfrac{5}{mp} * \dfrac{4}{p}$

$$\frac{5}{mp} * \frac{4}{p} = \frac{20}{mp^2}$$

26 – **B. 10 miles**

If you made a simple map with these three cities, it would look like this:

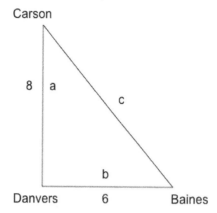

This is a right triangle. The longest side of a right triangle is called the hypotenuse. The two legs of the triangle are labeled *a* and *b*. The hypotenuse is labeled *c*. You can find the length of the hypotenuse (the distance between Caron and Baines) by using this equation:

$$a^2 + b^2 = c^2$$

In this case, the equation would be:

$$8^2 + 6^2 = c^2$$

or

$$64 + 36 = c^2$$

$$100 = c^2$$

To find *c*, ask yourself: What number times itself equals 100? The answer is 10.

---

27 – **C. 3/36**

When you roll a pair of 6-sided dice, there are 36 possible combinations of numbers (or outcomes) that can result. There are six numbers on each of the dice, so there are 6 * 6 possible combinations. Only three of those combinations will yield a total of 10: 4+6, 5+5, and 6+4. Much of the time, probability answers will be given in the form of simplified fractions. In this case, the correct answer could also have been 1/12.

---

28 – **A. $144**

When one person dropped out of the arrangement, the cost for the remaining three went up by $12 per person for a total of $36. This means that each person's share was originally $36. There were four people in the original arrangement, so the cost of the gift was 4 * $36, or $144.

Or alternatively:

Let 4x equal the original cost of the gift. If the number of shares decreases to 3, then the total cost is 3(x+12). Those expressions must be equal, so:

$$4x = 3(x+12)$$
$$4x = 3x +36$$

Subtracting 3x from both sides, we get:

$$x = 36$$

Then the original price of the gift was 4 times 36, or $144.

---

29 – C. 120

The factorial of a number is the product of all the integers less than or equal to the number. The factorial of 5 is 5 * 4 * 3 * 2 * 1 = 120. The factorial is written this way: 5!

---

30 – D. 7

In this number:
1 is in the thousands place.
2 is in the hundreds place.
3 is in the tens place.
4 is in the ones place
5 is in the tenths place.
6 is in the hundredths place.
7 is in the thousandths place.

---

31 – B. 4

The mode is the number that appears most often in a set of numbers.
Since 4 appears three times, it is the "Mode."

---

32 – C. 49

A perfect square is the product of an integer times itself. In this question, 49 is a perfect square because it is the product of 7 and 7.

---

33 – A. (14 + 24) * 8 * 5

In the correct answer, (14 + 24) * 8 * 5, the hourly wages of Amanda and Oscar are first combined, and then this amount is multiplied by 8 hours in a day and five days in a week. One of the other choices, 14 + 24 * 8 * 5, looks similar to this, but it is incorrect because the hourly wages must be combined before they can be multiplied by 8 and 5.

---

34 – D. 130,500

The population of Mariposa County in 2015 was 90% of its population in 2010. Convert 90% to a decimal by moving the decimal point two places to the left: 90% = .90. Now multiply .90 times 145,000 (the population in 2010).

$$.90 * 145,000 = 130,500$$

35 – C. 17/24

To add 1/3 and 3/8, you must find a common denominator. The simplest way to do this is to multiply the denominators: 3 * 8 = 24. Therefore, 24 is a common denominator. (This method will not always give you the <u>lowest</u> common denominator, but it does in this case.)

Once you have found a common denominator, you need to convert both fractions in the problem to equivalent fractions that have that same denominator. To do this, multiply each fraction by an equivalent of 1.

$$\frac{1}{3} * \frac{8}{8} = \frac{8}{24}$$

$$\frac{3}{8} * \frac{3}{3} = \frac{9}{24}$$

Now you can add 8/24 and 9/24 to solve the problem.

36 – B. Serena is 7, Tom is 4

Use S to represent Serena's age. Tom is 3 years younger than Serena, so his age is S–3. In 4 years, Tom will be twice as old as Serena was 3 years ago. So you can write this equation:

$$Tom + 4 = 2(Serena - 3)$$

Now substitute S for Serena and S–3 for Tom.

$$(S - 3) + 4 = 2(S - 3)$$

Simplify the equation.

$$S + 1 = 2S - 6$$

Subtract S from both sides of the equation. You get:

$$1 = S - 6$$

Add 6 to both sides of the equation. You get:

$$7 = S, \text{ Serena's age}$$

$$4 = S - 3, \text{ Tom's age}$$

37 – A. Length = 12, width = 4

Use w to represent the width of the rectangle. The length is three times the width, so the length is $3w$. The area of the rectangle is the length times the width, so the area is $w * 3w$, or $3w^2$.

$$3w^2 = 48$$

Divide both sides of the equation by 3. You get:

$$w^2 = 16$$

$$w = 4, \text{ the width of the rectangle}$$
$$3w = 12, \text{ the length of the rectangle}$$

38 – B. 24 = 2 * 2 * 2 * 3

The prime factors of a number are the prime numbers that divide that number evenly. The prime factorization of a number is a list of the prime factors that must be multiplied to yield that number.

The simplest method of finding the prime factorization is to start with a simple multiplication fact for that number. In this case, we could have chosen:

$$24 = 6 * 4$$

The prime factorization of 24 includes the prime factorization of both 6 and 4. Since $6 = 2 * 3$ and $4 = 2 * 2$, the prime factorization of 24 must be:

$$\underline{24 = 2 * 2 * 2 * 3}$$

39 – A. A number greater than x

When a positive number is divided by a positive number less than 1, the quotient will always be larger than the number being divided. For example, $5 \div 0.5 = 10$. If we solve this as a fraction, $5 \div (1/2)$ is the same as $5 * (2/1)$, which equals 10, since dividing by a fraction is the same as multiplying by the reciprocal.

40 – C. x = 11

Subtracting a negative number is the same as adding a positive number. So $8 - (-3)$ is the same as $8 + 3$, which equals 11.

41 – C. The square of a number is always a positive number.

When two numbers with the same sign (positive or negative) are multiplied, the product is always positive. When a number is squared, it is multiplied by itself, so the numbers being multiplied have the same sign. Therefore, the product is always positive.

The square of a number greater than 1 is always greater than the number. But the square of a positive number less than one (for example 0.5) is always less than the original number.

42 –   B. 515

Marisol scored higher than 78% of the students who took the test. Convert 78% to a decimal by moving the decimal point two places to the left: 78% = .78. Now multiply .78 times the number of students who took the test:

$$.78 * 660 = 514.8 \text{ or } 515 \text{ students (must be whole numbers)}$$

43 –   D. $12

Use the information given to write an equation:

$$530 = 40d + 50$$

When you subtract 50 from both sides of the equation, you get:

$$480 = 40d$$

Divide both sides of the equation by 40.

$$12 = d, \text{ Sam's hourly wage}$$

44 –   D. $r = \dfrac{p-3}{2}$

Begin by subtracting 3 from both sides of the equation. You get:

$$p - 3 = 2r$$

Now, to isolate r on one side of the equation, divide both sides of the equation by 2. You get:

$$r = \frac{p-3}{2}$$

45 –   B. 40

The least common multiple is used when finding the lowest common denominator. The least common multiple is the lowest number that can be divided evenly by both of the numbers.

Here is a simple method to find the least common multiple of 8 and 10. Write 8 on the left side of your paper, then add 8 and write the result, then add another 8 to that number and write the result. Keep going until you have a list that looks something like this:

8 16 24 32 40…

This is a partial list of multiples of 8. (If you remember your multiplication tables, these numbers are the column or row that go with 8.)

Now do the same thing with 10.

10 20 30 40 ...

This is the partial list of multiples of 10.

Eventually, similar numbers will appear in both rows. The smallest of these numbers is the least common multiple. There will always be more multiples that are found in both rows, but the smallest number is the least common multiple.

---

46 –   D. $x = 4$

When you multiply or divide numbers that have the same sign (both positive or both negative), the answer will be positive. When you multiply or divide numbers that have different signs (one positive and the other negative), the answer will be negative. In this case, both numbers have the same sign. Divide as you normally would, and remember that the answer will be a positive number.

---

47 –   A. $2\dfrac{5}{6}$

To convert an improper fraction to a mixed number, divide the numerator by the denominator. In this case, you get 2 with a remainder of 5. 2 becomes the whole number portion of the mixed number, and 5 becomes the numerator of the fraction.

---

48 –   B. –10

To find the value of q, divide both sides of the equation by –13. When a positive number is divided by a negative number, the answer is negative.

---

49 –   A. 12

Replace the letters with the numbers they represent, then perform the necessary operations.

$$3^2 + 6(0.5)$$

$$9 + 3 = 12$$

---

50 –   B. 32 inches

The radius of a circle is one-half the diameter, so the diameter of this circle is 8 inches. The diameter is a line that passes through the center of a circle and joins two points on its circumference. If you study this figure, you can see that the diameter of the circle is the same as the length of each side of the square. The diameter is 8 inches, so the perimeter of the square is 32 inches (8+ 8 + 8 + 8).

SCIENCE

1- B. Cilia

Cilia that are located on the outer membrane of bronchial epithelial cells are motile hairlike extension whose motion tends to move substances out of the airways toward the pharynx. Microvilli are found on the villi of intestinal epithelial cells. Flagella are found on sperm cells, but no other cells in the human body. Dendrites are thin branching cellular extensions of neuron cell membranes.

2- D. bile; small intestine

Fats molecules are primarily hydrocarbon in content and are therefore not soluble in water. To absorb fats the liver produces bile that is secreted into the duodenum. Fats are soluble in bile so bile is able to break large fat globules into smaller droplets which can be more easily absorbed into the body. The process of fat globule dissolution is call emulsification. Amylase is a digestive enzyme that breaks down certain carbohydrates.

3- D. intercellular membrane binding

The role of T-helper cells in immune responses involves the binding of membrane bound molecules, usually receptors or membrane bound antigens or antibodies between the T-helper cells and other immune system cells including B-cells and antigen-presenting cells, such as macrophages. T-helper cells can produce antibodies that bind to their own membranes, but do not produce antibodies that are released into the circulation (B-cells do this). T-helper cells do not directly cause lysis of other dells and do not engage in phagocytosis.

4- A. It passes through capillaries before returning to the internal chambers of the heart

Rationale: Blood is pumped out of the heart through either the pulmonic valve as deoxygenated blood to the pulmonary artery or secondly, through the aortic valve as oxygenated blood to the aorta. All blood, once it leaves the heart, must pass through capillaries before it returns to the internal chambers of the heart

5- D. continuously throughout the entire respiratory cycle

Deoxygenated blood is pumped through alveolar capillaries continuously throughout the respiratory cycle. If oxygen were not diffusing into the capillaries throughout each of the stages of the inspiratory cycle, the blood passing through the alveolar capillaries would not be oxygenated. This deoxygenated blood would return to the heart and mix with oxygenated blood, lowering the oxygen saturation level of the blood that is then pumped out of the heart through the aorta. Blood exiting the heart through the aorta is nearly 100% saturated so there is no inspiratory phase where oxygen is not passing into the circulatory system through the alveoli into their surrounding capillaries.

6- A. sensory input

The integrative functions of the nervous system occur in the brain, where sensory input is utilized to create memories and to help generate thought processes. This does not require hormonal regulation. Effector cells are cells that carry out instructions from the nervous system at locations throughout the body. This is not classified as integrative neurological function. Spinal cord reflexes are, for the most part, independent of the central nervous system and are not required for integrative functions.

7- B. CCK and secretin

Pepsinogen is a proenzyme released by the stomach and trypsinogen is a proenzyme released by the pancreas. CCK (cholecystokinin) is a hormone that stimulates the release of bile from the gall bladder and secretin is hormone that stimulates the release of bicarbonate from the pancreas. Both CCK and secretin are released by the duodenum.

8- C. production of antibodies

The innate immune system generates non-specific immune responses. Phagocytosis of foreign cells by macrophages, the stimulation of fever by the release of interleukins, and the release of and response to cytokines by cells involved in the innate immune responses is triggered by a wide variety of infectious agents or chemicals generated by tissue injury. the innate immune responses are then carried out through biochemical pathways and cell activities that do not require the participation of antibodies or the recognition of a specific antigens. Antibodies are produced by B-cells, which are required for activity of the humoral category of the body's adaptive immune system. B-cells do not participate in the innate immune responses.

9- A. The heart if ventral to the esophagus

The term ventral means toward the umbilical (belly button) abdominal wall versus the opposite direction, dorsal, which means, in this positional terminology, toward the spine. Proximal means toward the midline of the body, so it also can be interpreted as toward or closer to the spine, but this is contrasted with the opposite of proximal, which is described by the term distal, meaning away from the spine. Medial is used to describe relative locations toward any central axis of the body with the opposite relationship described by the term lateral, meaning to the side of that which is medial. Rostral indicates a relative position closer to the skull with the term caudal meaning a relative position that is closer to the base of the spine.

10- A. the liver

Urea is water-soluble, non-toxic molecule synthesized for the purpose of ridding the body of waste products generated by the catabolism of nitrogen containing compounds such as nucleic acids and proteins. Although urea is excreted through the kidneys it is synthesized by liver parenchymal cells.

11- D. the large intestine

All organs of the body must receive a direct arterial supply of oxygenated blood. The lungs also receive deoxygenated blood through the pulmonary artery, which is then oxygenated as it passes through alveolar capillaries. The heart receives deoxygenated blood through the superior and inferior vena cava veins which empty into the right atrium. The liver receives deoxygenated blood through the hepatic portal vein, which carries blood that has passed through capillaries in the small intestines. The large intestine, along with most of the other organs or organ regions of the body, receives supplies of oxygenated blood only.

12- B. the diaphragm

One is not expected to know the names of all of the voluntary muscles in the body, but the major voluntary muscles, such as the biceps are expected knowledge. the masseters are the muscles that cause the lower jaw to close. This is beyond expected knowledge but it is a higher level of anatomical knowledge that is not specifically, but as a category of superior mastery, included to distinguish the top levels of performance. At the expected knowledge level is that the diaphragm is the muscle that generates inhalation, that one can for brief periods of time voluntarily inhale or suppress inhalation but usually the inhalation process is involuntary, and always involuntary when one is asleep.

13- C. the small intestines

This question is often missed because most students know that the primary role of the large intestine is to absorb water. Nevertheless, 80% of water that passes through the digestive system is absorbed through the small intestine.

14- B. natural killer (NK) cells

Perforins are small molecules that are secreted by natural killer cells. They insert themselves into the cell membrane of the natural killer's target cell - the cell that the natural killer wants to kill - and arrange themselves to form a hole or perforation in the target cell's cell membrane. When sufficient quantities of these hole have been created. the target cell's internal contents leak away, its internal environment is increasingly diluted and its internal organelles are destabilized then rendered inoperable, and finally the target cell dies.

15- C. inadequate intake during childhood development can lead to the disease kwashiorkor

Kwashiorkor is a severe form of malnourishment which is usually fatal. It is specifically the result of inadequate protein intake that occurs children usually after the age of 18 months. Vegetarians can obtain all required dietary protein through non-animal or animal product sources -rice and legumes are sufficient for example. There are nine essential amino acids which must be obtained through the diet. The remaining amino acids can be synthesized by the body. The breakdown of proteins begins within the stomach.

16- A. Eubacteria and Archaebacteria

Before the introduction of the broadest category of living organisms, domains, kingdoms were the broadest category. Subsequently extensive genetic and biochemical analysis of species that had been classified as bacteria were found to differ from other bacteria in more fundamental ways that other bacteria differ from organisms in other kingdoms. This lead to the creation of the higher level category of "domain", with the Bacteria kingdom divided into two separate domains The Eubacteria and the Archaea or Archaebacteria. All other organisms are now assigned to the third domain, Eukarya.

17- B. Mutations in the germ line cells of the fertile members of the species must be able to occur

Without the possibility of the occurrence of mutations in DNA that can be passed to offspring, which is germline DNA found only in germline cells, no new genes or variations of genes in the form of alleles could be created. All offspring would have genes contained only in the genepool of the previous generation. One might argue that speciation could occur for a limited amount of time and to a limited extent by adaptation through natural selection for fitter combination of alleles that were already present in the previous generation's gene pool. This is actually an invalid argument however because it overlooks the fact that without germline mutations, there is no mechanism for the production of any alleles of genes to begin with.

18- C. a phosphate group, a pentose sugar and a nitrogenous base

In both RNA and DNA molecules, the backbone of a continuous single DNA or RNA molecular chain is an alternating sequence of cyclic 5-carbon sugars (pentoses) bonded to phosphate groups (PO4). each pentose sugar is also bonded to one of five possible nitrogenous bases. nitrogenous bases in nucleic acids are small, cyclic nitrogen-containing molecules consisting of either one or two rings. A nucleotide is defined as a molecular subunit consisting of one of these nitrogenous base that bonded to a nucleic acid pentose sugar and a phosphate group that is also bonded to the same pentose sugar. Any DNA or RNA segment can be built entirely from combinations of theses nucleotide subunits.

19- D. Some, but not all, eukaryotic cells have chloroplasts, but no prokaryotic cells have chloroplasts

Prokaryotic cells do not possess a nucleus. Prokaryotic cell DNA is organized into a structures called a nucleoid which analogous to a nucleus in eukaryotic cells. Cell walls are present in eukaryotic kingdoms of Plantae and Fungi and some organisms of the kingdom Protozoa, but not in any organisms in the kingdom Animalia. All organisms of the kingdom Plantae and some of the kingdom Protozoa have chloroplasts. No prokaryotes have chloroplasts. Every living cell contains ribosomes.

20- B. ribosomes

Ribosomes are protein complexes that may be free-floating within a cell's cytoplasm or, at times, attached to a cell's endoplasmic reticulum. It is simply a fact that they do not possess outer membranes, or, in fact, any membranes whatsoever. There is strong evidence that mitochondria, chloroplasts and the nuclei of eukaryotic cells evolved from prokaryotic cells that were ingested by other prokaryotic cells but survived and evolved to their present state within the evolutionary descendants of these cells. This is a compelling explanation for why these organelles possess encapsulating membranes.

21- D. The mRNA segment base sequence is identical to the complementary DNA strand segment of the gene base sequence except that uracil is substituted for thymine in the mRNA base sequence

An important and common misconception regarding RNA transcriptions of a gene is that the RNA transcription is a copy of the DNA gene segment except that uracil is substituted for thymine in the RNA sequence. In fact, the RNA segment is the compliment of the gene sequence, except that in the RNA transcript, uracil is substituted for by thymine.

22- A. Individual tissue layers begin to form

By definition, the gastrulation stage of development is the stage where individual tissue layers begin to form. The first multipotent stem cells begin to appear, and the four fundamental cell types begin to differentiate before the gastrulation stage. The organ differentiation stage occurs after the gastrulation stage

23- A. prophase, G1 and G2

The normal somatic cell cycle is divided into the mitotic and the non-mitotic stages. The non-mitotic stage is referred to as interphase. Interphase is divided into three subphases, G1, S, and G2. The mitotic stage of the cell cycle is divided into four stages; prophase, metaphase, anaphase and telophase. Cytokinesis refers to the physical separation of a cell into two daughter cells. This occurs during anaphase and telophase of mitosis in a normal somatic cell cycle and during anaphase and telophase of meiosis I and II of gamete cell production in the germ-line cell cycle.

24- B. individual tetrads align

Tetrads are formations of closely aligned homologous chromosome pairs where each chromosome is in the form where it consists of two identical sister chromatids. Tetrads only form during meiosis I. they can exchange chromatid segments as they are pulled apart during anaphase of meiosis I This is referred to as crossing over. When crossing over occurs, 2 new hybrid chromosomes are formed.

25- B. 6

During photosynthesis the following chemical reaction occurs:

$6CO_2 + 6H_2O + sunlight \rightarrow C_6H_{12}O_6 + 6O_2$. You should be able to balance simple chemical reactions and to know that photosynthesis uses carbon dioxide and water to produce glucose and oxygen. This gives an initial unbalanced reaction of $\_CO + \_H_2O \rightarrow C_6H_{12}O_6 + \_O_2$. There are 12 hydrogens in glucose so there must be $6H_2O$ molecules on the left side of the reaction. there are 6 carbon atoms in glucose so there must be 6 CO_2 molecules on the left side of the equation. The total number of Oxygen atoms required is 6 from 6 H_2O and 6x2=12 from $6CO_2$. This gives a total of 6+12=18 Oxygen atoms. Six oxygen atoms are used to form one glucose molecule leaving 12 or 12/2=6 O_2 molecules on the right side of the balanced equation.

26- B. A single, unique three-base codon will code for only one single, unique type of amino acid

This is a question that is commonly answered incorrectly. DNA is comprised, in part, of a linear sequence of nitrogenous base subunits. these subunits can be any of four different nitrogenous bases. These bases transmit genetic information in the form of 3-base unit sequences that are called codons. Statistically there are 64 possible 3-base sequences that can be constructed from a combination of these four different DNA bases.

27- B. identical genotypes only

Perfectly identical twins will have exactly the same genotypes. They may have different phenotypes because phenotypic expression is often dependent on the environment. Identical twins raised in different environments likely have obvious phenotypic differences.

28- B. H_2CO_3 is a weak acid

A strong base in that results from the deprotonation of an acid will strongly accept hydrogen ion, so the reverse reaction is favored, meaning the acid is preferentially more protonated than deprotonated at equilibrium This is the definition of a weak acid.

29- C. electromagnetic energy

Although the sun does emit vast amounts of electrons and protons in the form of the solar wind, the energy carried by the solar wind that reaches the earth is miniscule in comparison to the energy that is emitted by the sun in the form of electromagnetic waves that is received by the earth. The majority of this electromagnetic radiation is in the visible light wavelength spectrum.

30- A. a 5 kg mass, at rest, 10 m above the surface of the earth

Gravitational potential energy of an object is given by the equation Fg=mgh, where m is the object's mass and h is the object's height above the surface of the earth. The velocity of an object contributes nothing to the object's gravitational potential energy. For choice C, the object is actually below the surface of the earth so in a sense it actually has negative potential energy. For choice D, the object is at the surface of the earth so its potential energy is zero regardless of its mass. Between choices A and B, the mass of the objects is irrelevant because they are equal. The object in A has twice the potential energy compared to the object in B because object A's height above the earth's surface is twice that of object B's height.

31- B. connective tissue

An organized functional collection of a single type of cell is considered to be a tissue. Adipose cells (fat cells) are classified as a type of connective cell and therefore adipose cell tissue is connective tissue. A syncytium is a collection of cells that have to some extent fused such that cytoplasm can circulate throughout the entire collection of cells, A gland is an organized cell structure that secretes substance through a duct.

32- C. increases the rate of the reaction; increasing the activation energy

The efficiency of a reaction is the actual yield compared to the theoretical yield of products of the reaction. This is a function of the conditions under which the reaction occurs, but it is not affected by the presence of a catalyst. A catalyst increases the rate of a reaction by lowering the activation energy of the reaction. The activation energy is the difference between the energy of the reactants and the highest energy transition state between reactants and products. Lowering the energy of this transition state increases the probability that reactants will have sufficient energy to achieve the transition state so that the reaction can proceed to the final product state.

33- A. 1s2 2s2 2p6

The electron subshells of an atom beginning with the lowest energy subshells are the 1s, 2s, 2p, 3s, 3d and 3p subshells. The s subshells are filled when they contain 2 electrons. The p subshells are filled when they contain a total of 6 electrons. Neon, with an atomic number of 10 will in have neutral atoms with ten electrons and in the lowest energy state these will fill the lowest available energy levels. This corresponds to an electron configuration of 1s2 2s2 2p6

34- C. The enzyme has increased its effect on the rate of a chemical reaction

Enzyme activity is quantified, for the biochemical reaction that the enzyme catalyzes, as the amount of product generated per unit time. In general, it indicates how fast a reaction is occurring. The major factors that affect an enzyme's ability to increase the rate of a reaction are temperature, pH at which the reaction occurs and concentrations of the reactants and products of the reaction.

35- B. ammonia, blood, orange juice

Sulphuric acid is a strong acid so it will have a very low pH relative to either orange juice or vinegar which are weak acids. All acids by definition will have a pH that is lower than water. Water is neutral by definition, with a pH of 7.0. Blood is nearly neutral but slightly basic with a pH of 7.4 which is higher than any acid pH. Ammonia is a strong base so its pH will higher than any acid pH or any substances with a pH that is close to neutral pH.

36- A. The alkane contains 4 less hydrogen atoms than does the alkyne

Rationale: When an alkane is converted to an alkyne, two adjacent carbons in the alkane each break the bonds with two of their bonded hydrogens and then form two new carbon-carbon bonds between the two adjacent carbons resulting in the formation of a carbon-carbon triple bond. In the process the alkane loses the four hydrogens whose carbon-hydrogen bonds were broken during the triple bond formation process.

37- B. the adrenal gland

Steroid hormones are produced in the adrenal gland, in the gonads primarily. The pancreas produces insulin and glucagon which are peptide hormones. The thyroid hormones are also peptide hormones. The thymus is the site of T-cell maturation. It does not secrete any hormones.

38- B. $2O_2 + 8e- ---> 4O-2$

In oxidation-reduction reactions the reactants give product molecules that have covalent bonds, but there is a large difference in the electronegativities between the bonded atoms in the product molecules. The atoms in these molecules are not ions but they can be thought of as having strong ionic character, and that they undergo electron loss or electron acquisition as shown for the two molecules of oxygen in the answer choice B. Within a common solution environment these ions are never actually present, but if the reactants are separated into different reaction vessels and connected by an electrically conductive wire and a salt bridge, electrons will flow from the less electronegative species to the more electronegative species through the wire. This is how chemical batteries are constructed

39- B. The temperature of the liquid bromine will remain constant

The question describes a liquid that is undergoing a phase transition from liquid to gas. During phase transitions that require the input of energy (heat), the energy applied to the particles undergoing the transition does not result in any increase in temperature. Instead, the applied energy is consumed by the processes that allow particles to transition between the two phases.

40- A. the same type of

There are no different types of intermolecular bonding that occur among water molecules in the solid phase compared to the liquid phase. The difference is that the kinetic energy of water molecules in the solid phase is insufficient to overcome the intermolecular bonds that hold the water molecules in a fixed position relative to surrounding water molecules. In the liquid phase, water molecules have sufficient kinetic energy to change position within the liquid but insufficient energy to completely break free of intermolecular bonds and thus become gas phase water molecules.

41- C. class; order

The hierarchy of modern taxonomic classification categories, beginning with the broadest, most inclusive category is: domain, kingdom, phylum, class, order, family, genus and species.

42- C. every functional gene can be transcribed into a mRNA molecule

A single chromosome can exist in two different forms. In the singular form it contains a full set of genes, there may be more than one copy of a given gene and there may be more than one version of a given gene - which is called an allele located on the chromosome. It is not true that there are always two copies or two alleles of a gene on this version of a chromosome. In preparation for cell division, a copy of the single chromosome is made resulting in a version of the chromosome that consists of two identical sister chromatids. In this version there are always at least two copies of every gene, but not at least two alleles for every gene. Only one strand of a double -stranded DNA molecule contains genes. The other strand contains the complementary sequence of the DNA's genes, but this strand cannot be transcribed into RNA that will code for any gene proteins. By definition, a gene is a sequence of DNA bases that can be translated into a protein and this requires that every gene be capable of being first transcribed into a messenger RNA molecule.

43- B. UCG AUG GGC

In DNA, complementary base pairing occurs between adenine (A) and thymine (T) and between guanine (G) and cytosine (C). In RNA, the same complementary base relationship is true except that the complementary base of adenine is uracil (U) rather than thymine. The base sequence in choice B correctly identifies the complementary base sequence for RNA to the base sequence for DNA that is given within the question.

44- D. nucleoli

Nucleoli are located with the nucleus of cells. These are the organelles that are responsible for the construction of ribosomes. Peroxisomes and lysosomes are intracellular vesicles that contain specific types of substances, but they are not involved in ribosome construction. Ribosomes are attached to the endoplasmic reticular membranes in rough endoplasmic reticulum, but they are not constructed by the endoplasmic reticulum.

45- C. RNA polymerase

Ribosomes are the structures that physically assemble proteins by reading RNA base sequences and connecting amino acids to form a chain of amino acids, which is, by definition, a protein. RNA polymerase is the structure, in the form of an enzyme complex, that physically assembles messenger RNA molecules by reading DNA base sequences and connecting nucleotides to form a chain of nucleotides, which becomes the messenger RNA molecule.

46- D. Replication of both strands occurs simultaneously

The process of replication of double-stranded DNA begins with the breaking of hydrogen bonds between a small sequence of complementary base pairs at a single site on the DNA molecule This creates a gap within the DNA that allows a DNA polymerase enzyme complex to enter and to begin adding nucleotides with complementary bases to both the sense and antisense strands of the original DNA, The process differs somewhat between the two strands, but replication proceeds simultaneously on both strands.

47- B. centrosomes and chromosomes

The role of spindle fibers during mitosis is to separate the sister chromatids of each chromosome and then draw one of each chromatid pair to opposite sides of the dividing cell. This occurs by the connection of microtubules to the central region of the chromosome and then to either of the two centrosomes located on opposite sides of the cell. The microtubules then begin to shorten and move, along with an attached sister chromatid, towards either one or the other centrosomes. The process of cytokinesis follows and results in the production of two daughter cells, each containing one set of the sister chromatids.

48- B. absorption of sunlight

Chlorophyll molecules are located in the chloroplasts of cells that are capable of photosynthesis. Chlorophyll molecules absorb visible light wavelength photons and convert the photon energy into chemical energy stored in the bonds of carbohydrate molecules

49- A. purines and pyrimidines

Purines and pyrimidines are the two structural categories of nitrogenous bases that are found in DNA and RNA. The purines are guanine and adenine; the pyrimidines are thymine cytosine and uracil. The major structural difference between the two is that purines have a two-ring structure and pyrimidines have a one-ring structure.

50- A. 1 base error per 1000 genes

Without error correction mechanisms, this baseline level of error in DNA replication would result in extinction of a species within a few or possibly only one generation. Choice D is the final estimated error rate in human DNA after replication and subsequent error corrections of DNA by various repair mechanisms.

ENGLISH & READING

1. A. affected; effect; ought

Since a verb is needed in the first blank, "affected" not "effected" (a noun) will work; but the noun "effect" is correct in the second blank. "ought", meaning "should" correctly completes the sentence, indicating he should not drive. "aught", meaning zero, or nothing, or none, does not make sense in this context.

2. C. Hiking along the trail, we were assailed by the chirping of birds, which made our nature walk hardly the peaceful exercise we had wanted.

Who was hiking along the trail? "we" were, so only option C works. The other options are dangling participles: in option b, the birds were not attempting to hike, so that doesn't make sense; in option a, again, the birds were hiking along the trail, so that makes no sense; option d is just poorly constructed and makes the meaning overall unclear.

3. D. processed

"Processed" modifies "food products" so that is the adjective; "really" is an adverb modifying the adjective "serious"; "challenge" is a noun, which is a person, place or thing; "consume" is a verb, a word that shows action.

4. B. My husband and I attended my daughter's dance recital and were very proud when she received an award.

The most clear and concise sentence is option b; all the information is included, it is presented logically, it flows smoothly off the tongue, and it is not overly wordy.

5. D. Since the concert ended very late, I fell asleep in the backseat during the car ride home.

Option d is correct. "Since the concert ended very late" is a dependent clause which explains why "I fell asleep…"; since they are dependent, the only proper way to link them is with a comma.

6. D. they're

This question asks you make pronoun and antecedent agree; in this sentence the antecedent is "negotiations"; since this is a plural noun, the pronoun must also be plural, but the blank is also missing a verb. The only option with a plural pronoun and a verb is the contraction "they're".

7. A. is

"Group", a singular noun, is the subject of the sentence, so a singular verb is needed. Also needed is a present tense helping verb for "looking forward". The only option that satisfies both is "is".

8. C. Exclamatory

An exclamatory sentence is a type of sentence that expresses strong feelings by making an exclamation. Therefore, the above sentence is an exclamatory sentence.

9. A. Irregardless

"Irregardless" is incorrect as it is a double-negative: the suffix "less" already indicates a lack of regard, so the addition of the negative "ir" before the correct word, ***regardless,*** is unnecessary.

10. C. Between you and me, I brought back fewer books from my dorm room than I needed to study for my exam.

"Brought" is the correct past tense form of *bring*; "fewer" is the correct word to describe an exact number of items, whereas "less" is used to refer to an amount of something that cannot be exactly counted, like sand or air or water; and "than" is the correct spelling of the word that shows a comparison between two things.

11. D. us; was

Words that follow prepositions are considered to be in the objective case, therefore "us" is the correct word here; "Neither", a single pronoun, is the subject of the sentence, so a singular verb, "was" is needed to properly complete it.

12. C. books

A noun is a person, place or thing. While a "library" is usually used as a noun to denote a place where people can go to borrow books, or look up information, in this sentence it is used as an adjective to modify "books", which is the only true noun in the sentence.

13. A. Mary and Samantha ran and skipped and hopped their way home from school every day.

A *simple sentence* is one which has *one subject and one verb*, though both the subject and verb can be compound. In this case, option a is a simple sentence, with the one subject being compound ("Mary and Samantha") and the one verb also being compound ("ran and skipped and hopped"). The other options either have *more than one subject or more than one verb.*

14. B. Matthew was tall and shy, and Thomas was short and talkative.

A *simple sentence* is one which has *one subject and one verb*, though both the subject and verb can be compound. Linked by the conjunction "and", sentence B is the only compound sentence above because it links the first sentence "Matthew was tall and shy" with the second sentence "Thomas was short and talkative".

15. D. "There's a bus coming, so hurry up and cross the street!" yelled Bob to the old woman.

"There's" is the subject and verb of the sentence written as a contraction so the apostrophe is needed; a comma is needed before "so" because what follows it is a dependent clause which must be separated from the single sentence with a comma. When writing dialogue, the punctuation is included inside the quotation marks; in this case an exclamation is appropriate because Bob is warning the old woman to get out of the way of the oncoming bus; the use of the verb "yelled" is a clue that the statement by Bob is exclamatory.

16. C. It's a long to-do list she left for us today: make beds; wash breakfast dishes; go grocery shopping; do laundry; cook dinner; and read the twins a bedtime story.

"It's" is the subject and verb joined together in a contraction, so an apostrophe is needed. The sentence introduces a list, so it must be preceded by a colon; because the list is comprised of phrases instead of single words, a semicolon is needed to separate each item.

17. A. My room was a mess so my mom made me clean it before I was allowed to leave the house.

The use of the possessive pronoun "my" and the singular pronoun "I" indicates that the sentence is written from the first person perspective. "You" and "your" are second person; "her" or "him" are third person.

---

18. C. The president of France is meeting with President Obama later this week.

When referring to the "president of France", "president" is just a noun denoting his position, so it is not capitalized. In the case of "President Obama", "President" is the title by which he is addressed, so it is a proper noun and requires capitalization. The other options are incorrectly capitalized.

---

19. D. climb; creak

"Climb" is the proper spelling to denote ascending the stairs; "clime" refers to climate. "Creak" denotes a squeaky sound; "creek" denotes a stream or small moving waterway.

---

20. D. I will have completed

The FUTURE PERFECT TENSE indicates that an action will have been finished at some point in the future. This tense is formed with "will" plus "have" plus the past participle of the verb (which can be either regular or irregular in form). "By this time next summer" is the clue that lets you know the coursework will be done some time in the future.

---

21. A. assent; aide

The word "Assent" means approval, which is what the teacher wants to do to show encouragement to novice teacher who is currently her "aide" or assistance in the classroom. "Ascent" denotes a climb; "aid" is a verb denoting the action of helping.

---

22. D. No one has offered to let us use their home for the office's end-of-year picnic.

"No one", a singular pronoun, requires a singular verb, "has". "Us" is the objective case pronoun which is needed to follow the verb "to let"; "ourselves" is the reflexive case which is not needed in this sentence; "we" is subjective. "Their" shows possession of "home"; spelled "there", this word denotes location (e.g. here or there).

---

23. C. The tornado struck without warning and caused extensive damage.

Incorporating all of the information from the four sentences logically and concisely, option C is the best choice.

---

24. C. caused

"Caused" is the verb in this sentence; "Carrying" is the subject. Though it may look like a verb, it is actually a gerund (a verb acting as a noun) which is the subject. Deleting extraneous words will help see this, so let's rewrite the sentence in its most basic form: "Carrying caused her to throw out her back." This way it is clear to see that "carrying" is the subject, and is not a verb.

---

25. B. My eyelids drooping and my feet going numb, I thought his boring lecture would never end.

This sentence most clearly concisely conveys all of the information in the four above sentences; structure is parallel and no awkward or extraneous words are included.

---

26. D. Comets are balls of dust and ice, comprised of leftover materials that did not become planets during the formation of our solar system.

"Comets" (a plural subject requiring a plural verb) "are" "comprised of" (meaning: made up of) leftover materials that "did not" (in the past) become planets during the formation of "our" solar system.

27. B. Improvements in printing resulted in the production of newspapers, as well as England's more fully recognizing the singular concept of reading as a form of leisure; it was, of itself, a new industry.

The sentence is a compound sentence (two complete subject and verb phrases), so these should be separated by a comma after newspapers. The possession of recognition of the singular concept of reading by England needs to be shown with an apostrophe plus "s": "England's".

28. A. era

The Victorian Era is a two-word proper noun referring to a time period in history so "era" should be capitalized. The other words should not be capitalized.

29. C. coresponding

The correct spelling is *corresponding*.

30. D. market

"this demand" refers back to the "*market* (for cheaper literature)" in the last sentence of paragraph 2.

31. C. Working class boys who could not afford a penny a week often formed clubs that would share the cost, passing the flimsy booklets from reader to reader.

This sentence most clearly and concisely expresses the idea of book sharing amongst working boys who could not afford to spend a penny every week to buy the penny dreadfuls.

32. B. gothic

The word Gothic is a proper adjective referring to a specific genre of literature. None of the other words in this sentence should be capitalized.

33. D. The penny dreadfuls were influential since they were in the words of one commentator "the most alluring and low-priced form of escapist reading available to ordinary youth."

The independent clause "in the words of one commentator" needs to be set off by commas on either end; and since it is a direct quote, the last part of the sentence needs to be in quotation marks. The period at the end of the sentence needs to be inside the quotation marks.

34. B. novels

A noun is a person, place or thing. "Novels" is a plural noun which denotes a *thing* that can be read. "Serial" and "sensational" are adjectives; "generally" is an adverb.

35. D. greater

An adjective is a word which describes a noun. In this sentence, "greater" is an adjective describing *fear*. "Circulation" and "literature" are nouns; "however" is a pronoun.

36. C. Paragraph 3

Paragraph mentions that penny dreadfuls were often plagiarized versions of other popular literature at the time, so this would be the best place to add a sentence of supporting detail about this.

37. A. baptist

As the word identifies King's religion, "Baptist" should be capitalized.

38. A. His efforts to achieve racial equality in the United States, and his staunch public advocacy of civil rights are undoubtedly among the most important cultural contributions made to society in the last century.

Using parallel structure and no extraneous verbiage, option A is the most clear and concise of the versions.

39. D. I Have a Dream

"I Have a Dream" is the title of a speech and should therefore be put inside quotation marks.

40. B. Piece

In this sentence, "Piece" should be spelled *Peace*, as in harmony or an absence of fighting.

41. D. Metal

In this sentence, "Metal" should be spelled "Medal", as an award or honor, not "metal" as in a naturally occurring element or raw material.

42. C. This speech alienated many of his liberal allies in government who supported the war, but to his credit King never allowed politics to dictate the path of his noble works. (P. 3)

The phrase "to his credit" and the description of his works as "noble" provide clues that the author has a positive perspective about Martin Luther King and the role his activism played in American history.

43. C. No, because the passage is about King's public life and works, and information about his family would be irrelevant.

The focus of the passage is about King's work as a minister and activist, so details about his family are unrelated to this focus, and therefore should be left out.

44. C. "I am making pancakes for breakfast. Does anybody want some?" asked mom.

Only option C correctly includes sentence punctuation for quoted statements: punctuation for dialogue should be inside quotation marks, as is illustrated with mom asking if anyone wants pancakes; the question mark is within the quotation marks.

45. B. I woke up early that morning and began to do long-neglected household chores.

Option B contains two simple sentences, which when combined make a compound sentence:" I woke up early than morning" AND "I began to do long-neglected household chores."

46. D. A, C, E, D, B

The most logical progression of ideas is in option D. The topic of Disney's public persona is introduced, and is then contrasted with his treatment of people at work, and then the transformation of his persona from that of an American patriot to an imperialist. Finally, the paragraph is wrapped up with statements about the importance of his work and his current legacy in popular culture.

47. C. began to have

The sentence is discussing the contrast between Disney's private and public personas, stating that he *began to have* a public persona which was very different than the way he was in private.

48. A. You had better call and RSVP to the party right away before you forget.

Statements which show direct address, and use the pronoun "you" are referred to as the second person. Though the exclamation uses the pronoun you, it is a quoted statement, so it is really in the third person. Only choice A is an example of second person writing.

49. D. Parents are reminded to pick up their children from school promptly at 2:30.

Only D makes proper use of pronouns and their antecedents: in A, *novels* and *it* do not agree; in B, *everyone* is singular, so instead of *their*, the pronoun should be *him or her*; in C, *companies* and *it* do not agree.

50. C. Rice and beans, my favorite meal, reminds me of my native country Puerto Rico.

Choice C is the only sentence in which subject (*rice and beans/meal*) and verb (*reminds*) agree: in A, *one* and *have lived* do not agree; in B, *one* and *are going* do not agree; and in D, most (*of the milk* OR *it*) does not agree with *have gone*.

PRACTICE TEST 2

Round 2. You've been studying with Spire for
about a month — you're almost done!

Turn to the next page to begin.

MATHEMATICS

1 – Change to an improper fraction. 2 1/3
  A. 5/3
  B. 3/7
  C. 7/3
  D. 8/3

2 – Which of the following is equivalent to 60% of 90?
  A. 0.6 x 90
  B. 90 ÷ 0.6
  C. 3/5
  D. 2/3

3 – Convert the improper fraction $^{17}/_6$ to a mixed number.
  A. $1\,^7/_6$
  B. $2\,^5/_6$
  C. $^6/_{17}$
  D. $2\,^7/_6$

4 – The decimal value of 7/11 is _____?
  A. 1.57
  B. 0.70
  C. 0.6363…
  D. 0.77

5 – The decimal value of 5/8 is _____?
  A. 0.625
  B. 0.650
  C. 0.635
  D. 0.580

6 – The fractional value of 0.5625 is _____?
  A. 7/15
  B. 11/23
  C. 5/8
  D. 9/16

7 – The fractional value of 0.3125 is _____?
  A. 5/16
  B. 4/24
  C. 6/19
  D. 9/25

8 – What is the value of this expression if $a = 10$ and $b = -4$:
$$\sqrt{b^2 - 2 \bullet a}$$
  A. 6
  B. 7
  C. 8
  D. 9

9 – What is the greatest common factor of 48 and 64?

    A. 4

    B. 8

    C. 16

    D. 32

10 – Solve for x: $X = \frac{3}{4} \bullet \frac{7}{8}$

    A. 7/8

    B. 9/8

    C. 10/12

    D. 21/32

11 – Find the value of $a^2 + 6b$ when a = 3 and b = 0.5.

    A. 12

    B. 6

    C. 9

    D. 15

12 – What is the least common multiple of 8 and 10?

    A. 80

    B. 40

    C. 18

    D. 72

13 – What is the sum of 1/3 and 3/8?

    A. 3/24

    B. 4/11

    C. 17/24

    D. 15/16

14 – Solve this equation: –9 $\bullet$ –9 =

    A. 18

    B. 0

    C. 81

    D. –81

15 – Which of the following is between 2/3 and 3/4?

    A. 3/5

    B. 4/5

    C. 7/10

    D. 5/8

16 – Which digit is in the thousandths place in the number: 1,234.567

    A. 1

    B. 2

    C. 6

    D. 7

17 – Which of these numbers is largest?

    A. 5/8

    B. 3/5

    C. 2/3

    D. 0.72

18 – Which of these numbers is largest?

    A. −345

    B. 42

    C. −17

    D. 3^4

19 – Find 4 numbers between 4.857 and 4.858

    A. 4.8573, 4.85735, 4.85787, 4.8598

    B. 4.857, 4.8573, 4.8578, 4.8579,

    C. 4.8571, 4.8573, 4.8578, 4.8579

    D. 4.8572, 4.8537, 4.8578, 4.8579

20 – Which number is between 4 and 5?

    A. 11/3

    B. 21/4

    C. 31/6

    D. 23/5

21 – Which number is not between 7 and 9?

    A. 34/5

    B. 29/4

    C. 49/6

    D. 25/3

22 – If $\dfrac{4}{9}x - 3 = 1$, what is the value of x?

    A. 9

    B. 8

    C. 7

    D. −4½

23 – What value of q is a solution to this equation: $130 = q(-13)$

    A. 10

    B. −10

    C. 1

    D. 10^2

24 – Solve this equation: $x = -12 \div -3$

    A. $x = -4$

    B. $x = -15$

    C. $x = 9$

    D. $x = 4$

25 – Solve for r in the equation $p = 2r + 3$

    A. r = 2p – 3

    B. r = p + 6

    C. r = (p - 3) / 2

    D. r = p – 3/2

26 – Solve this equation: $x = 8 – (–3)$

    A. $x = 5$

    B. $x = –5$

    C. $x = 11$

    D. $x = –11$

27 – Evaluate the expression $7x^2 + 9x -18$ for x =7

    A. 516

    B. 424

    C. 388

    D. 255

28 – Evaluate the expression $x^2 + 7x -18$ for x =5

    A. 56

    B. 42

    C. 38

    D. 25

29 – Evaluate the expression $7x^2 + 63x$ for x =27

    A. 5603

    B. 4278

    C. 6804

    D. 6525

30 – Sam worked 40 hours at d dollars per hour and received a bonus of $50. His total earnings were $530. What was his hourly wage?

    A. $18

    B. $16

    C. $14

    D. $12

31 – The variable X is a positive integer. Dividing X by a positive number less than 1 will yield

    A. a number greater than X

    B. a number less than X

    C. a negative number

    D. an irrational number

32 – Amanda makes $14 an hour as a bank teller and Oscar makes $24 dollars an hour as an auto mechanic. Both work eight hours a day, five days a week. Which of these equations can be used to calculate how much they make together in a five-day week?

   A. $(14 + 24) \cdot 8 \cdot 5$
   B. $14 \cdot 24 \cdot 8 \cdot 5$
   C. $(14 + 24)(8 + 5)$
   D. $14 + 24 \cdot 8 \cdot 5$

33 – Seven added to four-fifths of a number equals fifteen. What is the number?

   A. 10
   B. 15
   C. 20
   D. 25

34 – If the sum of two numbers is 360 and their ratio is 7:3, what is the smaller number?

   A. 72
   B. 105
   C. 98
   D. 108

35 – Jean buys a textbook, a flash drive, a printer cartridge, and a ream of paper. The flash drive costs three times as much as the ream of paper. The textbook costs three times as much as the flash drive. The printer cartridge costs twice as much as the textbook. The ream of paper costs $10. How much does Jean spend altogether?

   A. $250
   B. $480
   C. $310
   D. $180

36 – The area of a triangle equals one-half the base times the height. Which of the following is the correct way to calculate the area of a triangle that has a base of 6 and a height of 9?

   A. $(6 + 9)/2$
   B. $\frac{1}{2}(6 + 9)$
   C. $2(6 \times 9)$
   D. $\dfrac{(6)(9)}{2}$

37 – Calculate the value of this expression: $2 + 6 \cdot 3 \cdot (3 \cdot 4)^2 + 1$

   A. 2,595
   B. 5,185
   C. 3,456
   D. 6,464

38 – A rectangle of length and width 3x and x has an area of $3x^2$. Write the area polynomial when the length is increased by 5 units and the width is decreased by 3 units. (3x+5) (x-3)

    A. $3x^2 + 14x - 15$

    B. $3x^2 - 4x - 15$

    C. $3x^2 - 5x + 15$

    D. $3x^2 + 4x - 15$

39 – A triangle of base and height 4x and 7x has an area of $14x^2$, which is equal ½ times the base times the height. Write the area polynomial when the base is increased by 2 units and the height is increased by 3 units. ½ (4x+2)(7x+3)

    A. $14x^2 + 14x + 6$

    B. $14x^2 + 14x + 3$

    C. $14x^2 + 13x + 3$

    D. $14x^2 + 28x + 3$

40 – Momentum is defined as the product of mass times velocity. If your 1,250 kg car is travelling at 55 km/hr, what is the value of the momentum?

    A. 68,750 kg m/s

    B. 19,098 kg m/s

    C. 9,549 kg m/s

    D. 145,882 kg m/s

41 – In her retirement accounts, Janet has invested $40,000 in stocks and $65,000 in bonds. If she wants to rebalance her accounts so that 70% of her investments are in stocks, how much will she have to move?

    A. $33,500

    B. $35,000

    C. $37,500

    D. $40,000

42 – Brian pays 15% of his gross salary in taxes. If he pays $7,800 in taxes, what is his gross salary?

    A. $52,000

    B. $48,000

    C. $49,000

    D. $56,000

43 – In a high school French class, 45% of the students are sophomores, and there are 9 sophomores in the class. How many students are there in the class?

    A. 16

    B. 18

    C. 20

    D. 22

44 – Marisol's score on a standardized test was ranked in the 78th percentile. If 660 students took the test, approximately how many students scored lower than Marisol?

    A. 582

    B. 515

    C. 612

    D. 486

45 – The population of Mariposa County in 2015 was 90% of its population in 2010. The population in 2010 was 145,000. What was the population in 2010?

    A. 160,000

    B. 142,000

    C. 120,500

    D. 130,500

46 – Alicia must have a score of 75% to pass a test of 80 questions. What is the greatest number of question she can miss and still pass the test?

    A. 20

    B. 25

    C. 60

    D. 15

47 – A cell phone on sale at 30% off costs $210. What was the original price of the phone?

    A. $240

    B. $273

    C. $300

    D. $320

48 – In the graduating class at Emerson High School, 52% of the students are girls and 48% are boys. There are 350 students in the class. Among the girls, 98 plan to go to college. How many girls do not plan to go to college?

    A. 84

    B. 48

    C. 66

    D. 72

49 – The number of students enrolled at Two Rivers Community College increased from 3,450 in 2010 to 3,864 in 2015. What was the percent increase?

    A. 9%

    B. 17%

    C. 12%

    D. 6%

50 – Produce is usually priced to the nearest pound. A scale for weighing produce has numerical values for pounds and ounces. Which of the following weights would you expect to be priced for 15 pounds?

    A. 15 pounds 14 ounces

    B. 15 pounds 10 ounces

    C. 14 pounds 4 ounces

    D. 14 pounds 14 ounces

51 – Which number is rounded to the nearest ten-thousandth?

    A. 7,510,000

    B. 7,515,000

    C. 7,514,635.8239

    D. 7,514,635.824

52 – Measuring devices determine the precision of our scientific measurements. A graduated cylinder is used that has a maximum of 10 cc's but has ten increments in between each whole number of cc's. Which answer is a correct representation of a volume measurement with this cylinder?

    A. 7 cc's

    B. 7.1 cc's

    C. 7.15 cc's

    D. 7.514 cc's

53 – If a man can unload about 50 pounds in a time of 15 minutes, estimate the time and labor force to unload 2.5 tons of 50 pound blocks from a truck working 8 hours per day.

    A. 1 man for 10 days

    B. 2 men for 1 day

    C. 4 men for 1 day

    D. 5 men for 5 days

54 – In rush hour, you can usually commute 18 miles to work in 45 minutes. If you believe that you can travel an average of 5 miles per hour faster in the early morning, how much time would you estimate for the early commute to work?

    A. 50 minutes

    B. 40 minutes

    C. 30 minutes

    D. 20 minutes

55 – You are taking a test and you are allowed to work a class period of 45 minutes. 20 problems are multiple choice and 30 of the problems are true / false. If they have equal value, how much time would you estimate for each type of problem if you believe you are twice as fast at multiple choice problems?

    A. 90 seconds per m/c; 45 seconds per t/f

    B. 60 seconds per m/c; 30 seconds per t/f

    C. 70 seconds per m/c; 35 seconds per t/f

    D. 80 seconds per m/c; 40 seconds per t/f

56 – Your interview is scheduled for 8:00 in the morning and you need to allow 20 minutes for your trip to the interview. You oversleep and leave 10 minutes late. How fast will you travel to get there on time?

    A. half as fast

    B. twice as fast

    C. three times as fast

    D. four times as fast

SCIENCE

1- Which of the following is a primary functional difference between smooth endoplasmic reticulum (SER) and rough endoplasmic reticulum (RER)?

    A. smooth endoplasmic reticulum does not participate in synthesis of products that are destined for external secretion.

    B. smooth endoplasmic reticulum does not participate in synthesis of proteins.

    C. Rough endoplasmic reticulum does not participate in synthesis of products that are destined for external secretion.

    D. rough endoplasmic reticulum does not participate in synthesis of proteins

2- Which of the following is a universal feature of all living cells?

    A. an external cell membrane

    B. an external cell wall

    C. a nucleus

    D. mitochondria

3- Which of the following terms would NOT be used to define the relative position of one body structure to another?

    A. caudal

    B. coronal

    C. ventral

    D. inferior

4- Which of the following identifies the type of intracellular filament that generates the whip-like motion of the flagellum of a human sperm cell?

    A. Thick filaments

    B. microfilaments

    C. microtubules

    D. intermediate filaments

5- Which of the following is NOT a characteristic of voluntary muscle tissue?

    A. synaptic muscle membrane interfaces with neurons

    B. high extracellular matrix volume

    C. high intracellular actin content

    D. electrically excitable cell membranes

6- Which of the following could be a nitrogenous base sequence of both a single codon and a single anticodon?

    A. ACG

    B. GCT

    C. UTC

    D. AGU

7- Which of the following is NOT a product molecule generated by a complete round of the Krebs (citric acid) cycle?

    A. CO_2

    B. acetyl CoA

    C. NADH

    D. $FADH_2$

8- Which of the following is an event that occurs during the successful maturation of a human primary follicle into a human secondary follicle?

    A. the corpus luteum degenerates

    B. a human sperm cell fertilizes the primary follicle

    C. a polar body is generated

    D. Increasing estrogen levels trigger a second luteinizing hormone (LH) peak.

9- Which of the following pairs of terms correctly completes the statement below?

In the human male reproductive system _____ cells produce _____.

    A. tunica albuginea; primary spermatids

    B. Sertoli; follicle stimulating hormone (FSH)

    C. spermatogonia; luteinizing hormone (LH)

    D. Leydig; testosterone

10- Which of the following pairs of terms correctly completes the statement below?

In humans, the _____ joint has a greater range of motion than the _____ joint.

    A. elbow; knee

    B. sacroiliac; atlanto axial

    C. elbow; shoulder

    D. knee; hip

11- Which of the following choices lists three organs that are all, to the greatest extent, derived from the same primary germ layer?

    A. heart, lung and kidney

    B. brain, heart and lung

    C. pancreas, liver, kidney

    D. lung, liver and pancreas

12- Which of the following is the primary function of pulmonary surfactant?

    A. prevention of rupture of alveoli during maximal inspiratory effort

    B. prevention of collapse of alveoli during exhalation

    C. increased solubility of oxygen in solution between alveoli and capillary endothelium

    D. decreased viscosity of bronchiolar luminal mucous secretions

13- Which of the following most likely does NOT increase during a maximal inspiratory effort compared to a normal (tidal) inspiratory effort?

    A. intrathoracic volume

    B. diffusion of CO_2 into alveolar airspaces

    C. pulmonary artery pressure

    D. diffusion of O_2 out of alveolar airspaces

14- Which of the following events occurs simultaneously with the end of systole?
   A. The aortic valve opens.
   B. The right ventricular pressure reaches a minimum value.
   C. The atrio-ventricular (A-V) node generates an electrical impulse.
   D. The mitral valve closes.

15- Among the choices below, within the cardiovascular system, which of the following in general has the lowest electrical conductivity?
   A. the atrioventricular septum
   B. intercalated discs
   C. Purkinje fibers
   D. The AV node

16- Which of the following is the most likely site for the origin of a blood clot that travels to and then lodges within the right main pulmonary artery?
   A. a peripheral vein located in the leg
   B. the aorta
   C. the left atrium
   D. a main pulmonary vein

17- Which of the following is by definition a lymphocyte lineage cell type?
   A. eosinophils
   B. plasma cells
   C. monocytes
   D. basophils

18- Dedicated or professional antigen presenting cells present antigens on their cell surfaces to T-cells in conjunction with which of the following types of cell membrane molecules?
   A. HLA class I antigens
   B. ABO glycoproteins
   C. Rh-factor proteins
   D. cadherin-class cell-adhesion molecules

19- Which of the following is NOT a cellular feature of enterocytes located in the small intestine?
   A. microvilli
   B. tight junctions
   C. desmosomes
   D. lacteals

20- Which of the following is most likely to lead to a suppression of the secretion of the hormone glucagon?
   A. high protein content of chyme in the stomach
   B. activation of the sympathetic nervous system
   C. a meal with high simple carbohydrate content
   D. the release of the hormone cholecystokinin (CCK)

21- Which of the following is a correct cause and effect sequence of events during the digestive process?

    A. CCK secretion→↑somatostatin secretion→↑pancreatic amylase secretion

    B. CCK secretion→↑bile secretion→↑fat emulsification

    C. secretin secretion→↑gastric mucous secretion→↑pepsin secretion

    D. secretin secretion→↑gastric HCL secretion→↑pepsin activation

22- Which of the following identifies the process responsible for the late hyperpolarization phase of an action potential?

    A. sodium ion ($Na+$) diffusion into a neuron

    B. sodium ion ($Na+$) diffusion out of a neuron

    C. potassium ion ($K+$) diffusion into a neuron

    D. potassium ion ($K+$) diffusion out of a neuron

23- Which of the following does not occur as a step in the physicochemical sequence that triggers sarcomere contraction within a myofibril?

    A. The release of norepinephrine (NE) into the neuron-myofibril gap of a neuromuscular junction

    B. The propagation of an electrical signal along a myofibril outer membrane into a T-tubule

    C. the release of $CA++$ ion from the sarcoplasmic reticulum of a myofibril

    D. the crosslink-binding of actin molecules and the "heads" of myosin molecules.

24- Which of the following pairs of cell types produce myelin sheaths?

    A. Schwann cells and oligodendroglia

    B. oligodendroglia and astrocytes

    C. astrocytes and Schwann cells

    D. microglia and neurons

25- Electrical signals to voluntary muscles most likely originate in which of the following locations in the central nervous system?

    A. the temporal lobes of the cerebral cortex

    B. the parietal lobes of the cerebral cortex

    C. the basal ganglia of the midbrain

    D. The cerebellum

26- Which of the following is most likely to directly result in the accumulation of lactic acid in muscle tissue?

    A. activation of the sympathetic nervous system

    B. depletion of glycogen stored in the liver

    C. inadequate amounts of O_2 delivered to muscle tissue

    D. inadequate levels of pyruvate within muscle tissue.

27- Which of the following is an effect of activation of the parasympathetic nervous system?

    A. increased activity of the sinoatrial node

    B. decreased activity of smooth muscle contractions in the wall of the digestive tract

    C. direct inhibition of deep tendon reflexes

    D. contraction of smooth muscle in the walls of arterioles in voluntary muscle tissue

28- On the outer membrane of a neuron, which of the following local regions would most likely contain the highest concentration of ligand-gated transmembrane ion channels?

    A. axon terminals

    B. junctional region of the axon and the main cell body (soma) of the neuron

    C. dendrites

    D. longitudinal mid-portion of the axon

29- Which of the following is the most precise anatomical location of the first stage of human spermatogenesis?

    A. the corpus spongiosum

    B. the seminiferous tubules

    C. the epididymis

    D. the seminal vesicles

30- Which of the following is the most precise location of the Bartholin's glands?

    A. immediately lateral to the labia majora

    B. medial to the labia majora and lateral to the labia minora

    C. medial to the labia minora and inferolateral to the vaginal introitus

    D. medial to the labia minora and superolateral to the urethral meatus

31- Which of the following correctly describes the course of a typical apocrine gland duct beginning at the duct's glandular origin and proceeding to the distal orifice of the duct?

    A. gland→hypodermis→basement membrane→dermis→shaft of hair follicle

    B. gland→dermis→basement membrane→epidermis→shaft of hair follicle

    C. a gland→hypodermis→basement membrane→dermis→external surface of the epidermis

    D. gland→dermis→basement membrane→epidermis→external surface of the epidermis

32- Which of the following describes the primary function of integumentary Langerhans cells?

    A. immune - antigen presentation

    B. somatosensory reception

    C. thermoregulation

    D structural adherence

33- Which of the following identifies the primary tissue type of the hypodermis and a primary function of the main cellular component of the hypodermis?

    A. epithelial; mechanical barrier

    B. epithelial energy storage

    C. connective; mechanical barrier

    D. connective; energy storage

34- Which of the following is NOT a hormone synthesized by the pituitary gland?

    A. prolactin

    B. melatonin

    C. oxytocin

    D. adrenocorticotropic hormones (ACTH)

HESI A² - Spire Study System

35- Which of the following hormones has rapid effects that are similar to effects associated with the activation of the sympathetic nervous system?
- A. insulin
- B. thyroid hormone (T3 and T4)
- C. testosterone
- D. aldosterone

36- Which of the following cell types initially secrets the majority of the hydroxyapatite component of lamellar bone?
- A. osteoblasts
- B. osteoclasts
- C. osteocytes
- D. fibroblasts

37- Which of the following is not a feature of or within trabecular (cancellous) bone?
- A. red blood cell progenitor cells
- B. white blood cell progenitor cells
- C. haversian canals
- D. adipocytes

38- Among the following, which choice identifies a join whose most general type is different from the other three?
- A. frontal-sagittal joint
- B. temporomandibular joint
- C. sternomanubrial joint
- D. sacroiliac joint

39- The initial filtration of blood by the kidney occurs at which of the following anatomical locations?
- A. the renal pelvis
- B. the adrenal cortex
- C. the collecting ducts
- D. the glomeruli

40- Which of the following is the kidney's response to exposure to antidiuretic hormone?
- A. increased secretion of urea
- B. decreased osmolality of extracellular fluid in the renal medulla
- C. Increased renal tubule permeability to water
- D. decreased secretion of glucose

41- Which of the following is the primary hormonal response of the central nervous system to an undesirably high plasma osmolarity?
- A. increased secretion of corticotropin releasing hormone
- B. decreased secretion of corticotropin releasing hormone
- C. increased secretion of antidiuretic hormone
- D. decreased secretion of antidiuretic hormone

42- Which of the following correctly completes the statement below?

The effect of _____ on the kidney is the release of _____ by the kidney.

   A. an undesirably low plasma sodium ion concentration; renin
   B. an undesirably high plasma sodium ion concentration; renin
   C. an undesirably low plasma sodium ion concentration; aldosterone
   D. an undesirably high plasma sodium ion concentration; aldosterone

43- Under normal physiological circumstances, which of the following is completely reabsorbed by the kidney?

   A. glucose
   B. sodium
   C. bicarbonate ion
   D. urea

44- Which of the following is a physiological purpose of the sodium ion reabsorption-secretion cycle in the loop of Henle?

   A. sodium ion conservation
   B. potassium ion excretion
   C. concentration of urine
   D. acidification of urine

45- Which of the following is a DIRECT consequence of decreasing blood pressure on kidney function?

   A. decreased reabsorption of sodium ions
   B. decreased glomerular filtration rate (GFR)
   C. decreased secretion of renin
   D. increased secretion of aldosterone

46- Which of the following is a DIRECT physiological effect of angiotensin II?

   A. increased blood pressure
   B. increased renal medullary osmolality
   C. decreased renal tubule permeability to water
   D. redistribution of gastrointestinal blood flow

47- Which of the following are structurally required for the formation of a membrane attack complex (MAC)?

   A. perforins
   B. antigen specific antibodies
   C. platelet adhesion factors
   D. complement proteins

48- Which of the following does not participate in the immune response to viral infection?

   A. T-cells
   B. interferons
   C. chief cells
   D. plasma cells

49- Which of the following describes the mechanism of action of antivenom in snakebite victims?

    A. blockade of cell membrane molecular targets of snake venom toxin

    B. proteolytic destruction of the snake venom toxin molecules

    C. Non-enzymatic deamination of the snake venom toxin molecules

    D. deactivation of the snake venom toxin molecules by antigen-specific antibody binding

50- Which of the terms below correctly completes the following sentence?

The influenza vaccine provides _____ immunity to the influenza virus.

    A. active innate

    B. active humoral

    C. passive cellular

    D. passive innate

51- Which of the pairs of terms below correctly completes the following sentence?

Human T-cells originate from cells located in the_____ and reach maturity in the_____

    A. bone marrow; cortex of the spleen

    B. bone marrow; thymus

    C. thymus; cortex of the spleen

    D cortex of the spleen, thymus

52- Among the four cardinal signs of localized infection, which of the following is/are NOT the DIRECT result of increased vascular permeability?

    A. redness and swelling only

    B. redness and heat only

    C. swelling and pain only

    D. pain and heat only

53- Which of the following is most clearly an autoimmune disease in humans?

    A. type 1 diabetes mellitus

    B. cystic fibrosis

    C. sickle cell anemia

    D. peptic ulcer disease

54- Which of the following identifies a direct causative sequence that results in the typical symptoms of seasonal pollen/mold allergies?

    A. antigen→mast cell release of peroxidase

    B. antigen→mast cell release of histamine

    C. antigen→Langerhans cell release of peroxidase

    D. antigen→Langerhans cell release of histamine

55- Which of the following diagrams the chemical reaction that results in the formation of a peptide bond between two amino acids, AA_1 and AA_2?

    A. $AA_1 + AA_2 \rightarrow AA_1\text{-}AA_2 + H_2O$

    B. $AA_1 + AA_2 \rightarrow AA_1\text{-}AA_2 + CO_2 + NH_3$

    C. $AA_1 + AA_2 \rightarrow AA_1\text{-}AA_2 + 2\ glucose$

    D. $AA_1 + AA_2 + NAD^+ \rightarrow AA_1\text{-}AA_2 + CO_2 + NADH$

ENGLISH & READING

Passage 1

The United States Treasury operates a subsidiary, the Bureau of Engraving and Printing (BEP), where the nation's supply of paper money is designed and manufactured. But to call American currency "paper" money is a slight misnomer that understates its unperceived complexity and intrinsic technological sophistication. The Treasury goes to extraordinary lengths to safeguard cash from counterfeiters. One of the most fundamental ways is by printing not on paper, per se, but on a proprietary blend of linen and cotton. American money is more akin to fabric than paper, and each bill that is printed is a phenomenal work of art and masterful craftsmanship.

The most frequently counterfeited denominations are the 20-dollar bill, preferred by domestic counterfeiters, and the 100-dollar note, which is the currency of choice for foreign forgers. To make the copying of twenties more difficult, the BEP uses color-shifting ink that changes from copper to green in certain lights. Evidence of this can be seen in the numeral "20" located in the lower right corner on the front of the bills. A portrait watermark – which is a very faint, rather ethereal image of President Jackson – is also juxtaposed into the blank space to the right to his visible and prominent portrait. Additionally, there is a security ribbon, adorned with a flag and the words "USA Twenty," printed on and embedded into the bill. When exposed to ultraviolet light, the thread glows with a greenish hue. Twenties also include an almost subliminal text that reads "USA20;" this micro-printed text is well-camouflaged within the bill. With the use of a magnifying glass, it can be found in the border beneath the Treasurer's signature.

The 100-dollar bill utilizes similar security features. These include color-shifting ink, portrait watermarks, security threads and ribbons, raised printing, and micro-printing. These units of currency, dubbed "Ben Franklins" in honor of the president whose face graces it, also boast what the BEP describes as a 3-D security ribbon. The ribbon has bells and numbers printed on it. When the currency is tilted it appears that the images of bells transform into the numeral 100 and, when tilted side to side, the bells and 100s seem to move in a lateral direction.

Security threads woven into each different denomination have their own respective colors, and each one glows a different color when illuminated with ultraviolet light. Fine engraving or printing patterns appear in various locations on bills too, and many of these patterns are extremely fine. The artists who create them for engraving also incorporate non-linear designs, as the waviness can make it exponentially more difficult to successfully counterfeit the currency. The surface of American currency is also slightly raised, giving it a subtly, but distinct, tactile characteristic.

1. Which of the following conclusions may logically be drawn from the first paragraph of the passage?
    A. Linen and cotton are more expensive printing materials than paper.
    B. The current process of printing money is reflective of decades of modifications.
    C. Counterfeiting of American money is an enormous problem.
    D. The artistry inherent in the making of American money makes it attractive to collectors.

2. What sentence, if added to the end of the passage, would provide the best conclusion to both the paragraph and the passage?
    A. It is clear from all these subtly nuanced features of the various bills that true artistry is at work in their making.
    B. Yet, despite all of these technological innovations, the race to stay ahead of savvy counterfeiters and their constantly changing counterfeiting techniques is a never-ending one.
    C. Due to the complexities involved in the printing of money, these artists are consequently well-paid for their skills.
    D. Thus, many other countries have begun to model their money-printing methods on these effective techniques.

3. The passage is reflective of which of the following types of writing?
    A. Descriptive
    B. Narrative
    C. Expository
    D. Persuasive

4. This passage likely comes from which of the following documents?
    A. A pamphlet for tourists visiting the United States Treasury
    B. A feature news article commemorating the bicentennial of the Bureau of Engraving and Printing
    C. A letter from the US treasury Secretary to the President
    D. A public service message warning citizens about the increased circulation of counterfeit currency

5. Which of the following is an example of a primary source document?
    A. A pamphlet for tourists visiting the United States Treasury
    B. A feature news article commemorating the bicentennial of the Bureau of Engraving and Printing
    C. A letter from the US treasury Secretary to the President
    D. A public service message warning citizens about the increased circulation of counterfeit currency

6. Which of the following describes the word *intrinsic* as it is used in the first paragraph of the passage?
    A. Amazing
    B. Expensive
    C. Unbelievable
    D. Inherent

Passage 2
In the Middle Ages, merchants an artisans formed groups called "guilds" to protect themselves and their trades. Guilds appeared in the year 1000, and by the twelfth century, analogous trades, like wool, spice, and silk dealers had formed their own guilds. _____, towns like Florence, Italy, boasted as many as 50 merchants' guilds. With the advent of guilds, apprenticeship became a complex system. Apprentices were to be taught only certain things and then they were to prove they possessed certain skills, as determined by the guild. Each guild decided the length of time required for an apprentice to work for a master tradesman before being admitted to the trade.

7. The topic sentence of the above passage is
    A. In the Middle Ages, merchants an artisans formed groups called "guilds" to protect themselves and their trades.
    B. Guilds appeared in the year 1000, and by the twelfth century, analogous trades, like wool, spice, and silk dealers had formed their own guilds.
    C. With the advent of guilds, apprenticeship became a complex system.
    D. Apprentices were to be taught only certain things and then they were to prove they possessed certain skills, as determined by the guild.

8. The main idea of the passage is that
    A. wool, spice and silk dealers were all types of merchant trades during the Middle Ages.
    B. Florence, Italy was a great center of commerce during the Middle Ages.
    C. merchant guilds originated in the Middle Ages and became extremely popular, eventually leading to a sophisticated apprenticeship system.
    D. apprenticeships were highly sought after, therefore merchants had many skilled workers to choose from to assist them in their trade.

9. From the content of the passage, it reasonably be inferred that
    A. prior to the inception of guilds, merchants were susceptible to competition from lesser skilled craftsmen peddling inferior products or services.
    B. most merchants were unscrupulous business who often cheated their customers.
    C. it was quite easy to become an apprentice to a highly skilled merchant.
    D. guilds fell out of practice during the Industrial Revolution due to the mechanization of labor.

10. As it is used in the second sentence, "analogous" most nearly means
    A. obsolete
    B. inferior
    C. similar
    D. less popular

11. Which of the following is the best signal word or phrase to fill in the blank above?
    A. Up until that time,
    B. Before that time,
    C. By that time,
    D. After that time,

Passage 3

Certainly we must face this fact: if the American press, as a mass medium, has formed the minds of America, the mass has also formed the medium. There is action, reaction, and interaction going on ceaselessly between the newspaper-buying public and the editors. What is wrong with the American press is what is in part wrong with American society. Is this, _____, to exonerate the American press for its failures to give the American people more tasteful and more illuminating reading matter? Can the American press seek to be excused from responsibility for public lack of information as TV and radio often do, on the grounds that, after all, "we have to give the people what they want or we will go out of business"?   --Clare Boothe Luce

12. What is the primary purpose of this text?
    A. To reveal an innate problem in American society
    B. To criticize the American press for not taking responsibility for their actions
    C. To analyze the complex relationship that exists between the public and the media
    D. To challenge the masses to protest the lack of information disseminated by the media

13. From which of the following is the above paragraph most likely excerpted?
    A. A newspaper editorial letter
    B. A novel about yellow journalism
    C. A diary entry
    D. A speech given at a civil rights protest

14. Which of the following is an example of a primary source document?
    A. A newspaper editorial letter
    B. A novel about yellow journalism
    C. A diary entry
    D. A speech given at a civil rights protest

15. As it is used in sentence 4, "illuminating" most nearly means
    A. intelligent
    B. sophisticated
    C. interesting
    D. enlightening

16. Which of the following is the best signal word or phrase to fill in the blank?
    A. so
    B. however
    C. therefore
    D. yet

17. What is the author's primary attitude towards the American press?
    A. admiration
    B. perplexity
    C. disapproval
    D. ambivalence

18. Which of the following identifies the mode of the passage?
    A. expository
    B. persuasive/argumentative
    C. narrative
    D. descriptive

19. Based on the passage, which of the following can most likely be concluded?
    A. The author has a degree in journalism
    B. The author has worked in the journalism industry
    C. The author is seeking employment at a newspaper
    D. The author is filing a lawsuit against a media outlet

Passage 4

The game today known as "football" in the United States can be traced directly back to the English game of rugby, although there have been many changes to the game. Football was played informally on university fields more than a hundred years ago. In 1840, a yearly series of informal "scrimmages" started at Yale University. It took more than twenty-five years, _____, for the game to become a part of college life. The first formal intercollegiate football game was held between Princeton and Rutgers teams on November 6, 1869 on Rutgers' home field at New Brunswick, New Jersey, and Rutgers won.

20. Which sentence, if added to the end of the paragraph, would provide the best conclusion?
- A. Despite an invitation to join the Ivy League, Rutgers University declined, but later joined the Big Ten Conference instead.
- B. Football was played for decades on school campuses nationwide before the American Professional Football Association was formed in 1920, and then renamed the National Football League (or the NFL) two years later.
- C. Women were never allowed to play football, and that fact remains a controversial policy at many colleges and universities.
- D. Football remains the national pastime, despite rising popularity for the game of soccer, due to increased TV coverage of World Cup matches.

21. Which of the following is the best signal word or phrase to fill in the blank above?
- 32. however
- 33. still
- 34. in addition
- 35. alternatively

Passage 5

Modernism is a philosophical movement that arose during the early 20th century. Among the factors that shaped modernism were the development of modern societies based on industry and the rapid growth of cities, followed later by the horror of World War I. Modernism rejected the science-based thinking of the earlier Era of Enlightenment, and many modernists also rejected religion. The poet Ezra Pound's 1934 injunction to "Make it new!" was the touchstone of the movement's approach towards what it saw as the now obsolete culture of the past. A notable characteristic of modernism is self-consciousness and irony concerning established literary and social traditions, which often led to experiments concerned with HOW things were made, not so much with the actual final product. Modernism had a profound impact on numerous aspects of life, and its values and perspectives still influence society in many positive ways today.

22. According to the passage, what is the overarching theme of the modernist movement?
- A. Rejection of the past and outmoded ideas
- B. Appreciation of urban settings over natural settings
- C. A concentration on method over form
- D. A focus on automated industry

23. As it is used in the passage, "touchstone" most nearly means
- A. Challenge
- B. Basis
- C. Fashion
- D. Metaphor

24. Which of the following statements from the passage can be described as an opinion?
   A. Among the factors that shaped modernism were the development of modern societies based on industry and the rapid growth of cities, followed later by the horror of World War I.
   B. The poet Ezra Pound's 1934 injunction to "Make it new!" was the touchstone of the movement's approach towards what it saw as the now obsolete culture of the past.
   C. A notable characteristic of modernism is self-consciousness and irony concerning established literary and social traditions, which often led to experiments concerned with HOW things were made, not so much with the actual final product.
   D. Modernism had a profound impact on numerous aspects of life, and its values and perspectives still influence society in many positive ways today.

Passage 6

The modern Olympics are the leading international sporting event featuring summer and winter sports competitions in which thousands of athletes from around the world participate in a variety of competitions. Held every two years, with the Summer and Winter Games alternating, the games are a modern way to bring nations together, _____ allowing for national pride, and sportsmanship on a global scale. Having withstood the test of time over many centuries, they are the best example of the physical achievements of mankind.

The creation of the modern Games was inspired by the ancient Olympic Games, which were held in Olympia, Greece, from the 8th century BC to the 4th century AD. The Ancient Games events were fewer in number and were examples of very basic traditional forms of competitive athleticism. Many running events were featured, as well as a pentathlon (consisting of a jumping event, discus and javelin throws, a foot race, and wrestling), boxing, wrestling, *pankration*, and equestrian events. Fast forward to the modern state of this ancient athletic competition, and we see that the Olympic Movement during the 20th and 21st centuries has resulted in several changes to the Games, including the creation of the Winter Olympic Games for ice and winter sports, which for climate reasons, would not have been possible in ancient Greece. The Olympics has also shifted away from pure amateurism to allowing participation of professional athletes, a change which was met with criticism when first introduced, as many felt it detracted from the original spirit and intention of the competition.

Today, over 13,000 athletes compete at the summer and Winter Olympic Games in 33 different sports and nearly 400 events. The first, second, and third-place finishers in each event receive Olympic medals: gold, silver, and bronze, respectively. And every country hopes to be able to go home with many of these medals, as they are truly still a point of pride for each nation to be recognized for some outstanding achievement on the world stage, however briefly.

25. Which of the following is the best signal word or phrase to fill in the blank in the first paragraph?
   A. despite
   B. however
   C. instead of
   D. as well as

26. Which of the following words from the last sentence of paragraph 2 has a negative connotation?
   A. Shifted
   B. Allowing
   C. Change
   D. Detracted

27. Which of the following statements based on the passage would be considered an opinion?
    A. The ancient Olympic games were held in Olympia, Greece.
    B. The Olympic games are the best example of humanity's physical prowess.
    C. When the games were changed from pure amateurism to allowing professional athletes to participate, this change displeased many people.
    D. Today, 33 different sports are represented at the Olympic games.

Passage 7

A day or two later, in the afternoon, I saw myself staring at my fire, at an inn which I had booked on foreseeing that I would spend some weeks in London. I had just come in, and, having decided on a spot for my luggage, sat down to consider my room. It was on the ground floor, and the fading daylight reached it in a sadly broken-down condition. It struck me that the room was stuffy and unsocial, with its moldy smell and its decoration of lithographs and waxy flowers – it seemed an impersonal black hole in the huge general blackness of the inn itself. The uproar of the neighborhood outside hummed away, and the rattle of a heartless hansom cab passed close to my ears. A sudden horror of the whole place came over me, like a tiger-pounce of homesickness which had been watching its moment. London seemed hideous, vicious, cruel and, above all, overwhelming. Soon, I would have to go out for my dinner, and it appeared to me that I would rather remain dinnerless, would rather even starve, than go forth into the hellish town where a stranger might get trampled to death, and have his carcass thrown into the Thames River.

28. Based on the passage above, the author's attitude toward his experience in London can best be described as
    A. Awe
    B. Disappointment
    C. Revulsion
    D. Ambivalence

29. Which type of document is this passage likely excerpted from?
    A. A travel guide
    B. A diary entry
    C. A news editorial
    D. An advertisement

30. Which of the following documents would likely NOT be considered a primary source document?
    A. A travel guide
    B. A diary entry
    C. A news editorial
    D. An advertisement

31. Based on the content of the passage, which of the following is a reasonable conclusion?
    A. The author is quite wealthy.
    B. The author has been to London before.
    C. The author is traveling to London based on the recommendation of a friend.
    D. The author will not be traveling to London again.

HESI A² - Spire Study System

32. Which sentence below illustrates proper use of punctuation for dialogue?
    A. "I have a dream", began Martin Luther King, Jr.
    B. "Can you believe that I have been asked to audition for that part," asked Megan excitedly?
    C. "You barely know him! How can she marry him?" was the worried mother's response at her teenager's announcement of marriage.
    D. "Remain seated while the seatbelt signs are illuminated." Came the announcement over the airplane's loud speaker system.

33. Which of the sentences below is NOT in the second person?
    A. "I have a dream", began Martin Luther King, Jr.
    B. "Can you believe that I have been asked to audition for that part," asked Megan excitedly?
    C. "You barely know him! How can you marry him?" was the worried mother's response at her teenager's announcement of marriage.
    D. "Remain seated while the seatbelt signs are illuminated." Came the announcement over the airplane's loud speaker system.

34. Which of the following sentences is an example of an Imperative sentence?
    A. "I have a dream", began Martin Luther King, Jr.
    B. "Can you believe that I have been asked to audition for that part," asked Megan excitedly?
    C. "You barely know him! How can she marry him?" was the worried mother's response at her teenager's announcement of marriage.
    D. "Please remain seated while the seatbelt signs are illuminated." Came the announcement over the airplane's loud speaker system.

35. Which of the following means "the act of cutting out"?
    A. Incision
    B. Concision
    C. Excision
    D. Decision

36. Which of the following refers to an inflammation?
    A. Appendectomy
    B. Colitis
    C. Angioplasty
    D. Dermatology

37. Which of the following refers to a cancer?
    A. Neuropathy
    B. Hysterectomy
    C. Oncology
    D. Melanoma

38. Which of the following conditions is associated with the nose?
    A. Hematoma
    B. Neuralgia
    C. Rhinitis
    D. Meningitis

39. Which of the following refers to the study of something?
    A. Gastroenterology
    B. Gastritis
    C. Psychosis
    D. Psychopath

ANSWERS PRACTICE TEST 2

MATHEMATICS

1 – C. 7/3

An improper fraction is a fraction whose numerator is greater than its denominator. To change a mixed number to an improper fraction, multiply the whole number (2) times the denominator (3) and add the result to the numerator. Answer C is the correct choice.

2 – A. 0.6 x 90

To find 60% of 90, first convert 60% to a decimal by moving the decimal point two places to the left. Then multiply this decimal, 0.6, times 90. Answer A is the correct choice.

3 – B. 2 $^5/_6$

To convert an improper fraction to a mixed number, divide the numerator by the denominator. In this case, you get 2 with a remainder of 5. 2 becomes the whole number and the remainder is the numerator. Answer B is the correct choice.

4 – C. 0.6363...

The ratio 7/11 implies division, so the decimal value can be determined by the long division problem of 7 divided by 11. The long division results in the repeating decimal 0.6363... There may be a simpler method to find this decimal. The ratio 7/11 is the product of 7 times 1/11. The ratio 1/11 is the repeating decimal 0.0909... so multiplying that decimal by 7 is 0.6363... provides the same answer. If it seems like the same amount of effort, remember that every fraction with 11 in the denominator can be determined in the same way. Answer C is the correct choice.

5 – A. 0.625

The ratio implies division, so 5/8 can be determined by the long division problem of 5 divided by 8. The long division results in the decimal 0.625. There is a simpler method to find this decimal. The ratio 5/8 is the product of 5 times 1/8. The ratio 1/8 is the decimal 0.125 so multiplying that decimal by 5 is 0.625, which is the same answer. If it seems like the same amount of effort, remember that every fraction with 8 in the denominator can be determined in the same way. Answer A is the correct choice.

6 – D. 9/16

The numerator in the correct ratio will be equal to the given decimal times the correct denominator. It is simply a result of cross multiplying. But first, these problems can be greatly simplified if we eliminate incorrect answers.

For example, answers A and B can both be eliminated because they are both less than 0.5 or ½. If you can't see that, then multiply .5 times 15 and .5 times 23. In answer A, .5 times 15 is 7.5 so 7/15 is less than the fractional value of 0.5625. In B, .5 times 23 is 11.5 so 11/23 is less than the fractional value of 0.5625.

Now, evaluating fractional answers this way, you may look at answer C and realize that since 0.6 times 8 equals 4.8. Since 4.8 is less than the numerator and 0.6 is larger than the given decimal value, C can be eliminated. Answer D is the correct choice.

7 – A. 5/16

The numerator in the correct ratio will be equal to the given decimal times the correct denominator. It is simply a result of cross multiplying. But first, the problem can be simplified if we eliminate impossible answers.

For example, answer B can be eliminated because it simplifies to 1/6 which is much less than 0.3125. If you can't see that, then divide 1 by 6 which becomes 0.167.

For answer D, the ratio 9/25 is a simplified form of 36/100 or 0.36. 0.36 is greater than 0.3125, so answer D can be eliminated.

Now, evaluating fractional answers this way, you may eliminate answer C for a very simple reason. 19 times 0.3125 will always leave a value of 5 in the ten-thousandths place because 19 times 5 equals 95. That means the product can never be the whole number 6, so answer C can be eliminated.

The correct answer is D because you have logically eliminated all the other possible choices.

8 – A. 6

If $a = 10$, then $2a = 20$.

Now compute the value of b^2

$b^2 = (b) \bullet (b)$
$b^2 = (-4) \bullet (-4)$
$b^2 = 16$

So now you have:

$$\sqrt{16 + 20} \; or \; \sqrt{36}$$

The square root of 36 is 6. Answer A is the correct choice

9 – C. 16

The greatest common factor of two numbers is the largest number that can be divided evenly into both numbers. The simplest way to answer this question is to start with the largest answer (32) and see if it can be divided evenly into 48 and 64. It can't. Now try the next largest answer (16), and you see that it can be divided evenly into 48 and 64. 16 is the correct answer. The other answers are also factors but the largest of them is 16. Answer C is the correct choice

10 – D. 21/32

To multiply fractions, multiply the numerators and the denominators. In this case, multiply 3 times 7 and 4 times 8. The answer is $^{21}/_{32}$. Answer D is the correct choice.

11 – A. 12

Replace the letters with the numbers they represent and then perform the necessary operations.

$3^2 + 6(0.5)$

$9 + 3 = 12$

Answer A is the correct choice.

12 – B. 40

The least common multiple is used when finding the lowest common denominator. The least common multiple is the lowest number that can be divided evenly by both of the other numbers.

Here is a simple method to find the least common multiple of 8 and 10. Write 8 on the left side of your paper. Then add 8 and write the result. Then add another 8 to that number and write the result. Keep going until you have a list that looks something like this:

8 16 24 32 40…

This is a partial list of multiples of 8. (If you remember your multiplication tables, these numbers are the column or row that go with 8.)

Now do the same thing with 10.

10 20 30 40…

This is the partial list of multiples of 10.

Eventually, the numbers will be found in both rows. That smallest common number is the least common multiple. There will always be more multiples that are common to both rows, but the smallest number is the least common multiple.

Answer B is the correct choice

13 – C. 17/24

To add 1/3 and 3/8, you must find a common denominator. The simplest way to do this is to multiply the denominators: 3 x 8 = 24. So 24 is a common denominator. (This method will not always give you the <u>lowest</u> common denominator, but in this case it does.)

Once you have found a common denominator, you need to convert both fractions in the problem to equivalent fractions that have that same denominator. To do this, multiply each fraction by an equivalent of 1.

$$1/3 \bullet 8/8 = (8 \bullet 1) / (8 \bullet 3) \text{ or } 8/24$$

$$3/8 \bullet 3/3 = (3 \bullet 3) / (8 \bullet 3) \text{ or } 9/24.$$
$$8/24 + 9/24 = 17/24$$

Adding 8/24 and 9/24 is the solution to the problem. Answer C is the correct choice.

14 – C. 81

When two numbers with the same sign (both positive or both negative) are multiplied, the answer is a positive number. When two numbers with different signs (one positive and the other negative) are multiplied, the answer is negative. Answer C is the correct choice.

15 – C. 7/10

The simplest way to solve this problem is to convert the fractions to decimals. You do this by dividing the numerators by the denominators.

$2/3 = 0.67$ and $3/4 = 0.75$, so the correct answer is a decimal that falls between these two numbers.

$$3/5 = 0.6 \text{ (too small)}$$
$$4/5 = 0.8 \text{ (too large)}$$
$$7/10 = 0.7 \text{ (correct choice between 0.67 and 0.75}$$
$$5/8 = 0.625 \text{ (too small)}$$

Answer C is the correct choice

16 – D. 7

In this number:

1 is in the thousands place.
2 is in the hundreds place.
3 is in the tens place.
4 is in the ones place
5 is in the tenths place.
6 is in the hundredths place.
7 is in the thousandths place.

Answer D is the correct choice.

17 – D. 0.72

The simplest way to answer this question is to convert the fractions to decimals. To convert a fraction to a decimal, divide the numerator (the top number) by the denominator (the bottom number).

$$5/8 = 0.625$$
$$3/5 = 0.6$$
$$2/3 = 0.67$$

So the largest number is 0.72. Answer D is the correct choice.

18 – D. 3^4

All positive numbers are larger than the negative numbers, so the possible answers are 42 or 3^4. 3^4 equals 81 (3 • 3 • 3 • 3). Answer D is the correct choice.

19 – C. 4.8571, 4.8573, 4.8578, 4.8579

The numbers **4.857 and 4.858** have an unlimited set of numbers between them and the simplest method is to start with another number after the last digit of 4.857. Therefore 4.8571 and 4.8572 are both greater than 4.857 and less than 4.858. Choices A, B, and D, include numbers that are equal to or greater than the larger of the two or less than the two numbers. Only C has all numbers between. Answer C is the correct choice

20 – D. 23/5

The numbers 4 and 5 can be multiplied by the denominators in the answer set to see which answers are correct. Only D is correct because 20/5 and 25/5 are the numbers that are less than and greater than the answer 23/5. Answer D is the correct choice.

21 – A. 34/5

The numbers 7 and 9 can be multiplied by the denominators in the answer set to see which answers are correct. A is correct because 34/5 is less than 35/5 and 45/5, so it can't be in between. Answer A is the correct choice.

22 – A. 9

Begin by subtracting –3 from both sides of the equation. (This is the same as adding +3). Then:

$$\frac{4}{9}X = 4$$

Now to isolate X on one side of the equation, divide both sides by $\frac{4}{9}$. (To divide by a fraction, invert the fraction and multiply.

$$9/4 * 4/9\ X = 4/1*9/4$$

You are left with $X = \frac{36}{4} = 9$. Answer A is the correct choice.

23 – B. –10

To find the value of q, divide both sides of the equation by –13. When a positive number is divided by a negative number, the answer is negative. Answer B is the correct choice.

24 – D. $x = 4$

When you multiply or divide numbers that have the same sign (both positive or both negative), the answer will be positive. When you multiply or divide numbers that have different signs (one positive and the other negative), the answer will be negative. In this case, both numbers have the same sign. Divide as you normally would and remember that the answer will be a positive number. Answer D is the correct choice.

25 – C. r = (p - 3) / 2

Begin by subtracting 3 from both sides of the equation. You get:

$$p - 3 = 2r$$

Now to isolate r on one side of the equation, divide both sides of the equation by 2. You get:

$$r = (p-3) / 2$$

Answer C is the correct choice

26 – C. x = 11

Subtracting a negative number is the same as adding a positive number. So $8 - (-3)$ is the same as $8 + 3$ or 11. Answer C is the correct choice.

27 – C. 388

The value can be expanded as 7 x 49 added to 9 x 7 with 18 subtracted from the total. That becomes 343 + 63 -18 with the answer equal to 388. Answer C is the correct choice.

28 – B. 42

The value can be expanded as 25 added to 5 x 7 with 18 subtracted from the total. That becomes 25 + 35 -18 with the answer equal to 42. There is another simple way to evaluate this expression. The expression can be rewritten as the product of two expressions (x+9)(x-2). If we substitute 5 for x then this product becomes 14 x 3 which is also 42. Answer B is the correct choice.

29 – C. 6804

The simplest way to evaluate this expression is to rewrite it as the product of two expressions. Factoring common factors out the given expression becomes 7x(x + 9). "7x" becomes 189 and x+9 becomes 36. The product of 189 and 36 becomes 6804. In the interest of eliminating incorrect answers, the product of the values in the "ones" column is 6x9 which is 54. The correct answer must end in 4 so the correct answer must be C. Answer C is the correct choice.

30 – D. $12

Use the information given to write an equation:

$$530 = 40d + 50$$

When you subtract 50 from both sides of the equation, you get:

$$480 = 40d$$

Divide both sides of the equation by 40.

$$12 = d,$$ Sam's hourly wage

Answer D is the correct choice.

---

31 – A. a number greater than X

When a positive number is divided by a positive number less than 1, the quotient will always be larger than the number being divided. For example, $5 \div 0.5 = 10$. If we solve this as a fraction, $5 \div (1/2)$ is the same as $5 \times (2/1)$ or 10 since dividing by a fraction is the same as multiplying by the reciprocal. Answer A is the correct choice.

---

32 – A. (14 + 24) • 8 • 5

In the correct answer, $(14 + 24) \cdot 8 \cdot 5$, the hourly wages of Amanda and Oscar are first combined, and the total amount is multiplied by 8 hours in a day and five days in a week. One of the other choices, $14 + 24 \cdot 8 \cdot 5$, looks similar to this, but it is incorrect because the hourly wages must be combined before they can be multiplied by 8 and 5. Answer A is the correct choice

---

33 – A. 10

Use the facts you are given to write an equation:
$7 + 4/5n = 15$

First subtract 7 from both side of the equation. You get:
$4/5n = 8$

Now divide both sides of the equation by 4/5. To divide by a fraction, invert the fraction (4/5 becomes 5/4) and multiply:
$(5/4)4/5n = 8 \cdot 5/4$

$n = 40/4$ or 10

Answer A is the correct choice

---

34 – D. 108

The ratio of the two numbers is 7:3. This means that the larger number is 7/10 of 360 and the smaller number is 3/10 of 360.

The larger number is $7 \cdot 360/10$ or $7 \cdot 36$ or 252
The smaller number is $3 \cdot 360/10$ or $3 \cdot 36$ or 108

Answer D is the correct choice.

---

35 – C. $310

The costs of all these items can be expressed in terms of the cost of the ream of paper. Use x to represent the cost of a ream of paper. The flash drive costs three times as much as the ream of paper, so it costs $3x$. The textbook costs three times as much as the flash drive, so it costs $9x$. The printer cartridge costs twice as much as the textbook, so it costs $18x$. So now we have:
$x + 3x + 9x + 18x = 31x$

The ream of paper costs $10, so $31x$, the total cost, is $310. Answer C is the correct choice

---

36 – D. $\dfrac{(6)(9)}{2}$

The area of a triangle is one-half the product of the base and the height. Choices A and B are incorrect because they add the base and the height instead of multiplying them. Choice C is incorrect because it multiplies the product of the base and the height by 2 instead of dividing it by 2. Answer D is the correct choice.

---

37 – A. 2,595

The steps in evaluating a mathematical expression must be carried out in a certain order, called the order of operations. These are the steps in order:

Parentheses: The first step is to do any operations in parentheses.
Exponents: Then do any steps that involve exponents
Multiply and **D**ivide: Multiply and divide from left to right
Add and **S**ubtract: Add and subtract from left to right

One way to remember this order is to use this sentence:
Please **E**xcuse **M**y **D**ear **A**unt **S**ally.

To evaluate the expression in this question, follow these steps:

Multiply the numbers in **Parentheses**: $3 \cdot 4 = 12$
Apply the **Exponent** 2 to the number in parentheses: $12^2 = 144$
Multiply: $6 \cdot 3 \cdot 144 = 2,592$
Add: $2 + 2,592 + 1 = 2,595$

Answer A is the correct choice.

---

38 – B. $3x^2 - 4x - 15$

The words in the problem tell us that the new expression for the length is $3x+5$ and the new width is represented by the expression $x-3$. The area is represented by the product of $(3x+5)(x-3)$. Multiplying the two binomials together with FOIL means that the first term is the product of x and $3x$ or $3x^2$. All of the multiple choices have the correct first term. However, the last term is the product of 5 and -3, or -15, which means that answer C is an incorrect answer.

Since the middle term is the difference of $5x$ and $-9x$, which is $-4x$, answer B is the only correct answer. If you choose to use the box method to solve these products, you will see the same results and the same factors. Answer B is the correct choice.

---

39 – C. $14x^2 + 13x + 3$

The words in the problem tell us that the new expression for the base is $4x+2$ and the new height is represented by the expression $7x+3$. The area is represented by the product of $1/2(4x+2)(7x+3)$. Multiplying the two binomials together with FOIL means that the first term is the product of $4x$ and $7x$ and ½ or $14x^2$.

However, the last term is the product of 2 and 3 and 1/2, or 3, which means that answer A is an incorrect answer.

The middle term is ½ the sum of 14x and 12x which is 26/2 x or 13x. Therefore answer C is the only correct answer.

40 – B. 19,098 kg m/s

Momentum is defined as the product of mass times velocity. The conversion of 55 km/hr to meters per second means multiplying by one thousand and dividing by 3600. (seconds per hour). That value,15.28, must be multiplied by the 1,250 kg mass. That answer is 19,098 kg m/s. Answer B is the correct choice.

41 – A. $33,500

Janet has a total of $105,000 in her accounts. 70% of that amount, her goal for her stock investments, is $73,500. To reach that goal, she would have to move $33,500 from bonds to stocks. Answer A is the correct choice.

42 – A. $52,000

Convert 15% to a decimal by moving the decimal point two places to the left: 15% = 0.15. Using x to represent Brian's gross salary, you can write this equation:

$0.15\,x = \$7,800$

To solve for x, divide both sides of the equation by 0.15. $7,800 divided by 0.15 is $52,000. Answer A is the correct choice.

43 – C. 20

To solve this problem, first convert 45% to a decimal by moving the decimal point two place to the left: 45% = .45. Use x to represent the total number of students in the class. Then: $.45x = 9$

Solve for x by dividing both sides of the equation by .45. 9 divided by .45 is 20. Answer C is the correct choice.

44 – B. 515

Marisol scored higher than 78% of the students who took the test. Convert 78% to a decimal by moving the decimal point two places to the left: 78% = .78. Now multiply .78 times the number of students who took the test:

.78 x 660 = 514.8 or 515 students (whole number answers)

Answer B is the correct choice.

45 – D. 130,500

The population of Mariposa County in 2015 was 90% of its population in 2010. Convert 90% to a decimal by moving the decimal point two places to the left: 90% = .90. Now multiply .90 times 145,000, the population in 2010.

$.90 \cdot 145{,}000 = 130{,}500$

Answer D is the correct choice.

46 – A. 20

Alicia must have a score of 75% on a test with 80 questions. To find how many questions she must answer correctly, first convert 75% to a decimal by moving the decimal point two places the left: 75% = .75. Now multiply .75 times 80:

$.75 \cdot 80 = 60.$

Alicia must answer 60 questions correctly, but the question asks how many questions can she miss. If she must answer 60 correctly, then she can miss 20. Answer A is the correct choice.

47 – C. $300

If the phone was on sale at 30% off, the sale price was 70% of the original price. So

$\$210 = 70\% \text{ of } x$

where x is the original price of the phone. When you convert 70% to a decimal, you get:

$\$210 = .70 \cdot x$

To isolate x on one side of the equation, divide both sides of the equation by .70. You find that $x = \$300$. Answer C is the correct choice

48 – A. 84

First, find the number of girls in the class. Convert 52% to a decimal by moving the decimal point two places to the left:

$52\% = .52$

Then multiply .52 times the number of students in the class:

$.52 \cdot 350 = 182$

$182 - 98 = 84$

Of the 182 girls, 98 plan to go to college, so a total of 84 do not plan to go to college. Answer A is the correct choice

49 – C. 12%

To find the percent increase, you first need to know the amount of the increase. Enrollment went from 3,450 in 2010 to 3,864 in 2015. This is an increase of 414. Now, to find the percent of the increase, divide the amount of the increase by the original amount:

$$414 \div 3{,}450 = 0.12$$

To convert a decimal to a percent, move the decimal point two places to the right:

$$0.12 = 12\%$$

When a question asks for the percent increase or decrease, divide the amount of the increase or decrease by the original value. Answer C is the correct choice.

50 – D. 14 pounds 14 ounces

When rounding measurements to the whole number value, the measurement is usually rounded up to the next larger whole number if that measurement is halfway or closer to the next higher value. In this case, since there 16 ounces in a pound, D is the correct answer.

51 – C. 7,514,635.8239

When rounding a number to a given place value, the next lower place value is used to determine if the number is rounded up or down. The rounded value has its last significant digit in that place. Answer C has a number 9 in the ten thousandths place. Notice the difference between ten-thousands and ten-thousandths. Answer A is rounded to the ten-thousands place!

52 – C. 7.15 cc's

When rounding a measurement, the value includes a precision of plus or minus half of the smallest increment measured. The lines on the cylinder would have the values of 7.00, 7.10, 7.20, or each tenth of a cc. The actual value of the meniscus that reads between tenths would be 7.15 cc. Answer C has a number with the correct precision.

53 – C. 4 men for 1 day

When estimating, it is helpful to round before estimating. The summary of this problems solution includes a rate of 200 pounds per hour (15 minute each). Two and one-half tons is 5000 pounds. 5000 pounds divided by 200 pounds per hour means 25 hours of labor is required. Answer C is the best estimate of 25 hours of labor (32). Answer A is 800 hours, B is 16 hours, and D is 200 hours.

54 – B. 40 minutes

When estimating this answer, the basic formula of distance equal to rate multiplied by time applies. So the time required for the trip is the distance divided by the rate. 18 miles divide by ¾ (45 minutes is ¾ of an hour), is 24 miles per hour. The new rate would be 29 miles per hour (increase of 5). 18 divided by 29 is about 60% of an hour or close to 40 minutes. 30 minutes is a close answer, but that is only possible if the rate is 36 miles per hour! Estimating may require that you eliminate answers that are close to the correct answer. Answer B is the correct choice

55 – C. 70 seconds per m/c; 35 seconds per t/f

An estimate often means that you will need to check possible answers to see if they are correct. In this example, the basic assumption is that the time for m/c problems will be twice the value for the t/f. Trying one minute for m/c and one half minute for t/f comes out to 35 minutes. So answer B is not correct. The next closest one is answer C which comes out to 1400 seconds and 1050 seconds for the total 2450 seconds. That is close to the allowable 2700 seconds (45 minutes). If you try answer

D, the total comes out to 1600 plus 1200 or a total of 2800 seconds. That's more than the allowable total of 2700. Answer C is the correct choice.

56 – B. twice as fast

When estimating this answer, the formula of distance equal to rate multiplied by time applies. So the speed required for the trip is the distance divided by the time. In this example 10 minutes late means half the amount of time. Dividing by one-half means that the rate must be doubled. Answer B is the correct choice.

SCIENCE

1- B. smooth endoplasmic reticulum does not participate in synthesis of proteins.

Smooth endoplasmic reticulum does not contain ribosomes. Rough endoplasmic reticulum does contain ribosomes. Ribosomes are required to synthesize proteins. Both RER and SER may be involved in the synthesis of products that are destined for transport and secretion out of the cell into the external environment.

2- A. an external cell membrane

An external cell membrane is a feature of all living cells. Many cells such as plant fungi and bacterial cells also possess at least one outer cell wall, but human and other animal cells do not. Bacterial cells do not possess a nucleus or mitochondria.

3- B. coronal

Coronal refers to an axial plane of the body. The other axial planes are the sagittal and the cross sectional planes. Caudal means nearer to the tail or the posterior part of the body. Ventral means at or nearer to the frontal surface of the body. The term inferior means near to the feet.

4- C. microtubules

Human sperm flagellum are constructed from and internal bundle of microtubules that interact with a microtubule organizing structure at the base of the flagellum. The individual microtubules sequentially slide back and forth within the outer envelope of the flagellum causing a whipping motion that generates a forward motion of the sperm cells. Thick or myosin filaments are critical elements of muscle contraction and actin microfilaments are involved in many functions that require active purposeful movement of cells and within cells but neither are elements of the flagellum of human sperm cells. Intermediate filaments are generally structural elements of the cytoskeletal framework of a cell and do not contribute to the functioning of flagellum of human sperm cells.

5- B. high extracellular matrix volume

Muscle and nerve tissue have high cell volume compared to extracellular matrix volumes. In voluntary muscle the neuromuscular junction is an interface between the terminal endings of axons of neurons and cell membranes of muscle fibrils. Actin filaments are a component of the thin fibers of sarcomeres in voluntary muscle tissue. All muscle cells have electrically excitable membranes that can conduct electrical signals along the surface of muscle outer cellular membranes

6- A. ACG

The nitrogenous base thymine (T) occurs in DNA molecules but not in RNA molecules. The nitrogenous base uracil (U) occurs in RNA molecules but not in DNA molecules. The remaining nitrogenous basis of nucleic acids, adenine (A), cytosine (C) and guanine (G) occur in both RNA and DNA. Codons are DNA 3-base sequences and anticodons are RNA 3-base sequences. Among the choices only choice A has a three base sequence that does not include thymine or uracil. Therefore, this is the only choice that could occur in both an RNA and a DNA sequence.

7- B. acetyl CoA

Acetyl CoA is generated by conversion of pyruvate -an end product of glycolysis and by many other chemical pathways including the metabolism of lipids. It is a starting reactant molecule that enters at the beginning of a Krebs cycle. Two CO_2 molecules, 2 NADH molecules and one $FADH_2$ molecules are among the product molecules generated by each round of a Krebs cycle.

8- C. A polar body is generated

The successful maturation of a human primary follicle into a human secondary follicle occurs in response to the LH peak in the ovulatory cycle. During this maturation phase, the primary oocyte of the primary follicle undergoes a meiotic division resulting in a secondary oocyte and a polar body. The formation of the corpus luteum occurs after the rupture of the secondary follicle and the release of the secondary oocyte. Degeneration of the corpus luteum occurs a few days after ovulation if the secondary oocyte is not fertilized. Increasing estrogen levels trigger an initial luteinizing hormone (LH) peak during an ovulatory cycle but a second peak does not occur during a cycle.

9- D. Leydig; testosterone

Leydig cells of the testes produce testosterone in the male reproductive system. The tunica albuginea is a fibrous outer membrane of the testis and does not directly participate in the production of any particular type of cells. Sertoli cells produce various substances that support the development of sperm cell precursor cells, but they do not produce FSH. Spermatogonia are cells that are progenitors of mature sperm cells. Spermatogonia do not produce LH.

10- A. elbow; knee

The elbow and knee joints are both synovial hinge joints which allow flexion and extension. The elbow joint is a complex hinge joint that also allows the head of the radius to pivot at the articulation of the distal end of the humerus. This allows for additional range of motion in the form of supination and pronation of the lower arm and hand. This additional range of motion is much greater than that allowed by the knee joint. The sacroiliac joint connects the sacrum (triangular bone at the bottom of the spine) with the pelvis (iliac bone that is part of the hip joint) on each side of the lower spine. It is a non-synovial ligamentous joint that has very little range of motion, less than any of the other joints listed in the choices above. The elbow and shoulder joints are both synovial ball-and-socket joints which have a much greater range of motion than hinge joints such as the knee and elbow.

11- D. lung, liver and pancreas

The lung, liver and pancreas are all primarily derived from endoderm. The heart and the kidney are primarily derived from mesoderm. The brain is primarily derived from ectoderm.

12- B. prevention of collapse of alveoli during exhalation

Pulmonary surfactant decreases the surface tension of the fluid layer overlying the internal surfaces of alveoli. The surface tension of fluid layers of a concave surface such as the internal surface of a sphere increases as the radius of sphere decreases. Without pulmonary surfactant the surface tension of the aqueous layer within alveoli would increase as the alveoli deflate during exhalation to a point where the alveoli would completely collapse. This event would prevent reflation of the alveoli on a subsequent inspiratory effort.

13- C. pulmonary artery pressure

A maximal inspiratory effort increases intrathoracic volume by maximally decreasing the convexity of the diaphragm and by lifting the ribs upward and outward through contraction of intercostal muscles (accessory muscles of inspiration). Maximal inspiration increases the volume of lung that is both perfused and ventilated therefore the diffusion of CO_2 into the alveolar airspaces and the diffusion of O_2 out of alveolar airspaces will increase. With additional regions of the lung perfused during maximal inspiration, the total cross sectional area of the pulmonary outflow tract of the heart increases. The total resistance to a fixed amount of blood delivered by the contraction of the right ventricle decreases and the pulmonary artery pressure most likely will decrease rather than increase.

14- B. The right ventricular pressure reaches a minimum value.

Systole is the portion of the cardiac cycle where the ventricles are contracting. The end of systole corresponds with the completion of ventricular contraction. The pressures within ventricle reach a minimum value at the end of their contraction cycles. The aortic valve opens and the mitral valve closes at the beginning of systole. The AV node does not generate electrical impulses but will conduct electrical signals across the AV septum at the beginning of systole.

15- A. the atrioventricular septum

The AV septum tissue is non-conductive and prevents the propagation of electrical signal from the atrium to the ventricles. The exception occurs at The AV node where electrical signals are intercalated discs possess gap junctions that allow electrical signals to propagate through cardiac muscle tissue. Purkinje fibers act as electrical conduction wires within the walls of ventricles.

16- A. a peripheral vein located in the leg

The pulmonary arteries are components of the right cardiovascular circulation system. Blood clots of the pulmonary arteries (thrombotic pulmonary embolisms) must originate from sites within the right heart circulation unless there is an abnormal pathway from the left to the right circulation pathways such as a direct connection between the left and right atrium. Most commonly, thrombotic pulmonary embolisms originate as blood clots in large deep veins of the lower leg. The origins listed in the other choices are all located on the left side of the heart circulation.

17- B. plasma cells

White blood cells or leukocytes include lymphocytes and non-lymphocytes Lymphocytes include T-cells, B-cells and the activated form of B-cells - the plasma cell Eosinophils, basophils, monocytes and polymorphonuclear leucocytes (PMNLs) are all non-lymphocyte lineage white blood cell types.

18- A. HLA class I antigens

The major histocompatibility complex (MHC) class I human leukocyte antigens (HLA) are generally restricted to the cell membranes of dedicated or professional antigen presenting cells of the immune system. T-cells are activated when they bind with a class I molecule and an antigen on the surface of an antigen presenting cell. ABO and Rh factor molecules are generally restricted to red blood cell (RBC) membranes and can be a antigen that is identified as foreign by the immune system. Cadherin class cell adhesion molecules are involved primarily with structural functions related to binding with extracellular matrix molecules.

19- D. lacteals

A common feature of non-glandular epithelial tissues, including the primary cell type of the epithelial lining of the intestines, is polarity. This refers to the separation of structure and functions of the top or apical region of the epithelial cell from lower or basal regions of the cell. Enterocytes at their apical surface (the surface exposed to the contents of the lumen of the intestinal tract) have dense hair like extensions called microvilli. These microvilli vastly increase the surface area of the enterocytes that is exposed to the contents of the lumen of the intestines. This increases the efficiency of the enterocytes ability to absorb water and nutrients from the intestine. Tight junctions and desmosomes knit adjacent enterocytes together at or near their apical surfaces. This creates are relatively impermeable barrier to contents of the intestine, preventing the contents from diffusing between enterocytes. Lacteals are sealed terminals of lymphatic vessels that are located in the cores of intestinal villi that underlie enterocytes. They are responsible for receiving lipids from overlying enterocytes. Theses lipids are derived from lipids absorbed by the enterocytes from the intestine.

20- C. a meal with high simple carbohydrate content

The most common stimulus for the release of the hormone glucagon is low levels of glucose in the bloodstream. The primary effect of glucagon is on the liver, where it induces the liver to break down stored glycogen molecules into glucose molecules. The glucose molecules are secreted into the bloodstream and restore the blood glucose levels toward normal. Conversely, high blood glucose levels have the opposite effect, namely the suppression of the release of glucagon. A meal high in carbohydrates will generally result in high levels of blood glucose, because carbohydrates are composed primarily of glucose monomers. Simple carbohydrates are easily hydrolyzed by enzymes in the digestive tract to glucose molecules which in turn are rapidly absorbed into the circulation. This increases blood glucose levels and consequently tends to suppress glucagon secretion.

21- B. CCK secretion→↑bile secretion→↑fat emulsification

Cholecystokinin release from the duodenum triggers the release of bile from the gallbladder into the duodenal lumen. Bile emulsifies collections of lipids in the duodenum. Somatostatin is a hormone secreted by the duodenum and the pancreas (and anterior pituitary gland) that inhibits HCL secretion and gastrin secretion in the stomach. Secretin is a hormone released by the duodenum that inhibits HCl secretion in the stomach and stimulates the release of bicarbonate by the pancreas.

22- D. potassium ion (K+) diffusion out of a neuron

As the transmembrane potential reaches a positive peak during an action potential, voltage-gated potassium ion channels are activated and K+ ions, which have a higher intracellular concentration compared to extracellular concentration, diffuse out of the cell. This rapidly reverses the peak positive transmembrane potential of the action potential and generates a negative transmembrane potential that is more negative than the normal resting transmembrane potential. This is referred to as hyperpolarization. The effect of hyperpolarization is to cause the local cell membrane to become less likely to generate another action potential. The short period of time that corresponds to the persistence of the hyperpolarization of the local membrane region is called the refractory period of an action potential.

23- A. The release of norepinephrine (NE) into the neuron-myofibril gap of a neuromuscular junction

The choices from A through D summarize the process of contraction that occurs in sarcomeres within a myofibril beginning with the release of a neurotransmitter at a neuromuscular junction. The incorrect step is that the neurotransmitter that is released is not norepinephrine (NE). Acetylcholine (ACh) is the neurotransmitter released at neuromuscular junctions.

24- B. oligodendroglia and astrocytes

Both Schwann cells - in the peripheral nervous system - and oligodendroglia - in the central nervous system - produce myelin sheaths for axons of neurons. Astrocytes contribute to the blood-brain barrier of the central nervous system. Microglia provide metabolic support functions to neurons in the CNC. The axons of neurons can have myelin sheaths, but neurons do not produce myelin themselves.

25- B. the parietal lobes of the cerebral cortex

The primary motor cortices of the parietal lobes contain upper-motor neurons that initial the electrical signal sequence that ultimately triggers voluntary muscle movement. The parietal cortex processes auditory information. Both the basal ganglia and the cerebellum provide additional processing of voluntary muscle signals, but they do not initiate voluntary muscle movement signals.

26- C. inadequate amounts of O_2 delivered to muscle tissue

Lactic acid (lactate) production in muscle tissue results from the anaerobic conversion of pyruvate (predominantly as a product of glycolysis) to lactic acid. This process generates energy but is very inefficient compared to oxidative metabolism of glucose. Inadequate oxygen supplies shift energy production to the anaerobic pathway that generates lactic acid. Additionally, oxygen is required to reduce lactate back to pyruvate. In an oxygen deficient environment, muscle tissue cannot convert lactate back to pyruvate and consequently lactate levels rise within muscle tissue.

27- D. contraction of smooth muscle in the walls of arterioles in voluntary muscle tissue

Parasympathetic nervous system activation produces physiological changes that are associated with resting and digestive functions. Contraction of smooth muscle in the walls of arterioles in voluntary muscle tissue redirects blood flow from voluntary muscles where it can be utilized by the digestive system. Increased sinoatrial node activity results in an increase in heart rate; decreased activity of smooth muscle contractions in the wall of the digestive tract slows peristalsis and inhibits digestive processes. Both of these effects are the opposite one would expect of parasympathetic effects. There are no direct autonomic effects on deep tendon reflexes. These are independent reflex arc consisting of only a sensory receptor cell and one or two neurons in a sequence terminating on a voluntary muscle.

28- C. dendrites

Ligand-gated ion channels respond to the binding of a substance to it membrane receptor. In neurons, these ligands are usually neurotransmitter molecules. The site of release of neurotransmitters by neurons is usually at the synapse of two neurons or at a neuromuscular junction. Neurotransmitters are released by axon terminals of the presynaptic neuron into the synaptic cleft. The neurotransmitters diffuse across to the adjacent membrane region of the postsynaptic neuron. Most often this is the terminal region of a dendrite of the postsynaptic neuron. This is the reason that ligand-gated ion channels are usually most highly concentrated in the dendrites of neurons.

29- B. the seminiferous tubules

The first stage of spermatogenesis occurs in the walls of seminiferous tubules in the testis. Later stages of spermatogenesis occur within the lumen of the convoluted vessels that is the epididymis. The corpus spongiosum is highly vascularized region of the penis that comprises most of the tissue mass of the penis. The seminal vesicles are internal gland of the male reproductive system that provides most of the seminal fluid that nourishes and transports sperm within the genitourinary system. Neither the corpus spongiosum nor the seminal vesicles contain any sperm cells or progenitors of sperm cells.

30- C. medial to the labia minora and inferolateral to the vaginal introitus

The Bartholin's glands or greater vestibular glands are 1 to 2 cm length glands with a terminal ductal orifice located immediately inferolateral (one gland to the left and one to the right) to the vaginal introitus (external entrance). Bartholin's glands secrete mucus which provides lubrication of the vagina.

31- D. gland→dermis→basement membrane→epidermis→external surface of the epidermis

There are two general types of sweat glands located in human integument, apocrine and eccrine sweat glands. The eccrine sweat glands are by far the most numerous and excrete sweat onto the outer surface of the skin. The apocrine sweat glands are located in the lower dermis near the interface with the underlying hypodermal layer of the integument (also called the subcutaneous layer) apocrine sweat gland duct beginning at the origin to the body of the gland must sequentially pass through the overlying region of the dermis and then pass through the basement membrane which separates the dermis from the more superficial epidermis. In the epidermis the duct inserts into a hair follicle and excretes the apocrine glandular oily sweat solution into the space between the keratigenous hair shaft and the outer wall of the hair follicle.

32- A. immune - antigen presentation

Langerhans cells are a form of dendritic cell that are located primarily in the epidermis (except for the most superficial layer - the stratum corneum) regions of the epidermis and superficial regions of the dermis. Langerhans cells are antigen presenting cell. In the integument they ingest debris resulting from skin infections and present them on their cell membranes for interaction with other immune system cells.

33- D. connective; energy storage

The hypodermis is the deepest of the three layers of the human integument. It is primarily loose connective tissue with a high content of adipocytes. One of the primary functions of the adipocytes is the storage of fat which serves as an energy reserve for the body. The adipocytes also provide some mechanical cushioning properties to the integument but they allow interstitial fluids and cells to freely pass through the hypodermis. This is the opposite of a barrier function

34- B. melatonin

There are no obvious methods to determine if a hormone is produced by the pituitary other than to memorize which are and which are not. Often this type of question can be answered by recognizing a hormone that is easily identified as the product of another endocrine gland. In this case, melatonin is the only significant hormone produced by the pineal gland and it is not a significant product of any other gland.

35- B. thyroid hormone (T3 and T4)

At the most general level the activation of the sympathetic nervous system induces a high level of overall alertness and priming of the body for high energy activities. Among these effects is an elevated metabolic state. Thyroid hormones in general also induce increased metabolic activity. It is often difficult to distinguish the difference is symptoms between persons with excessive levels of thyroid hormone (hyperthyroidism) and those with extreme activation of the sympathetic nervous system, as occurs with general anxiety disorders, and panic attacks.

36- A. osteoblasts

The non-cellular structural components of bones consist of a matrix of a calcium and phosphorous containing mineral called hydroxyapatite and collagen fibers. Collagen is produced by fibroblasts and the hydroxyapatite that is laid down during bone formation is secreted by osteoblasts. In mature bone, some osteoblasts differentiate into osteocytes' which are sparsely distributed within the center of osteons of bones. Osteocytes secrete small amounts of hydroxyapatite but this is after the bone has been formed. Osteoclasts break down bone matrix - usually during bone remodeling activities. Lamellar bone has well organized arrangements of collagen fibers within the bone matrix. In contrast, woven bone has randomly arranged collagen fibers. Lamellar bone possesses significantly greater mechanical strength compared to woven bone.

37- C. haversian canals

Trabecular or cancellous bone is one of two general types of bone, the other being cortical or hard bone. In contrast to cortical bone, trabecular bone has a porous, irregular structure that forms extensive cavities that contain adipocytes and the progenitor cells of both red blood cells (hematopoietic stem cells). Trabecular bone is diffusely and heavily vascularized. Compact bone is comparatively poorly vascularized, with blood vessels primarily limited to haversian canals. Haversian canals are features of compact bone. Haversian canals are longitudinal passages that contain blood vessels that branch into smaller vessels that provide blood supplies to osteocytes located in lacunae (small hollow spaces) located in the center of osteons (structural subunits) of compact bone.

38- B. temporomandibular joint

Of the four choices, three are completely fused or relatively immobile non-synovial joints. The temporomandibular joint is a highly mobile synovial joint which allows for the chewing motions of the lower jaw (mandible).

39- D. the glomeruli

Arterial blood arrives for filtration by the kidney via the renal artery. The renal artery undergoes several branching to eventually form renal arterioles that extend throughout the renal cortex. Branches of these arterioles form tufts of capillaries that occupy an invagination of Bowman's capsule. Bowman's capsule is a balloon-like expansion of the proximal renal tubule. The combined region of capillary tufts and Bowman's capsule is called a glomerulus. There are over one million glomeruli in the renal cortex. The walls of the capillary tufts are uncharacteristically permeable to water and dissolved solutes such as electrolytes, urea and other substances. The blood pressure inside the capillaries exceeds the pressure of the surrounding extracellular space and of the fluid within the lumen of Bowman's capsule. This pressure gradient drives water and dissolved solutes out of the capillary tufts and into the lumen of Bowman's capsule. The solution that enters the capsule lumen is referred to as a filtrate.

40- C. Increased renal tubule permeability to water

Rational: The effect of antidiuretic hormone on the kidney is to increase the permeability of the renal tubules and collecting ducts to water. This results in the diffusion of water out of the filtrate solution and into the renal medulla where it can be reabsorbed into the circulation by renal capillaries within the renal medulla. This concentrates urine and reduces the loss of additional water from the body that occurs through the excretory system.

41- C. increased secretion of antidiuretic hormone

Osmoreceptors in the hypothalamus and the pituitary gland directly detect plasma osmolality from adjacent capillaries. When plasma osmolality is undesirably high, the osmoreceptors relay this information to the pituitary. The pituitary response is to release antidiuretic hormone (ADH). As discussed in the rationale for question 40, the effect of antidiuretic hormone on the kidney is to increase the permeability of the renal tubules and collecting ducts to water. This results in the diffusion of water out of the filtrate solution and into the renal medulla where it can be reabsorbed into the circulation by renal capillaries within the renal medulla. This concentrates urine and reduces the loss of additional water from the body that occurs through the excretory system.

42- A. an undesirably low plasma sodium ion concentration; renin

The kidney is able to directly detect the sodium ion concentration of plasma within renal arterioles. A response of the kidney to an undesirably low plasma sodium ion concentration (and also to low blood pressure) is the release of the hormone renin. Renin in the bloodstream leads to the production of angiotensin II. Angiotensin II is a potent vasoconstrictor and also stimulates the release of aldosterone from the adrenal gland. The adrenal gland is not part of the kidney - although it does rest upon the superior pole of the kidney. Aldosterone causes the kidney to increase the reabsorption of sodium ion thereby helping to restore plasma ion concentrations to normal levels.

43- A. glucose

Under normal circumstances, glucose molecules that are filtered from the blood into a renal tubule are 100% reabsorbed from the filtrate. This process can be overwhelmed when blood levels of glucose are abnormally high. Glucose in the urine is an abnormal finding and often indicates the presence of type 1 or type 2 diabetes mellitus. The presence of sodium, urea and bicarbonate ion in the urine is normal so clearly these are not completely reabsorbed from renal tubule filtrates

44- C. concentration of urine

The loop of Henle is a U-shaped segment of the renal tubules. It is the mid-portion of the renal tubule - located between the proximal convoluted tubule segment and the distal convoluted tubule segment of the renal tubules. The bottom of the "U" in the loops of Henle are located in the renal medulla. The distal or ascending limb of the loop excretes sodium ion from the tubule into the adjacent interstitium of the medulla. This creates a very high osmolality of the interstitial fluids in the adrenal medulla. The renal collecting tubules pass through the renal medulla on their pathway to the sinuses of the renal pelvis. The permeability of the renal collecting tubules to water can be adjusted by various hormonal influences. The collecting tubules are impermeable to sodium and other solutes. When the tubules are maximally permeable to water, water diffuses out of the tubules into the adrenal medulla interstitium. Since this is a process of diffusion, the maximal concentration of urine or the maximum osmolality of the urine that can be produced is slightly lower than the osmolality of the interstitium of the adrenal medulla. As water diffuses out of the tubule solution, the osmolality of the solution increases. When the osmolality of the two regions are nearly equal the driving force of the diffusion of water disappears as the concentration gradient between the two regions is eliminated.

45- B. decreased glomerular filtration rate (GFR)

The glomerular filtration rate of the kidney is the volume of fluid that is driven out of glomerular capillaries and into the lumen of Bowman's capsule per unit time. This rate is determined by the blood flow rate to the glomerular capillaries and the pressure gradient between blood within glomerular capillaries and the pressure within Bowman's capsule - the greater the pressure gradient the greater the filtration rate. Decreasing blood pressure decreases the magnitude of the pressure gradient and therefore reduces the kidney's glomerular filtration rate.

46- A. increased blood pressure

Angiotensin II is the activated form of angiotensin hormone. Activation of angiotensin begins with the release of the hormone renin from the kidney. Angiotensin II has a direct effect on circulatory vessels causing contraction of smooth muscle cells located in the walls of arteries and veins. This increases the force of the vessel walls on the blood within the vessels resulting in increased blood pressure. Angiotensin II has a direct effect on the proximal tubules to increase Na+ reabsorption. But this is not one of the answer choice options. Angiotensin II also stimulates the release of the hormone aldosterone which has additional effects on the kidney. These effects are indirect effects on the kidney.

47- D. complement proteins

The membrane attack complex is a multiprotein structure that attaches to the exterior cell membrane of disease causing bacteria that have invaded the human body. The MAC punctures the cell membrane allowing contents of the cell to escape and external substances to enter the interior of the cell (cell lysis). This results in the death of the cell. The MAC is formed from activated protein fragments of the complement proteins (the C5b-C6-C7-C8-C9 complement proteins and protein fragments). Complement proteins circulate continuously throughout the body. Over 30 proteins and protein fragments make up the complement system When the either the innate or active immune system is activated, complement proteins may be activated in a sequential cascade, where one activated complement protein or protein fragment catalyzes the activation of the next set of complement proteins. The activation of the complement cascade also produces activated proteins and protein fragment that the phagocytosis of cells and other substances and also act as cell signaling molecules that recruit immune cells to the site of an infection

48- C. chief cells

Chief cells are cells located in the stomach that secrete pepsinogen - a digestive proenzyme. The immune response to viral infection is generally an active immune response requiring the activation of B-cells by T-cells and the differentiation of B-cells -into plasma cells. Plasma cells then produce circulating antibodies that target the specific viral associated antigens. Interferons are circulating proteins that suppress the intracellular replication of viruses and have several other important antiviral functions.

49- D. deactivation of the snake venom toxin molecules by antigen-specific antibody binding

Antivenom to snake venom (and other biological venoms) is created by injecting the venom into lab animals and collecting the animal's blood serum afterwards. The injected animal will generate an active immune response to the venom that includes the production of antibodies that are targeted to antigens present on the venom molecules. In human patients, these antibodies bind to the venom molecules and in the process disrupt the venom's ability to cause injury either by altering the active sites of the venom molecule or by sequestering the venom molecules within antigen-antibody complexes which neutralize the antigen and enhance the clearance of the venom molecules from the body.

50- B. active humoral

The influenza virus contains viral shell proteins of the influenza virus that are recognized upon injection into the body by T-helper cells that have receptors complementary to the injected antigens. The T-cells activate B-cells with complementary antibody capability. Activation induces B-cell differentiation into plasma cells which actively release antigen specific antibodies into the circulation. These antibodies are short lived and will not protect against influenza infection after a few days. The exposure to the vaccine proteins antigens also results in the differentiation of some of the activated B-cells into long-lived memory cell that can generate a much stronger and more rapid antibody response to a subsequent encounter with infectious influenza viral particles. This rapid response is sufficient to prevent the viral particles from infecting significant numbers of cells in the body. The antibody response is part of the active immune response (vs. the innate immune response) and is categorized as the humoral division of the active immune response (vs. the cellular cell-dependent active immune response).

51- B. bone marrow; thymus

All circulating red and white blood cell types of the human body originate from hematopoietic stem cells located in the bone marrow (and a few other regions in some circumstances in some individuals). Immature T-cells then migrate to the thymus early in life. These immature T-cells, as a group, have at least a few T-cells have the ability to respond to almost any possible specific molecular antigen including all of the antigens that are present in the host body. In the thymus, those T-cells that are capable of reacting to host antigens are detected and eliminated. Without this vital selection process, these T-cells would trigger immune system attacks against the body's own cells. This T-cell screening process continues into the early- to mid-teenage years. Afterwards the thymus progressively decreases in size and functionality.

52- B. redness and heat only

The four cardinal signs of localized infection are the result of the effects of various molecules that are generated by injured and infected cells and by immune cells that migrate to the site of infection. The most important of these molecules are histamines and prostaglandins. One of the effects of these molecules is to induce dilation of the local blood vessels - resulting in redness and increased heat due to increased local blood flow. Swelling is due to the accumulation of fluids and other substances that leak from the local blood vessels due to the increased permeability of the vessels induced by the infection-associated molecules. The pain associated with a localized infection is in part indirectly due to vascular permeability since increased swelling can trigger pain receptors. Pain is also a direct effect of the infection-associated molecules.

53- A. type 1 diabetes mellitus

Type 1 diabetes is a disease where the body produces either inadequate amounts of insulin or more commonly no insulin. In diabetes type 1, the immune system attacks the insulin-producing beta cells in the pancreas and destroys them. Cystic fibrosis and sickle cell disease are classic genetic diseases characterized by dysfunctional alleles of specific genes. Peptic ulcer disease is usually a result of chronic infection of the stomach by the bacteria H. pylori. The Nobel Prize in medicine was awarded to the physician who proved this was true.

54- B. antigen→mast cell release of histamine

Seasonal pollen and mold allergies (hay fever) are a type I hypersensitivity reaction. Hypersensitivity reactions are caused by activation of the immune system in response to relatively harmless substances or excessively strong immune responses to relatively minor infectious or toxic chemical exposure. Hay fever is a hypersensitivity to airborne pollen or molds that are otherwise not harmful to the mucosal tissue of the upper airway epithelium. Mast cells are immune response cell that contain large amounts of histamine and other substances that can trigger inflammation processes. Mast cells are located within or just deep to the epithelial tissue of respiratory airways. Pollen or mold antigens that are inhaled subsequently diffuse into upper respiratory epithelial tissue and bind to receptors on mast that are complementary to these antigens. This triggers the release of histamine into the surrounding tissue. The effects of histamine are dilation and increased blood flow in local blood vessels, increased permeability of local blood vessels and direct and indirect chemical irritation of local sensory nerve fibers and adjacent cells within the epithelia tissues. These effects generate the typical signs and symptoms of hay fever including itching, nasal congestion sneezing, watery eyes and increased watery mucous secretion within the upper airways.

55- A. $AA_1 + AA_2 \rightarrow AA_1\text{-}AA_2 + H_2O$

Single chain proteins are linear amino acid polymers that are synthesized by formation of peptide bonds between individual amino acid monomers. Amino acids contain an amine group (-NH2) and a carboxylic acid group (-COOH) bonded to a central carbon atom. Peptide bonds are formed between adjacent amino acids in a polypeptide chain through a dehydration (condensation) reaction of the amine group of one amino acid and the carboxylic acid of an adjacent amino acid. Dehydration reactions produce a one or more H_2O molecules as a product of each individual dehydration reaction. Amino acids can form two peptide bond with other amino acids by forming one peptide bond through a dehydration reaction with their carboxylic acid group and the amine group of an adjacent amino acid and a second peptide bond through a dehydration reaction with their amine group and the carboxylic acid group of an adjacent amino acid.

ENGLISH & READING

1. C. Counterfeiting of American money is an enormous problem.

C is the best option as we are told that "The Treasury goes to extraordinary lengths to safeguard cash from counterfeiters."

2. B. Yet, despite all of these technological innovations, the race to stay ahead of savvy counterfeiters and their constantly changing counterfeiting techniques is a never-ending one.

B is the best as the main point of the passage is to emphasize the extent of counterfeiting and detail the technology used to counteract such constantly changing fraudulent activity.

3. C. Expository

An expository essay is one in which an idea is investigated and expounded upon, and an argument is set forth presenting evidence concerning that idea in a clear and concise manner. In this case the idea being investigated and expounded upon is anti-counterfeiting techniques.

4. A. A pamphlet for tourists visiting the United States Treasury

The style and specific subject matter all indicate that it is most likely from an informational pamphlet written for visitors to the Bureau of Engraving and Printing.

5. C. A letter from the US treasury Secretary to the President

A primary source document is one which was created and serves as a first-hand source of information or evidence about a particular time period. Only the personal letter would meet the criteria of a primary source.

---

6. D. Inherent

Technological sophistication is inherent, (or naturally found) in the making of American money, so much so that to call it "paper" does not fully reveal how complex a product it really is.

---

7. A. In the Middle Ages, merchants an artisans formed groups called "guilds" to protect themselves and their trades.

The first sentence is the topic sentence because it introduces the main idea of the paragraph.

---

8. C. merchant guilds originated in the Middle Ages and became extremely popular, eventually leading to a sophisticated apprenticeship system.

The guild system's origins and development is the main idea of the paragraph. The other options are too narrow to constitute a main idea.

---

9. A. prior to the inception of guilds, merchants were susceptible to competition from lesser skilled craftsmen peddling inferior products or services.

It can be inferred that if guilds were instituted, there must have been a need for merchants to safeguard themselves from threats to their livelihood.

---

10. C. similar

The sentence conveys to us that the spice, silk and wool dealers were similar tradesman to that of other merchants who had set up guilds.

---

11. C. By that time,

The passage introduces the inception of guilds and their development over time, chronologically. From the previous sentence, it is clear that guilds grew in popularity over the centuries, until towns like Florence had 50 guilds by the twelfth century. "By that time" most clearly states this increase and development over time.

---

12. B. To criticize the American press for not taking responsibility for their actions

Luce is clearly criticizing the press for not taking responsibility to disseminate enlightening information to the public, and instead are blaming the public for not asking for reading matter which is "tasteful and more illuminating".

---

13. A. A newspaper editorial letter

Given the paragraph's opinionated style and serious, critical tone, it most likely excerpted from a longer letter printed in the op/ed section of a newspaper.

---

14. C. A diary entry

The diary entry (which would likely provide firsthand thoughts, feelings and opinions about current life or world events as witnessed by the author) would qualify as a primary source document of evidence or information of a particular time period.

---

15. D. enlightening

Illuminating reading matter is that which would be enlightening and provide necessary information to the public.

---

16. C. therefore

Luce is using a cause and effect argument here, but she is questioning the excuse of the press to not do their job as a result of certain demands of the public, which would "therefore exonerate the American press for its failures to give the American people more tasteful and more illuminating reading matter".

17. C. disapproval

Luce clearly disapproves of the press and their practice of serving up a lack of news to the public, "on the grounds that, after all, "[they] have to give the people what they want or [they] will go out of business".

18. B. persuasive/argumentative

Luce utilizes several modes of writing here, but overall, she is critical of the American press, and is *arguing* that they are at fault for not giving the American public useful information or "illuminating reading matter".

19. B. The author has worked in the journalism industry

The author clearly has an understanding of the business of the media, as well as its public responsibility to inform citizens, so it can be concluded that she likely has worked in the journalism industry. None of the other statements can reasonably be concluded based on the content of the passage.

20. B. Football was played for decades on school campuses nationwide before the American Professional Football Association was formed in 1920, and then renamed the National Football League (or the NFL) two years later.

This statement adds additional information to the paragraph about the progression of the game of football in the US and therefore, appropriately concludes the paragraph. The other statements discuss topics not directly related to football, or add additional information that is slightly off topic.

21. A. however

The sentence is explaining that, despite the appearance of football as a sport on some college campuses, and annual scrimmages occurring at Yale, 25 years passed before it became a regular activity in college life. "However" shows this contrast best.

22. A. Rejection of the past and outmoded ideas

From the paragraph it is clear that modernism is mainly concerned with rejecting the ideas of the past -- like the science of the enlightenment, and old ideas about religion –and instead focusing on creating what was "New".

23. B. Basis

Pound's suggestion to "Make it new" was the basis, or *touchstone* of the Modernist movement's outlook and approach to interpreting the world and society.

24. D. Modernism had a profound impact on numerous aspects of life, and its values and perspectives still influence society in many positive ways today.

The author's description of Modernism's influence as being "positive" is clearly an opinion about the nature of the influence. The other statements are factually based, providing general information about the Modernist movement.

25. D. as well as

This sentence discusses all of the positive benefits that result from the continuation of the Olympic games in the present day, so "as well as" is the correct signal phrase to convey this idea, in a list form.

26. D. Detracted

The idea that allowing professional athletes to participate in the games would cause people to believe it "detracted" from the intentions of the original, is a negative notion, as it suggests that this would *take away from* the games, instead of adding something positive.

27. B. The Olympic games are the best example of humanity's physical prowess.

This statement is the opinion of the author, as there is no indication that this idea has been tested or proven in any way, but is simply what the author believes or feels.

28. C. Revulsion

The author uses words like "moldy smell" and "black hole" to describe his rented room in the inn, and "heartless" and "hideous" to describe the environment of London, adding that he "would rather even starve" than go out to find himself a meal in the "hellish town where a stranger might get trampled to death". These are very strong negative sentiments that clearly indicate his *revulsion* to the city.

29. B. A diary entry

The personal and frank tone that the author uses to describe his hotel room and his private fears about going out into the city of London for dinner suggest that this would have been written in a journal or diary.

30. D. An advertisement

A primary source document is one which was created from first-hand experience under a period of study of a particular event, moment in time, situation etc. A travel guide, diary entry and news editorial could all potentially be primary sources which chronicle one of the aforementioned. The only one that would likely NOT qualify as a primary source is the advertisement, as usually advertisements are meant to persuade one to engage in an experience, purchase a product or the like, and are often not completely based in personal experience and may not even be factual.

31. D. The author will not be traveling to London again.

It is clear that the author is unhappy with his lodging and finds London a generally disagreeable place, so it is likely that he would not travel to London again. The other statements are not reasonable conclusions which can be made from the content of the passage.

32. C. "You barely know him! How can she marry him?" was the worried mother's response at her teenager's announcement of marriage.

Sentence punctuation always is inside quotation marks; therefore, option C is punctuated correctly for dialogue.

33. A. "I have a dream", began Martin Luther King, Jr.

Second person uses the pronoun "you" or features direct address. Though punctuated incorrectly, it is clear that only the first sentence is not written in the second person; the use of "I" illustrates first person.

34. D. "Please remain seated while the seatbelt signs are illuminated." Came the announcement over the airplane's loud speaker system.

An Imperative statement is one which gives a command. Though punctuated incorrectly, it is clear that option D is imperative: the announcement is commanding the passengers to remain seated.

35. C. Excision

The prefix "ex" means out, so that is our clue here. "Excision" refers to a surgical procedure done to cut out something unwanted or unnecessary.

36. B. Colitis

The suffix "itis" is one which refers to inflammation, so "colitis" is an inflammation of the colon.

37. D. Melanoma

The suffix "oma" refers to a tumor or cancer, so "melanoma" refers to a cancer of the skin (coming from melanin, that which gives our skin its color). "Oncology" is the *study* of cancer, but it does not refer to cancer itself.

38. C. Rhinitis

The root "rhino" refers to the nose or nasal area, so "rhinitis" is an inflammation of the nasal passages.

39. A. Gastroenterology

The suffix "logy" refers to the study of some discipline or area, therefore gastroenterology is the study or examination of the gastrointestinal area of the body.

HESI A^2 - Spire Study System

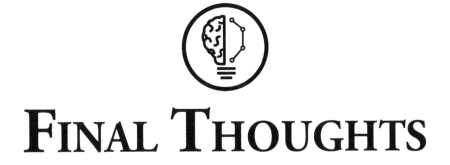

FINAL THOUGHTS

Congratulations!

If you're reading this, that means you have successfully completed your first experience with the Spire Study System, a fresh new approach to studying. You've proven that you're one of the free thinkers of the world, willing to try new things and challenge the conventional wisdom.

We sincerely hope you enjoyed the Spire Study System for the HESI A^2 (...well, as much as anyone can enjoy studying — you know what we mean).

If we succeeded and you're impressed with the Spire Study System, or if you have suggestions about how we can improve, we'd love to hear from you! Our inbox is always open: contact@spirestudysystem.com.

Better yet, tell your friends about us. And be sure to look for our upcoming books. We can't wait to bring the Spire Study System to more students!

Best Wishes,

Your study partners at Spire